First we make our habits,
then our habits make us.

—Charles C. Noble

Dr. A's HABITS of HEALTH

The Path to Permanent
Weight Control & Optimal Health

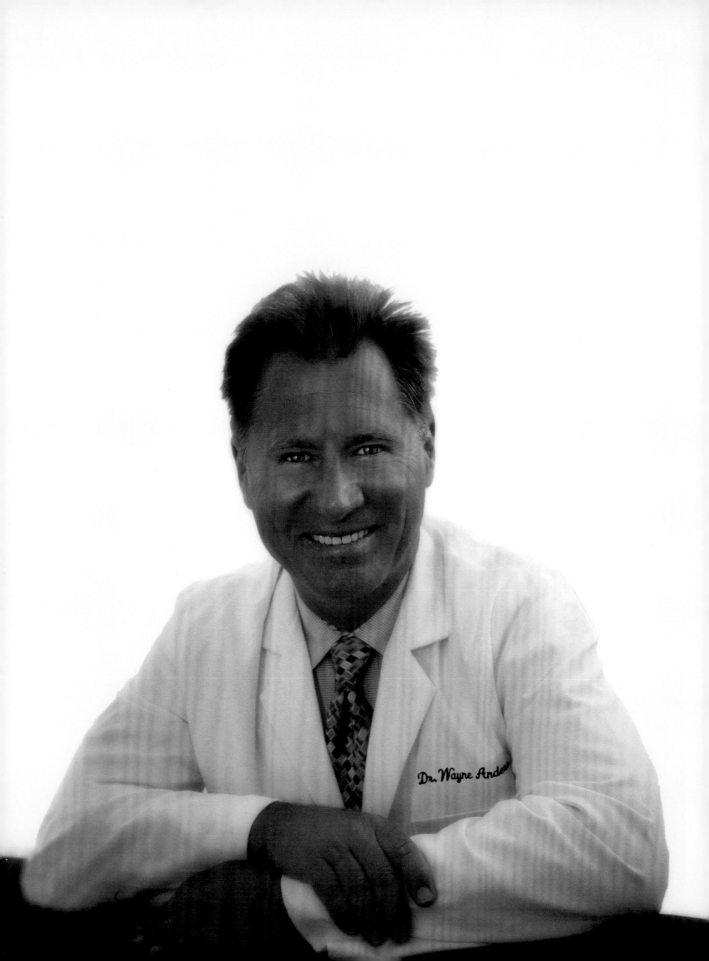

DR. A'S
HABITS
of HEALTH

·····················>

The Path to Permanent
Weight Control & Optimal Health

Dr. Wayne Scott Andersen

HABITS OF HEALTH PRESS • ANNAPOLIS, MD/USA

Dr. A's
HABITS OF HEALTH

P.O. Box 3301
Annapolis, Maryland 21403
www.drwayneandersen.com

Printed in the United States of America

40 39 38 37 36

ISBN
978-0-9819146-0-2 paperback
978-0-9819146-1-9 hardcover

Design by Dede Cummings and Ryerson Kipp
Production by Aleta Alcorn-Coursen, Carolyn Kasper, and Maggie Schiele Sullivan
DCDESIGN / BRATTLEBORO, VERMONT

Front/back cover family photo and author photo by Linda Shaffer.

First Edition

To my wife, Lori . . .

you are the essence of everything that is right in the world,

and each morning I wake up excited to have another day

with you and the two wonderful girls we have created.

Savannah and Erica, I love you more than life itself.

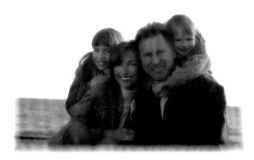

. . . .

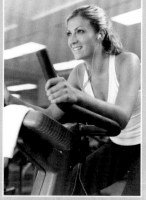

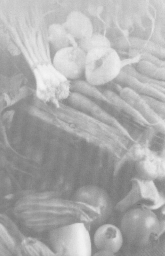

"... in the last six years, I have redirected my full-time focus to bring together medical science and daily choices into a practical system that will empower you to turn your life from surviving to thriving!"

Contents

Part Three **The Path to Longevity** 275

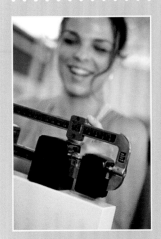

Probably you have tried to lose weight before and failed. You are not alone. Anyone who goes on a diet without behavioral support has an 85% chance of failure.

At the very essence of this book, and the path it describes, is the union of two powerful forces: medical science and the personal drive for fulfillment. For this reason, I have asked two important thinkers in their respective fields—**Robert Fritz,** international best-selling author and leading authority on the creative process, and **Dr. Lawrence Cheskin,** founder and director of the Johns Hopkins Weight Management Center—to share their unique perspectives and insights by contributing forewords to this text.

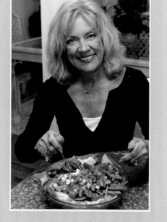

Foreword BY ROBERT FRITZ

Dr. A's Habits of Health may be one of the most important books you will ever read. By following Dr. Wayne Andersen's advice, you'll be able to re-direct lifelong patterns that are leading you down the wrong path and replace them with new, helpful practices that will enable you to build better and better health over time.

But this isn't yet another book trying to motivate change through fear, warnings, shame, and images of disaster. Dr. A knows the difference between a process that allows you to create the state of health you truly want and a process that merely addresses health problems.

There's a profound difference between architecture and building demolition. Creating, like architecture, involves taking action to have something you want come into being. Problem solving, like building demolition, involves taking action to have something you don't want go away.

Most of the medical establishment today is problem-driven, not outcome-driven. They're against illness, but ironically they don't think in terms of creating health in the first place. And therefore they have to wait for you to get sick before they can begin their work. Yes, there are a slew of pharmaceutical and medical advances that help slow the progression of heart disease, high blood pressure, high cholesterol, and other life-threatening conditions. But while we're all grateful that this technology exists, it's a product of this very same problem orientation—an orientation that has profound limitations when it comes to actually creating optimal health.

Treating illness surely has an important place in our lives, but doesn't it make sense, too, for each of us to create the highest level of health possible before we face life-threatening problems? While the logic of this is non-arguable, many in the medical community think that it's virtually impossible for people to change their ways, that people simply aren't able to develop new habits. And while, as this book will show, these opinions are false, they're clearly steeped in physicians' own experiences. Throughout the years, their warnings have gone unheeded by patients. What are they left with but an ongoing search for therapies that address the consequences of destructive habits?

What's unique about this book is that Dr. A understands how to help people accomplish real and lasting change. He understands that it's not a matter of willpower, or reactions to dire warnings. He knows that if it's hard to change a habit, people won't do it. So he's developed processes that are easy to adopt. And he knows that even if the process is easy, if the logistics surrounding that habit are challenging, change won't happen either. So he's developed straightforward, manageable, and clear logistics that anyone can handle.

Dr. A isn't going to give you a pep talk or a gloom-and-doom tirade. Instead, he'll show you how to design an overall strategy to accomplish one of the most important goals you will ever have: optimal health. And his approach isn't ivory tower theory, either. He's already helped thousands of people create optimal health in their lives.

You'll find that one of the nicest things about this book is Dr. A's down-to-earth voice, which is fun, friendly, warm, and personable. The material he presents is full of critical insights, science, wisdom, and practical advice, all brought to light in a highly readable and thoroughly enjoyable style.

I've known Dr. A for a number of years, and I'm privileged to call him a friend. He's highly creative, open, quick-witted, upbeat, and truly interested in other people's success. As you read *Dr. A's Habits of Health,* you'll find yourself developing a personal relationship with him. He'll become your health coach, your guide, your teacher, and your friend.

Dr. Wayne Scott Andersen has had a remarkably distinguished career that ideally positions him to forge new territory in the realm of creating optimal health. A board-certified anesthesiologist and critical care specialist, he has served as chairman of the Department of Anesthesiology and director of critical care at Grandview Medical Center, one of the top 100 hospitals in the country. He graduated first in his class from medical school and completed postdoctoral work that included residency training at the Cleveland Clinic in cardiovascular anesthesiology and fellowship training at the University of Miami in surgical critical care medicine. As the tenth board-certified physician in the nation in critical care, he helped pioneer the emerging subspecialty of intensive care medicine. It was in the course of this work, upon observing the pivotal role that nutrition plays in recovery from illness, that Dr. A determined to redirect his focus into the preventative arena of nutritional intervention and lifestyle management.

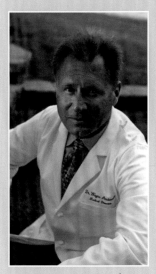

Dr. Wayne Scott Andersen,
author

What's unique about this book is that Dr. A understands how to help people accomplish real and lasting change.

> ix

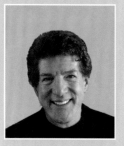

Robert Fritz, composer, filmmaker, and organizational consultant, is the author of the international best-seller *The Path of Least Resistance*.

Dr. A's life is about helping you create the highest state of health available to you. He can help you just as he's helped thousands reach a healthy weight, one of the first building blocks for creating optimal health. But his goal isn't merely to help you reach your desired weight. It's to instill in you the habits that support a lifetime process of achieving the highest state of health possible—and making it last.

This book can be a major contributor to the goal of creating optimal health, if you allow yourself to study it, follow its design and insights, and let it be your manual for reaching your health goals. So prepare yourself to transform your life, learn profound life-changing lessons, and reach a higher state of health than you ever thought possible!

Robert Fritz

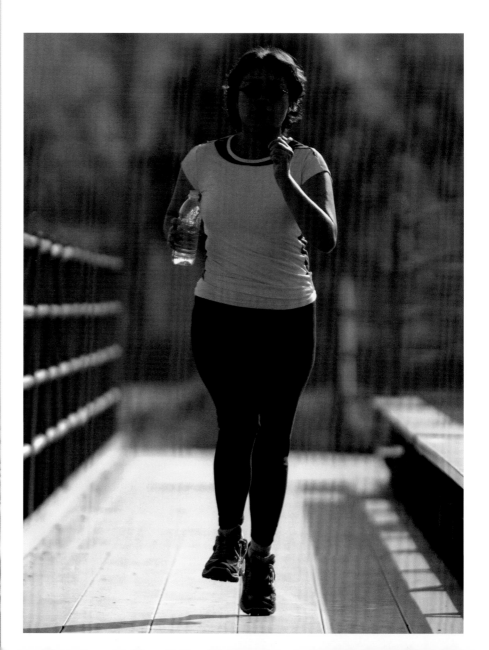

Foreword

BY LAWRENCE J. CHESKIN, MD, FACP

Let's start with the stark facts:

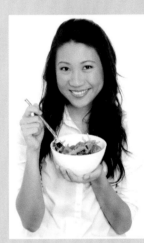

- In the U.S. alone, excess weight, obesity, and inactivity are reportedly responsible for about 300,000 deaths every year.
- Complications from obesity, including increased risk of coronary heart disease, type 2 diabetes, stroke, osteoarthritis, and certain cancers, now account for over 9 percent of all health care costs.
- Surveys indicate that at least 66 percent of American adults are now overweight or obese, and that obesity is increasing at an even faster pace among children. As a result, the coming generation may actually have a shorter life span than their parents for the first time in American history.

Undeniably, we have a collective problem building in the U.S. today, and one that we're rapidly exporting around the world.

While the underlying causes of this epidemic rise in obesity are still much debated, behavioral factors appear to be the number one contributor. What causes someone to make poor decisions about food in today's obesity-generating environment? Genetics, socioeconomic factors, and learned behaviors all play a role. But of these, only learned behaviors can be altered in any meaningful way—in particular, what we eat and how we respond to stress and other triggers that lead to inappropriate eating.

According to research, adults make at least 200 food choices every day. Learning to make better choices in terms of specific foods, portion size, and physical activity could maximize our ability to counter the pervasive environmental influences that make attaining and maintaining a healthy, stable weight so difficult.

In the end, though, hard facts and theoretical concepts like these aren't really all that useful or motivating for those of us who struggle daily with the battle against weight gain.

What is useful, then?

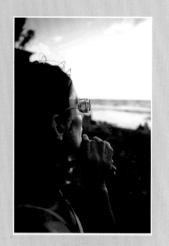

The goal of Dr. Andersen's groundbreaking new book is to shift the emphasis away from passive reaction to disease and toward individual responsibility for health—to encourage people to create health in the first place, rather than stand by while the negative forces of our society erode their health.

As the founder and director of the Johns Hopkins Weight Management Center in Baltimore, a clinical and research program devoted to helping people who are obese, I've treated thousands of individuals with weight problems. I have also been associated with Medifast, its programs, and its dedicated leaders for the past twenty years. In the course of this work, I've become convinced that we must move toward a new era of medicine, one that focuses on fostering optimal health and preventing health problems before they appear. Dr. Andersen shares this vision.

Unfortunately, we are still in the minority in our current health care system. Ironically, patients rarely receive financial coverage for weight-control services, despite ample coverage for all the medical consequences of obesity that could be avoided by losing weight to begin with!

Dr. Andersen's book offers a new paradigm—a simple, practical way for people to change their habits and lifestyle by building on small, easy, almost imperceptible steps. While this may go against our tendency to view change as a dramatic break from the past, change is in fact often easiest, and easier to make permanent, when it's gradual—a journey.

In the journey that you're about to take, reaching a healthy weight is a starting point, not an end point, and this in itself helps create the momentum that moves you forward toward change, rather than backward into old behaviors. The ultimate goal is to continue this forward movement toward optimal health. As Dr. Andersen explains, that goal will look different for each of us, but the decision to take our health into our own hands is the critical first step.

You'll find his book replete with all the tools that will help you on this journey to a new, better approach to health and a more fulfilled life. These include a variety of revealing self-assessment techniques and questionnaires, and exercises to help you change those ingrained, lifelong habits that make it so hard to break free. You'll learn to make daily choices that support your goals through a healthy eating system, a movement plan, and strategies for invigorating rest and sleep. Dr. Andersen reveals tested dietary tools that can serve as an important shortcut to healthy weight, and explains how the support of a like-minded community of people can help you reach and maintain your goals.

The book also contains a series of innovative ways to reflect on your goals and monitor how you respond to life's changes and stresses. After all, it's often not so much what we face that stymies us, but rather our reactions to these challenges. Dr. Andersen is a master at helping you look at situations in the most positive way possible—a valuable tool indeed in your journey toward optimal weight and health.

I urge you to look at this journey you're about to embark upon under Dr. Andersen's guidance with eager anticipation. Facing and overcoming something that has challenged you, perhaps for your whole life, with an open mind and heart, with determination and conviction, is a wonderful gift that only you can give yourself. I invite you now to take the first step of your journey, and enjoy!

Lawrence J. Cheskin, MD, FACP

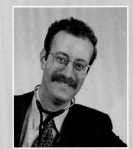

Lawrence J. Cheskin, MD, FACP, is director and founder of the Johns Hopkins Weight Management Center.

REFERENCES

Allison, D. B., et al., "Annual Deaths Attributable to Obesity in the United States," *Journal of the American Medical Association* 282 (16): 1530–8.

Colditz, G. A., "Economic Costs of Obesity and Inactivity," *Medical Science Sports Exerc* 31 (11 Suppl, 1999): S663–7.

Ogden, C. L., et al., "Prevalence of Overweight and Obesity in the United States, 1999-2004," *Journal of the American Medical Association* 295 (13, 2006): 1549–55.

Wansink, B., et al., "Exploring Comfort Food Preferences across Age and Gender," *Physiology and Behavior* 79 (4–5, 2003): 739–47.

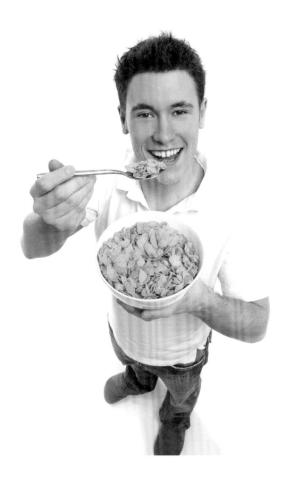

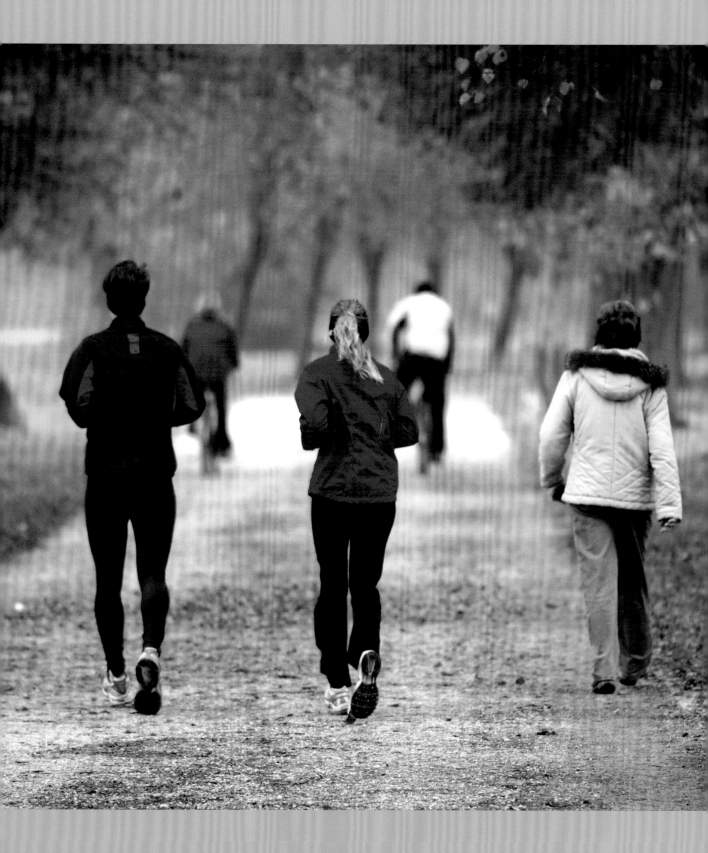

Preface

· ·

Obesigenic:
Likely to cause
someone to become
excessively fat

We live in an obesigenic world.

We're surrounded by seductively tasty, cheap, convenient, but oh-so-un-healthy food. Combine this with our many energy-saving devices and lack of activity, and our own way of life may soon kill us. We're supersizing ourselves to death!

If you're like most of us, this unhealthy environment is already taking a toll. It's affecting how you feel, what you're able to do, maybe even the state of your health. Every day, it seems, we hear about how fat we have become, how badly we're eating, how little we're exercising, and how much it's hurting us. We read about breakthrough research that might someday lead to a cure for obesity. We're exposed to a multitude of diet books, self-help books, diet programs—and yet the reality is that Americans keep getting bigger and bigger.

The fire hose of weight-loss information out there is conflicting, over-whelming, and confusing. Like many, you've probably tried to lose weight and failed. You are not alone. Even most of those who are successful initially fail eventually.

It's no wonder you're struggling. It's likely that your life is full of never-ending things to do, longer hours of work, more chores, less sense of meaning and purpose, and less fun—and on top of it all, that creeping weight gain is draining your battery and making everything feel like a battle for survival.

I know how you feel, because I once lived that way, too. As a critical care physician, I spent over eighty hours a week in the intensive care unit, scram-bling to keep patients alive—many of whom were suffering the ravages of obesity-induced disease. Lack of sleep combined with terrible eating habits caused my waistline to grow. Only the drawstring of my scrubs hid the reality that I was becoming the very thing I was treating.

Today, those thirty pounds of belly fat—along with all that stress and fatigue—are in the distant past. I now have a 32-inch waist with very low body fat, I sleep well, and I get out of bed every day with energy and enthusiasm. The best part is that I've redirected my focus. Over the past six years I have developed a practical system—based on bringing together medical science and everyday choices—that will empower you to turn your life around.

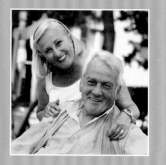

Go from barely surviving to effortlessly thriving!

In those six years I've helped countless people lose weight and create health in their lives. More importantly, I've shown them how to make those changes last. In fact, the National Weight Control Registry, which tracks long-term, successful weight loss, designates many of the people I've helped—including myself—as masters of weight loss.

This book is a journey. Your destination is nothing short of optimal health. Along the way you'll be adopting new and healthy habits—habits that will bring you a lifetime of health and well-being. One of my proudest achievements is to have cofounded the Take Shape for Life™ Health Network (TSFL), which has helped over 100,000 individuals improve their health. As a tribute to all of those who have taken the journey to optimal health, we will feature some of those successes throughout the book.

Dr. Wayne Scott Andersen
October 2008

"Getting healthy was easier than we ever imagined!"
DOMINIC AND RITA TARINELLI
Over four years at optimal health

Stressed out, weighing 242 pounds, I didn't know where to turn. Then I started on the path to optimal health, and I lost inches from my waist and I dropped 70 pounds—just where I was in high school! My wife came along on my journey too, and she's lost over 30 pounds and gone from a size 12 to a size 4. But the best part of all is that we've kept the weight off and are much stronger, healthier, and happier.

Today, I feel like I have a whole new life. Dr. A and Take Shape for Life have given us the plan, the tools, the strategy, and the knowledge to continue our path toward optimal health. This advice is simple, practical, and easy to follow for anyone who wants to take control of their health and their life. In fact, getting healthy was easier than we ever imagined! ∎

The Tarinellis: before and after
Results vary. Typical weight loss is 2-5 lbs per week for the first 2 weeks and 1-2 lbs per week thereafter.

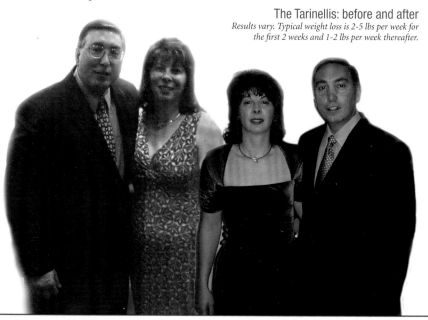

Introduction

Beating the Odds

Eighty-five percent of people who go on a diet without behavioral support gain the weight back within two years.

History of Dieting?

According to studies, you are likely to gain more weight in the end than your non-dieting friend—and have poorer health.

Those are lousy odds!

If that isn't enough to convince you to abandon the dieting circus, let's look at a recent study out of UCLA. In the largest, most comprehensive and rigorous analysis to date, investigators reviewing thirty-one long-term dieting studies discovered (to no one's surprise) that the dieters gained their weight back and then some. In fact, several studies indicated that dieters are actually more likely to gain weight in the future and to suffer from poorer long-term health than non-dieters.*

Ironic, isn't it?

I know what you're thinking . . . there's no point in dieting, so you're off the hook! Not so fast, my friend.

Dieting on its own may not be the answer, but neither is the status quo. Being overweight increases the likelihood that you'll suffer from overall poor health and eventually become sick. Medical literature is teeming with studies that confirm it. And you don't even have to be obese to be at risk. As your weight rises, so do your health risks.

Extra weight around the middle is a harbinger of poor health to come. As body fat gathers around our organs, it sends out ever larger quantities of dangerous substances that increase blood pressure, cholesterol, triglycerides, and blood sugar, turning on a cascade of inflammatory pathways that erode the body's defenses. This cluster of symptoms, called *metabolic syndrome,* is currently attacking the health of over 70 million Americans.

*Mann, T., et al., "Medicare's Search for Effective Obesity Treatments: Diets Are Not the Answer." *American Psychologist* 62 (April 2007): 220–233.

Some physicians don't think patients have it in them to lose weight. Just read what one writer in the *Journal of the American Medical Association* had to say about patient motivation: "Many believe humankind does not have the self-control to counterbalance the forces that create a predictable wave of obesity in a technologically advancing society."* When I read this, it made my skin crawl. It's a bunch of hogwash!

*Dansinger, M. L., and Schaefer, E. J., "Low-Fat Diets and Weight Change." *Journal of the AMA* 295: 94–95.

So diets alone don't work, but it's dangerous to be overweight. . . what can we do?

We need go beyond simple dieting. Medical and pharmaceutical companies are working overtime to treat symptoms caused by excessive weight gain. But the cure will never come from medication or from focusing on treating disease. The cure will come by helping people reach and maintain a healthy weight and by equipping them with the habits to make it last.

Physicians tend to ignore this simple fact—it's almost as if they think their patients just can't do it. And yet, with understanding, support, proper motivation, and a long-term plan to follow, it is straightforward and very doable. It's what this book is all about!

Unlike a diet book, this book helps you sort through your life choices to make sure they're positioning you for success. We'll look at your current health and your daily habits, determine what you need to move forward, and create an individualized, step-by-step plan to support what I call your Habits of Health.

This plan is about much more than weight loss. It's about reaching and maintaining optimal health. If you had the chance to live your best, in the very best health possible, would you grab it? Of course you would. And I'm going to help you get there!

Maybe you're already at a point where you're feeling unwell—gaining weight, spinning out of control, even developing symptoms of metabolic syndrome. Or maybe you're on medication, or have undergone angioplasty for a blocked coronary artery. If so, you may be asking yourself why. Why is this happening to me?

The reason is simple: your daily choices. Small errors of judgment in what you eat, in how much you move or don't move, and other habits that seem insignificant but that snowball, until one day you realize that you feel heavy, tired, and sick. But you can stop this out-of-control scenario dead in its tracks. I'm going to give you the knowledge, skills, and support to put you back in the driver's seat.

Working Together

You and I are going to build a different kind of relationship than you may have experienced in your past medical treatments. I'm not going to use prescriptions, warnings, or fear tactics. Instead, I'll be your coach, your guide. Together, we'll put you on the path to taking permanent charge of your health.

Changing lifelong habits takes effort and can be stressful at times, especially in the beginning. Just remember, this book isn't the product of medical research alone, or of my thirty years as a physician. It was forged through real life experience—from the experiences of the thousands of people I've helped to reach a healthy weight and live a healthy life. I've fought alongside my patients and the people I have coached as they worked to create health. I've joined them in celebrating their successes. And with each and every one, I have listened and learned what works and what doesn't, what's easy and what's hard.

This book is the culmination of those experiences. It's about good habits and bad ones—about making a fundamental choice to create optimal health. I've made that choice, and I know that you can, too.

Think of this as the roadmap for your journey to optimal health.

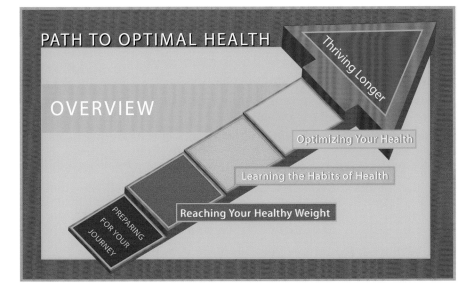

We begin in Part One by teaching you the knowledge you need to prepare for your journey. After all, getting where you want to go depends on knowing where you are right now, and understanding what you're up against. Part Two takes you through three distinct phases that help you master practical tools for long-term health. And in Part Three we will study the principles of longevity—ways to extend your life and enjoy your newfound health with every step.

Let's take a closer look.

Dr. A Says . . .

This plan is about much more than weight loss. It's about reaching and maintaining optimal health.

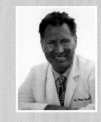

Part One   Preparing for Your Journey

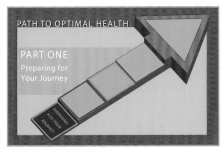

Did you know that ours is the first generation whose quality of life is actually less than that of our parents? It's a fact: our technologically advanced society is no longer serving our best interests.

In Part One, we'll examine how today's world, with its nutritional pollution, too little movement, and way too much stress, is affecting our weight and health. We'll take a close look at how the basic design of the human body, once key to our survival, is now helping to accelerate our weight gain. And we'll see why the institutions we once depended on to keep us healthy are now the very ones driving us toward sickness.

You'll come to understand why it's not your fault that you're overweight and unhealthy. You'll learn what I mean by "optimal health," "non-sick," and "sick," and discover how your choices are leading you down this continuum, eroding your health. And we'll help you change the very way you look at your weight and your health by exploring your motivation and learning how to make the fundamental choice to be healthy—a choice available to each and every one of us. Together, we'll outline a specific path that will bring you to a state of health you never thought possible, and we'll do it in baby steps.

Part One concludes with an in-depth assessment of your current state of health. We'll explore aspects of your life beyond just lab results and blood pressure, to paint a complete picture of your current habits and lifestyle—to make sure we're touching on all the factors at work in your journey to optimal health.

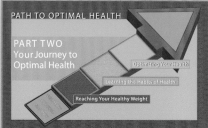

Part Two — Your Journey to Optimal Health

Phase I: Reaching Your Healthy Weight

This is where we'll help you reach a healthy weight, and transform your tired days with restful sleep and new energy. But we'll do it through the science of proper weight loss, quickly and consistently. Tailored with options that fit your needs and lifestyle, our plan will help you lose two to five pounds each week for the first two weeks and one to two pounds each week thereafter, while taking you to a healthier place on your path.

How? Through a tool I have found to be a powerful ally in our time-starved world—medically formulated, low-calorie portion-controlled meal replacements (PCMRs). Created through advanced nutrition technology, PCMRs are a proven, safe way to help you start losing weight quickly. As part of a comprehensive system, they can be an invaluable support, providing proper fuel in a hectic schedule. They're a great example of harnessing technology to help overcome weight challenges—just one of many of the tools we'll be giving you as you build your foundation for a life of health.

In fact, meal replacements have been so integral in helping me help others to reach optimal health that I decided to join the industry leader in the development of medically based, low-calorie portion-controlled meal replacements, Medifast®, as their medical director. This wonderful relationship has given me the opportunity to help thousands of people lose weight, and to learn what works and what doesn't.

I'll help guide you into the fat-burning state, where you'll experience rapid, safe weight loss. Soon you'll be feeling better, sleeping better, and have so much more energy that you'll be ready to take your next step. You'll be ready to feel this way for the rest of your life by learning the Habits of Health, the fundamental building blocks of optimal health.

And during this period I will teach you my healthy eating strategy that will help you develop healthy eating habits for life. I'll take you shopping and teach you techniques that fit seamlessly into your busy lifestyle. Soon you'll be equipped with a complete eating strategy to support a lifetime of health.

Phase II: Learning the Habits of Health

Now that you're firmly on the path to optimal health, with a healthy weight in reach, you're ready to build on that foundation. As I teach you key Habits of Health—including how to eat healthy for life, how to integrate movement into your daily routine, how to harness the power of restorative sleep, and how to develop an individualized support system—you'll model each example in your own life, internalizing the strategic choices that are critical to long-term success. You'll gain control over your health and find that over time these habits become automatic.

They'll help you develop a new lifestyle that will shield you from the obesigenic world out there! As you gain health, who knows what thriving new life awaits you?

Phase III: Optimizing Your Health

You've graduated from the fundamentals of health and are ready for your master's degree!

Now that your health is improving and you're practicing daily behaviors that support permanent weight loss, I'll introduce you to up-to-date strategies and technologies to enhance your healthy new body. We'll explore ways to remove potent health-robbers and equip you with strategies to protect and enhance your health, including anti-inflammatory foods and optimizing supplements. You'll discover the value of antioxidants and eicosanoids, and learn age-specific strategies for each point on your biological passage.

Best of all, I'll protect you from snake-oil remedies by equipping you with scientifically validated recommendations, based on peer-reviewed research, to maximize your health for life.

Part Three The Path to Longevity

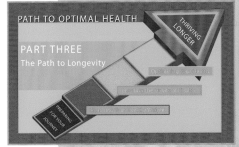

Phase IV: Thriving Longer

Finally, in Part Three, we enter the final phase, Phase IV, in which you'll find out how to extend your healthy new life beyond what's considered a normal lifespan. After all, now that you're enjoying optimal health, you might as well stick around! We'll fine-tune your energy control, adding new techniques to help you live longer and healthier, and we'll introduce ways to keep you Ultrahealthy as an extension of your new Habits of Health.

• •

Before you start your journey, let me summarize why this book can help you succeed where others have failed.

Losing weight is only half the battle. Our goal is to help you *create permanent optimal health*. I want you to enjoy radiant health, more energy, restful sleep, and a body that supports you in living not only a longer life, but one that's focused around what matters most to you. With my Habits of Health, this isn't as hard as it may seem.

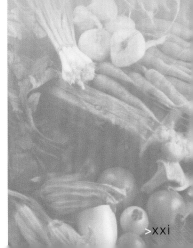

I know that this book can help you take control of your health and your life. In it, you'll find stories about people from every walk of life—people who were where you are now and who are thriving today, thanks to our formula of success. They didn't get there overnight, though they probably reached their healthy weight quicker than they expected. Notice that these are people who have remained healthy for many years. They succeeded by taking a series of simple steps that showed them how to create lifelong Habits of Health.

Come walk with us up the path to optimal health!

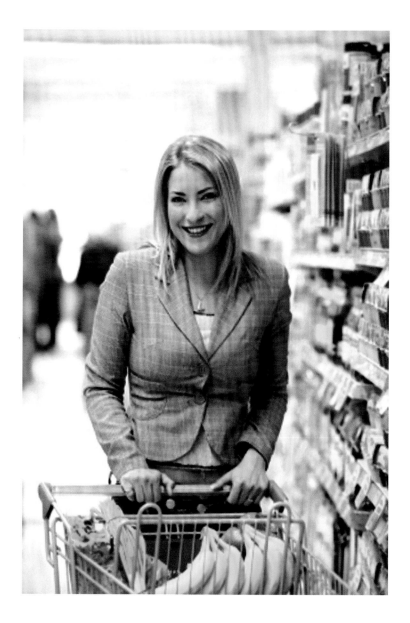

Part One

· ·>

Preparing for Your Journey

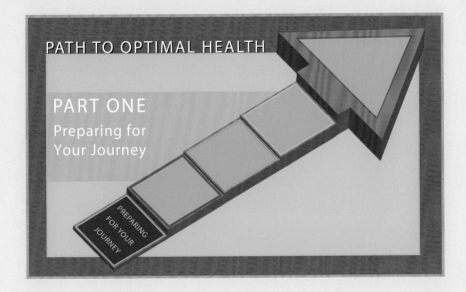

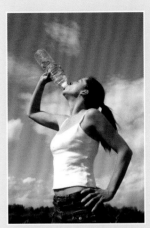

Achieving optimal health in today's world requires us to do something most of us have never had to—take charge of our own health. Ironically, the very places we normally turn to for help are actually making it harder for us to get healthy. The food industry offers us tasty, cheap products that are addictive and unhealthy. The medical and pharmaceutical industries are more intent on curing sickness than on promoting health. Even the preventative health care movement takes an all-too-passive approach, focusing on avoiding disease rather than on helping people achieve the best health they can.

My approach, by contrast, is about actively creating health. If you're willing to invest the time and energy, I can teach you specific steps to move you from where you are right now to a state of optimal health.

Let's start by going back in time. . .

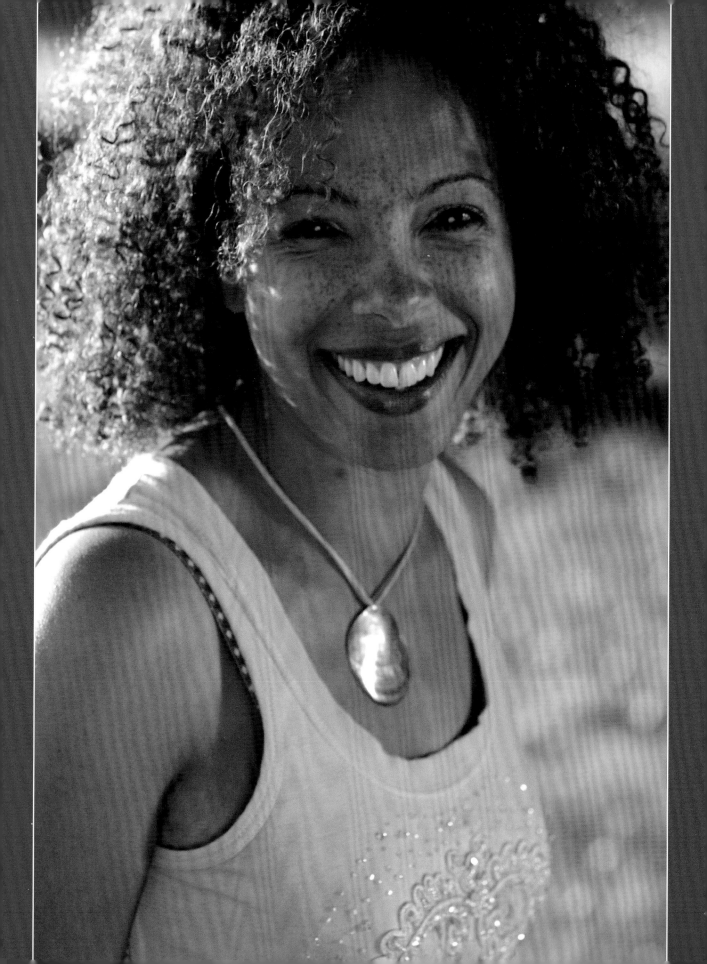

Chapter 1

It's Not Your Fault

That You're Struggling with Your Weight

Your 10,000-Year-Old Body

Ten thousand years ago, there was no obesity, heart disease, or Type 2 DM diabetes. Just getting enough to eat was a struggle. We had to forage most of the day for food—some roots here, vegetables and berries there. So naturally if you found a whole bush full of ripe berries, you ate them right away. Who knew when, or even if, there would be more? And if you were fortunate enough to catch an animal, you and your clan ate the whole thing then and there. In those days, being overweight would have meant you were an extremely successful member of the tribe—in fact, your ancestors may have made you their leader. It would have taken a lot of ambition back then to have a body mass index (BMI) above 25!

Today, when I hear someone say, "I went to a party, and suddenly I'd eaten a whole bag of potato chips" or "I was watching TV and I ate a whole pint of ice cream," I think. . . well, of course you did. Your body was designed that way. Faced with so much nutritional energy right in front of you, your 10,000-year-old biological programming insisted that you eat it all, especially with your conscious mind distracted by television or a party.

Ancient humans used all their energy just staying alive. If they wanted to get somewhere, they had to walk or run or paddle a canoe. If they wanted to eat, they had to gouge out roots or find vegetables and fruits or grind up grasses and grains. Cooking meant carrying water, gathering wood, and building a fire. So our bodies evolved to be extremely efficient at using energy. If they hadn't, none of us would have survived. To this day, our bodies fight to hold onto every calorie of energy we take in, because that's how we're programmed—as if our survival is still in question.

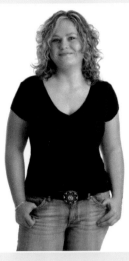

Our bodies are programmed to hold onto calories for the sake of survival. So when you try to "diet," you're really fighting your own nature.

The Storage Factor

Our bodies are designed to store and conserve fat and calories for those times when we can't find food—all too often the case 10,000 years ago. Our energy storage system is made up of over 40 billion adipose (fat) cells, providing a virtually unlimited storehouse to keep us alive. We also store small amounts of carbohydrates in our liver and muscles, *but the ability to stockpile precious energy as fat is our most critical survival mechanism.* We're here today because our ancestors' bodies stored fat so well 10,000 years ago.

Now let's jump ahead to today. What happens when this perfect, biologically balanced creation, with its complex system of cells, organs, and tissues designed

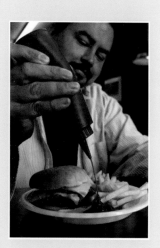

to conserve energy, is plunked down in the twenty-first century? Today, getting food takes almost no effort at all—drive to the supermarket, throw packages into a cart, roll the cart to your car, and drive home. OK, maybe you have to carry your groceries into the house. How much energy does that take?

Or how about hunting and gathering at your local fast food restaurant, say McDonald's, Burger King, or Taco Bell? You pull up to the drive-thru and roll down your window—no, actually you take your finger and simply toggle the switch. That takes about two calories. Shout into the speaker and place your order—that's another two to four calories—and drive to the pick-up window. Then you take your supersized burger, supersized fries, and supersized drink and perform some heavy lifting as you place them on the seat next to you. Maybe eight calories for that. And in about three minutes or so, it's all eaten.

So let's do the math. Calories consumed: 1,500. Calories expended as energy: 12. What's wrong with this picture?

The Supersized Generation

You've probably noticed that in the past twenty years serving sizes have gotten bigger and bigger. Restaurant portions are now as much as eight times the standard serving size in the FDA's dietary guidelines. *Eight times!*

At Outback Steakhouse, they take a 70-calorie, truly wonderful, nutritious root vegetable full of vitamin C, antioxidants, and healthy phenols and transform it into a 2,400-calorie, 134-grams-of-fat cardiac stress test called a Bloomin' Onion. And that's just the appetizer!

Calories consumed versus calories used are way out of whack in our world. *Dangerously* out of whack! Today we're surrounded by food that's larger portioned and more calorie dense than anything imagined even fifty years ago. At the same time, our labor-saving devices let us conserve energy at an unprecedented rate. No wonder over two-thirds of Americans take in more calories than they can ever use.

It's not your fault that you were born in a time of unparalleled plenty and physical ease, with a body that stores and conserves energy. It's not your fault that you're confronted by food that's more plentiful and addictive than at any time in history, with a day-to-day lifestyle that most often finds us in a chair at our desk or on the couch in front of the television.

Living with a 10,000-Year-Old Body in the Twenty-first Century

So you see, there's a lot more going on inside of you than weak willpower or lack of resolve. Our bodies inherited a number of instincts that are no longer useful but are still a force to be reckoned with. How do you manage two competing tendencies: the ancient instinct to eat whenever you can and the modern aspiration to live a long and healthy life? And what happens when this balance tips? You yo-yo. You go through periods when you lose weight and periods when you put it back on. This is critical to understanding why it's not your fault that you're overweight.

And one thing's for sure—all the pep talks in the world won't help you.

Your doctor may say, "Lose weight, go on a diet, exercise." Sound advice, but it's not terribly useful without a specific road map to guide you, especially long term. Or your family, who loves you and wants the best for you, may give you the latest diet books, many of which you've probably already tried. If you take their advice but then fall into a yo-yo pattern, what then? You probably conclude that, much as you might agree with them, you just can't pull it off in the real world.

Then there's old-time positive thinking. "If you think you can, you can!" So what happens one day when your boss has been screaming at you, and you find yourself in front of a pint of Ben and Jerry's fantastic chocolate cherry butternut marshmallow fudge ripple ice cream? Your 10,000-year-old biological instinct says *Eat it all right now!* while your brain tries to repeat, "I am a positive and healthy person." Soon enough the Ben and Jerry's is completely devoured. You end up feeling guilty—and powerless to change your life.

You're not powerless. You don't have a willpower problem, or a negative thinking problem. You have a simple conflict between two real desires: the desire to achieve your health goals, and the desire to satisfy your instincts. Dr. A's Habits of Health takes this conflict into consideration and empowers you to take charge successfully, safely, and permanently.

How the Food Industry Sabotages Your Health

The food industry isn't your friend. Between sodas, snacks—even an innocent-looking slice of bread—the average American consumes twenty-six spoonfuls of refined sugar every day. Yet your body only needs the equivalent of one teaspoon of sugar to operate your entire bloodstream.

Americans now consume an average of 135 pounds of sugar each year. That's an increase of 26 pounds per person in just the past twenty years! And to think that a century ago our average consumption was only 5 pounds per year. So why does twenty-first-century food have so much sugar in it? Because sugar makes food taste good, and food companies want to produce food that sells.

In the old days, businesses made profits by offering high-quality food that earned customer loyalty. If the local butcher sold you a bad piece of meat, you stopped using him and let everyone in town know about it. If the green grocer sold you rotten vegetables, you didn't go back to him. Back then, the food industry was run by professionals who took pride in their products. The butcher knew his beef, lamb, and pork; the green grocer knew his fruits and vegetables, as well as the farmers who supplied them. The food industry was very personal. But as food became big business, the focus moved from quality to cost.

Who's running the food industry now? Accountants, mostly. They don't love food, they love numbers. And the numbers they love most are the ones they can control—costs. Lower costs mean bigger profits. One way to cut costs is to get a better deal from suppliers by buying in larger quantity. That's how big companies like Amazon can offer the same book at lower prices than the corner bookstore. Another way to cut costs is to use cheaper ingredients. In the mind of an accountant, the way to success is very simple: buy cheap stuff at high volume.

To reach and maintain your ideal weight, you need to get on top of the inherent battle between your 10,000-year-old biological predisposition and your desire to be healthy.

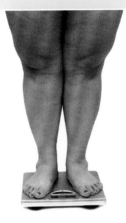

5

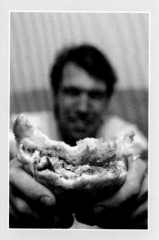

High-glycemic carbohydrates: starchy foods and sugars that quickly raise your blood sugar to a high level.

In the early 1980s, high-fructose corn syrup replaced sugar in Pepsi and Coke. Why? Because it was cheaper. Now soft drink companies could super-size their 8-ounce bottles and offer 64 ounces *for the same price!* That's a great value for you—or is it? You see, sugar or sucrose can be metabolized by any cell in the body, while high-fructose corn syrup can only be processed by your liver, after which it's turned into triglycerides and then laid down as fat.

On top of that, high-fructose corn syrup is addictive. Your body gets used to it, and starts to crave it. If I were an accountant thinking of ways to sell more Coke or Pepsi or cakes or hot dogs or even bread, I would probably decide that adding something that creates a demand for more of my product makes good business sense. And unfortunately, it does make sense—to Wall Street.

A sweet tooth may be good for business, but it's not good for your health and well-being. Your 10,000-year-old biological instrument, with its insatiable lust for energy, can't handle this fire hose of sugar and other high-glycemic carbohydrates indefinitely. And high-fructose corn syrup is even worse than sugar, because it keeps your body from producing key hormones that regulate your energy cycle and inhibit hunger—so your body can't even sense when it's full. But it all catches up to you. One day you go to the doctor and discover that you're prediabetic or, worse, already have diabetes or liver disease.

So our 10,000-year-old body must deal with a modern world that profits by selling us the most addictive and unhealthy food there is. It's easier to go to a fast food chain than to a healthier, more expensive restaurant or to prepare a healthy meal at home. And when we do go to the supermarket, we're confronted by products that are so overly processed they have limited nutritional value. They taste great, they're convenient, they're cheap and easy to prepare—and they're so bad for you!

High-Fructose Corn Syrup: Padding the Pockets of the Food Industry, Paving the Path to Disease

Here's a little experiment: try reading the labels on the products you eat. Notice how many contain high-fructose corn syrup. If you look at the original recipes for these same foods, you'll see that very few of them even contain sugar, much less high-fructose corn syrup.

Why is our food so full of this stuff? Because when high-fructose corn syrup is added to salty foods like catsup and lunch meats, we eat more—and that means more money for the food industry. Your internal appetite control center, called the appestat, is designed to tell you you're full once it senses specific quantities of certain nutrients in your blood. But food scientists, working for food companies, manipulate the ingredients in processed foods to prevent you from getting that "I'm full" feeling. Is it working? Well, when the art of food science began in the 1970s, Americans were spending 6 billion dollars a year on fast food. Today, we're spending 130 billion. Do the math!

A Habit of Disease: The Fast Food Habit

Did you know that eating too much unhealthy fast food—even for a single week—can cause noticeable damage to your body?

In a recent study published online in *Gut,* the international journal of gastroenterology and hepatology, eighteen healthy adults ate at least two fast food meals a day, doubling their daily intake of calories. They also limited their exercise. In just one week, half of the group began experiencing elevated levels of ALT enzymes—a common indicator of liver damage. And by the end of the study, the entire group had gained an average of fourteen pounds. The conclusion? Our bodies just aren't made to handle more than an occasional indulgence in fast foods.

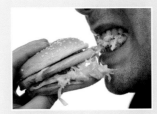

There's been an alarming increase in our daily ingestion of calories since the early 1980s. Coupled with lifestyles that are becoming ever more sedentary, the result is a rise in fat accumulation leading to pre-obesity and obesity. As you can see in the chart below, this trend is expected to accelerate into the next decade. According to a 2003 Baylor University study, over 90 percent of us will be overweight or worse by 2032 unless we significantly change our behaviors.

How did this happen? First, the overworked, time-starved workforce of the early 1980s spurred the food industry to begin producing convenient, prepared products and easy-access, affordable restaurants. This brought more variety—but also more calories. Add to this the Reagan Administration's hasty deregulation of the agriculture industry, which made cheap food abundant and more energy dense. Finally, continued demand for higher short-term return on investment by Wall Street's stockholders forced food companies to expand their reach into schools, bookstores, and just about any other location frequented by humans. I can just hear a marketing director standing up and saying to his board, "If we can introduce a delivery system to feed our customers while they sleep, we can tap into a seven-hour-a-day niche that no one owns!"

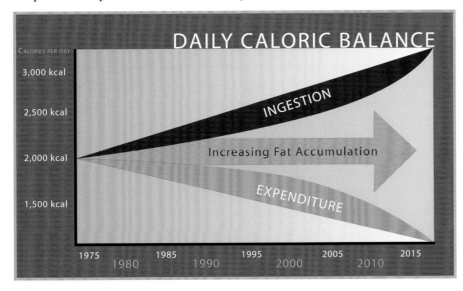

DAILY CALORIC BALANCE

CALORIES PER DAY

3,000 kcal

2,500 kcal

INGESTION

2,000 kcal

Increasing Fat Accumulation

1,500 kcal

EXPENDITURE

1975   1985   1995   2005   2015
  1980   1990   2000   2010

Daily Caloric Balance. Since the early 1980s, we've been increasingly taking in more calories (ingestion) than we're using (expenditure). If this trend continues, 90 percent of us will be overweight by the year 2032.

The doctor of the future will give no medicine but will interest his patients in the care of the human frame, in diet and in the cause and prevention of disease.

—Thomas Edison

Dr. A Says. . .

Our plan is about creating health to help prevent disease from occuring.

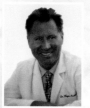

The food industry lobbies hard in Washington, sponsoring journals and special interest groups to market favorable viewpoints of their goods. And today's great common marketplace, the supermarket, where consumers go for sound nutritional advice, has become a for-profit enterprise guided by its need to return profit to its stockholders.

These factors aren't your fault. But by their very structure, these institutions are in conflict with your desire for health. It's important to know what we're dealing with as we turn our focus from fighting disease to creating optimal health.

The Numbers Tell the Story

The math couldn't be simpler or more deadly: consume more caloric energy than you use and the excess must be stored as fat. Keep that up for years, or decades, and those extra pounds quickly lead to pre-obesity and obesity—an insidious disease that leads directly to premature death.

So where is medical technology in all this? Sadly, it's focused on *sick* care, not *health* care. Exactly where I used to be focused—on new technologies and life-saving breakthroughs in operating rooms and intensive care units, too far downstream from the source of the problem.

Part of the blame lies in the medical model itself, which is geared to curing illness rather than creating health and well-being. The fact is that most of us won't even have access to medical services under the current model until we're exhibiting symptoms and are well down the path to disease. While healing the sick is a noble cause, it comes too late in the process. Why is disease present in the first place? More importantly, *how do we create health so that diseases don't occur?* Medical science, with its emphasis on fighting disease rather than preventing it, just isn't prepared to answer these questions.

And it's totally understandable. It's in our nature to be problem solvers. In fact, society encourages it. Ten thousand years ago, our hostile world presented one life-threatening problem after another, from saber-toothed tigers to nasty snakes. In order to survive, we had to think in terms of threats, hazards, dangers, risks.

Of course we're all against the idea of disease. But unfortunately that doesn't mean we're necessarily doing what's needed to create health and well-being. And most of the medical profession hasn't made this critical distinction either. True, today's medications and surgery are helping to control the symptoms of more and more people who are already sick, but modern medicine is doing very little to stop the progression from health to non-sickness and disease. In

---

What Is a Calorie?

Calories are used to measure the amount of energy we get from our food. While different types of calories appear in scientific contexts, in the fields of nutrition and food labeling, a calorie refers to the amount of energy needed to increase the temperature of one kilogram of water by 1 degree centigrade—hence the abbreviation kcal. For our purposes, we'll use the terms calorie and kcal interchangeably.

fact, the vast majority of us—90 percent—are currently in a less than optimal state and headed in the wrong direction.

The reality—that the current health plan isn't working—is nowhere more apparent than in today's disturbing increases in obesity, diabetes, and hypertension among our youth. Even the term *adult-onset diabetes* has become obsolete. Renamed type 2 diabetes, this debilitating disease is reaching epidemic proportion among people of all ages, attacking children as young as ten.

The chart below illustrates the effect that the current medical model is having on our health. As you can see, the forecasted path indicates that in the future more people are expected to become sick at a younger age. Life expectancy is forecasted to shorten as well. By contrast, my health plan is helping thousands of people take control of their health and forge a new health path—one of optimal health and longevity.

And it's not just our health that's suffering—it's our pocketbooks as well. Despite the fact that we spend more than any nation in the world on health care, we're not even in the top twenty-five in terms of the health of our citizens. Not that we haven't made great strides. Our directive on curing heart disease, for example, brought about many new advancements, including noninvasive diagnostics and clot-busting medications. The death rate from heart disease has decreased dramatically as a result. But the cost of these Star Wars–type devices and advances is bankrupting our health care system. In the U.S., we spend 50 percent of our $2 trillion health care budget taking care of people who are sick, while less than 3 percent is spent on helping people stay healthy in the first place. On top of which, the medications we're using to treat symptoms caused by excess weight and lack of exercise are making us sicker yet.

So I think it is clear that the institutions we depend on to keep us safe are letting us down. If that's the case, what can you do for yourself to combat an ever-increasing waistline and avoid the slippery slope toward disease?

Are we on the path to health or disease? According to a study published in the *New England Journal of Medicine,* as a result of the growing obesity epidemic, the "youth of today may, on average, live less healthy and possibly even shorter lives than their parents."*

*Olshansky, S. J., et al., "A Potential Decline in Life Expectancy in the United States in the Twenty-first Century," *New England Journal of Medicine* 352 (March 17, 2005): 1138–1145.

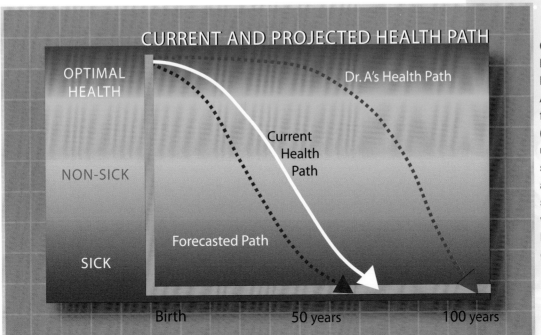

CURRENT AND PROJECTED HEALTH PATH

OPTIMAL HEALTH

Dr. A's Health Path

Current Health Path

NON-SICK

Forecasted Path

SICK

Birth   50 years   100 years

Current and Projected Health Path. According to the forecasted path (in red), more of us will be getting sicker younger and dying sooner—unless we adopt a new health path (in green).

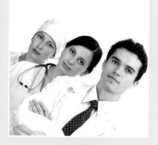

Diets that put your
nutritional balance out
of whack nearly always
fail and can actually
make it harder to lose
weight in the future.

The Failure Pattern: Diet vs. Exercise

Your doctor tells you to lose weight and sends you off to the hinterlands to look for answers. *It's like sending the lamb to the wolves.* There are a million "miracle" weight-loss products out there, and just as many opinions on how to lose weight. We're told every day on TV, in the papers, in the tabloids how heavy we are and how the latest breakthrough weight-loss cure will save us. Just about every one of those cures has its proponents. Forget for now the cabbage diet, the lemon juice diet, the water diet, colonics, purging, and other unhealthy methods, and let's just take a look at the two major schools of thought: diet and exercise.

In moving you toward your goal, most diet pundits tell you to focus on diet and most exercise pundits tell you to focus on exercise. Of course, both sides pay lip service to the other, but ultimately they're invested in supporting their own interests.

The fad diet folks tell you to lower your calorie intake and manipulate macronutrients (protein, fat, carbohydrates). That's where we get the "low-fat diet," "low-carb diet," and "high-protein diet"—all of which create an abnormal ratio of nutritional intake. But in fact, the food fight among these diet gurus as to who's right and who's wrong is an exercise in futility, because at the end of the day your body doesn't quite work the way they think it does.

If you lower your carbohydrates, fat, or protein by the wrong percentage, your body will develop cravings, and your chance of maintaining that weight loss is like a dog trying to stay away from a juicy porterhouse steak. To paraphrase Abraham Lincoln, "You can manipulate some of the people's percentage of nutrients some of the time, but you can't do it long term."

If you make it through this first phase of weight loss—and many people don't—the irony is that you will have lowered your total energy expenditure per day and therefore lowered your metabolic rate. Or, by not picking precisely the right fuels and foods, you'll lose muscle—the bane of periodic cycling (yo-yoing). Your body's furnace has been reset at a lower level than it was when you began your diet. This can actually lead to obesity. Without going through a recalibration process, you're likely to slip into your old eating habits and gain back the weight—but with a metabolic furnace that doesn't burn as well. The result? More weight, a higher percent of body fat versus muscle, a lower

---

Medication: A Double-Edged Sword

Did you know that medications are now among the leading causes of death in the nation? According to a study in the *Archives of Internal Medicine,* the number of serious adverse drug events (those resulting in disability, hospitalization, birth defects, etc.) more than doubled between 1998 and 2005, and the number of adverse drug events resulting in death nearly tripled.*

*Moore, T. J., et al., "Serious Adverse Drug Events Reported to the Food and Drug Administration, 1998–2005," *Archives of Internal Medicine* 167 (September 10, 2007): 1752–1759.

metabolic rate, and less inclination to be active—all of which makes it even harder to lose weight next time.

Imagine what happens after many repetitions of this cycle. After a while, your food intake just can't be lowered enough to have any effect on weight loss. That's when people become a fat factory, much to their disgust and frustration.

The exercise enthusiasts try to exercise themselves to a healthy weight. But people who focus on exercise tactics will find themselves as disappointed as the dieters. Although there are health benefits associated with exercise, it's hard to lose much weight through exercise alone.

To really lose weight, you would need ninety minutes of strenuous exercise a day, according to the U.S. Institute of Medicine. That's a daunting task for most of us to fit into our schedules! So while exercise is critical for long-term success, it needs to be part of a comprehensive process of building optimal health—and it should be deployed in baby steps. Once we have you losing weight, you'll naturally become more active. At that point, we'll increase your activity incrementally through fun choices that increase muscle mass and can last you a lifetime.

To lose weight through exercise alone, you'd need to work out strenuously for ninety minutes every day.

· ·

So now you can see why you gain back weight after dieting alone. There's just no simple solution to reaching and maintaining a healthy weight. That's not to say it's difficult to do, but there's a lot more to it than just diet or exercise.

Instead, there's a different path that will teach you how to create permanent health—the path to optimal health. And it's paved with the Habits of Health.

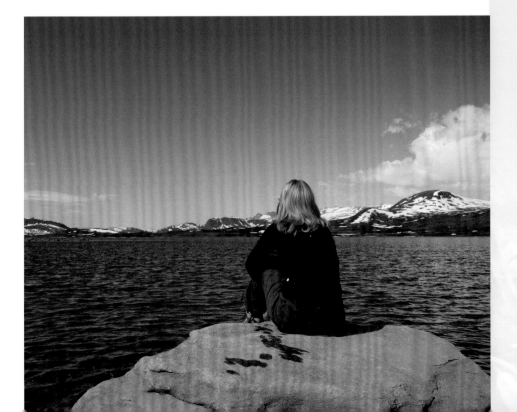

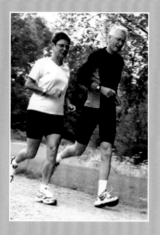

What do we mean by
optimal health? It's
different for everyone.
Optimal health is the
highest degree of health
that's possible for you
to achieve.

Chapter 2

The Path: The Creation of Optimal Health

If I were a genie in a bottle and could grant you the proverbial three wishes, I'll bet one of them would be for optimal health for you and your family. The good news is that this is one wish you can accomplish yourself—you just need to know how.

Is "Non-Sick" Your Way of Life?

If you're not sick, you're healthy, right? That's often how the medical world sees it. But in reality, these two states—*non-sick* and *healthy*—are vastly different.

Non-sickness is like purgatory—simply surviving, as opposed to a healthy state of thriving. It is caused by eating an excess quantity of nutritionally barren food, which overworks the pancreas and facilitates your body's storage of fat. Non-sickness is a state in which your muscles become weak and flabby, a state of not enough sleep and way too much stress. It's a state that leads you to progressive dependence on medications to relieve your symptoms—symptoms that are merely your body's way of telling you you're not healthy.

Being non-sick often leads to life-threatening illness over time, as when excess weight eventually takes its toll and leads to metabolic syndrome. This state on the road to obesity is what I call *pre-obesity*—a more apt description of the corresponding negative health effects than the innocuous-sounding *overweight*.

In a state of non-sickness, time is against you. It may go unnoticed until one day you're so fatigued that you finally go to your doctor and find out you have diabetes. Your health path has led you from non-sick to sick.

The bad news is that close to 90 percent of us fall into this non-sick category. The good news—or shall I say great news?!—is that the non-sick can usually reach optimal health in a relatively short amount of time.

Choosing Your Health Path

Let's look at the health path that most people find themselves on. Too often, it leads from non-sickness to sickness and disease—a descent accelerated by our modern lifestyle, as described in chapter 1.

Fortunately, this type of decline isn't inevitable. There's another way. But choosing the direction your path takes begins by understanding that life isn't a reality show—it's real, and it's the only life you've got. You can't wait passively for doctors, weight gurus, or drug companies to come up with a solution. Your health isn't a spectator sport!

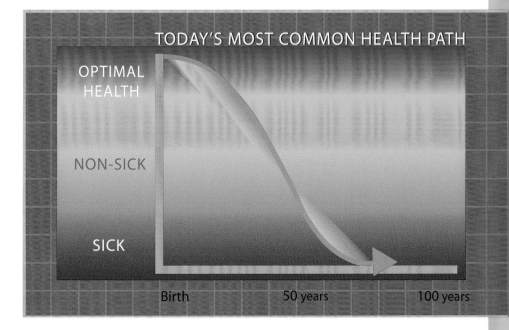

TODAY'S MOST COMMON HEALTH PATH

OPTIMAL HEALTH

NON-SICK

SICK

Birth — 50 years — 100 years

Today's Most Common Health Path. Today's most common health path descends steeply from optimal health at birth, to an unhealthy state of "non-sickness" by age fifty, to sickness and disease.

Start by asking yourself a few questions:

- Is my health improving every day?
- Are my daily habits creating greater health and vibrancy, or are they draining my battery and putting me on an accelerating path toward disease?
- Am I already in a non-sick or sick state?

Your answers will tell you whether you're on the path toward illness or toward health.

What if you find that you're already on the path to disease? Is it too late for you? Not at all. Even if you've tried time and again to lose weight and create good health—only to fail—your future is far from determined. You can change your path. And best of all, you don't even need to believe that optimal

Are You Non-sick?
When you're non-sick you're neither healthy nor ill, but somewhere in between. You may be non-sick if you're:
- Overweight (pre-obese)
- Not sleeping well
- Fatigued
- Weak or flabby
- Stressed out
- Taking lots of over-the-counter medications

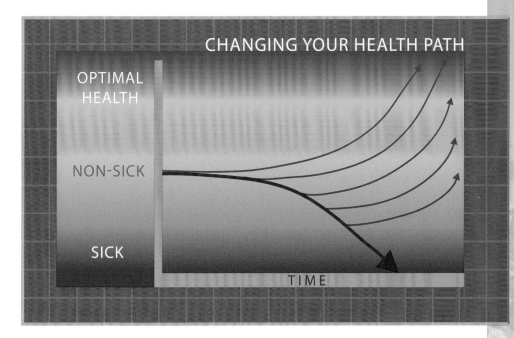

CHANGING YOUR HEALTH PATH

OPTIMAL HEALTH

NON-SICK

SICK

TIME

Changing Your Health Path. Your health path isn't predestined to be a steady decline. By adopting Habits of Health, you can change your path at any point and go from a state of sickness to one of thriving optimal health.

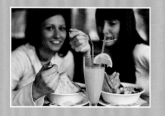

**Global Drug
Companies:
Selling Sickness?**
They're justifiably
applauded for saving
lives and reducing
suffering—but the
global drug giants
are no longer content
selling medication just
to the ill. There's much
money to be made
convincing healthy
people that they're
sick, and Wall Street
knows it. So successful
are pharmaceutical
companies' saturation
advertising and slick
awareness campaigns
that the U.S. currently
makes up 50 percent
of the global market for
pharmaceuticals, even
though we account for
less than 5 percent of the
world's population.

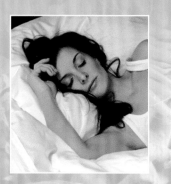

health is possible. You just need to take the right actions, begin to adopt new healthy habits, and build momentum. Your path can change at any point on your journey, and that change can occur almost instantaneously. *You're not predestined to get sick. That's the drug companies' message, not ours.* In fact, as you can see from the chart at the bottom of page 13, the further you are from optimal health, the more dramatic your change in health is likely to be.

Remember, our goal for you is to be much more than "non-sick": it's to be healthy. And it's your daily habits—your Habits of Disease or Habits of Health—that determine that direction.

The Habits of Health: An Overview

So what exactly are these Habits of Health? Let's take a closer look.

Habits of healthy eating. I'll teach you how to lose weight safely—about two to five pounds a week for the first two weeks and then one to two pounds a week thereafter—until you reach a healthy weight. At that point, we'll shift to helping you maintain your ideal weight for good. This eating plan is specifically designed to move you through a fat-burning stage to a recalibration stage to an optimizing stage, in which your metabolism is working at its most efficient. It's easy to do, and you won't have hunger pangs or food cravings.

Habits of moving your body. We'll ease you into the right amount of physical activity at the right moment in your development. While your movement plan may include formal exercise, it's more often made up of fun activities and clever strategies that make moving your body easy and fun—including some you've probably never even considered.

Strategic behavioral habits. Your long-term success depends on choosing the best strategic actions to support your health. These include examining how you make choices, understanding your patterns and triggers, and helping you establish support systems. As in any good strategy, the first steps make the next steps easier to do.

The habit of support through vitanutrients. Feeding the body with the right nutrients is one of the most helpful habits you can adopt. Food is the major source of these vitanutrients, but sometimes additional support is needed in the form of vitamin and mineral supplements.

The habit of reducing dangerous inflammation. Inflammation is systemic. When you're overweight, a higher level of inflammatory substances are released from your fat and circulate through your body, raising havoc. Traditional medicine treats this inflammation separately, as if it were isolated from the rest of the body's functioning. But because the body works as a whole system, it's critical to address the root causes of inflammation in order to ensure good heart health and longevity. I'll teach you the types of foods that fuel the inflammatory process as well as those that can calm this dangerous state. And through a variety of easy daily activities, we'll turn down your hyperactive immune system and help you attain optimal health.

Habits of good sleep. The effect of regular sleep patterns on health is often underestimated—but sleep is one of the most critical factors in creating overall health and well-being, and surprisingly has a direct impact on losing weight and keeping it off.

The habit of creating a positive environment. Your environment can enhance or diminish the success of your other health habits. I'll show you how to build a "health bubble" that will help you take control of your personal environment and create conditions that support long-term health.

Habits of support. It's important to create a structure to assist you in your quest for optimal health. I'll help you build the support system that works best for you, whether that's me, a friend, a group of friends, a coach, or a whole network of people!

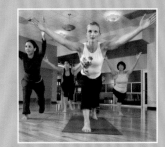

Changing just one or two habits isn't enough—all the Habits of Health need to work together to harness the power to create optimal health.

All Together Now

You may have tried to improve a few of these habits in the past, but with limited success. You may even be doing some of them really well. Maybe you've reduced your daily intake of calories, but you haven't gotten into the habit of putting your body in motion every day. Or you're exercising and taking vitamins, but you're not getting enough sleep. We're after much more: we want to harness all of the recuperative power of your body. And for that to happen, *it's essential that all the habits work together.*

To make this all a little easier and less overwhelming, we'll introduce our new habits in baby steps, little by little, through a plan that's logical, doable, and effective. One step will lead to the next, and soon you'll have a firm foundation for optimal health.

Now, if you're like most of my patients, you probably have some questions by this point.

Can I adopt these Habits of Health? Yes.

Will they work for me? Better than you can imagine at this point.

Is it hard? No. In fact, because of the way this approach is structured, and because of the science behind it, you'll find it much easier than you may have expected.

Do I need willpower? Not in the usual sense. You won't be manipulating yourself through willpower or pressure. Instead, you'll learn how to make strategic choices that support your highest aspirations.

If I lose weight, will I yo-yo and gain it back? No. Most programs can get you to lose weight. But what they're missing is the crucial way these Habits of Health work together to reinforce long-term success and sustainability.

Dr. A Says . . .

We're going to introduce these new healthy habits in baby steps to make them easier to adopt. Soon, you'll have a solid foundation for a life of optimal health.

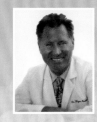

Your Daily Choices and Your Current Health

Like most of us, you probably haven't escaped the effects of too much food and too little activity. Today, over two-thirds of Americans are either pre-obese or obese. But just by deciding to read this book and make a change, you're about to experience a powerful impact on your life.

At each phase of your journey, you'll be making choices that fit your lifestyle—whatever your current reality may be. Whether you're twenty years

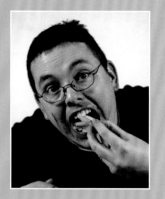

One cheeseburger doesn't kill you. It's making those negative choices day after day, year after year, that add up to poor health, disease, and premature death.

Time and daily choice are our most powerful agents of change. Our choices can be powerful allies or an erosive force that takes our health from us.

old and not eating right, forty years old and seriously overweight, or sixty years old with diabetes, high blood pressure, and a previous heart attack, the habits I'm about to teach you will create a blueprint for your daily life, advancing you from your current state of health toward optimal health. And as you lose weight and increase your energy, you'll find that it gets easier and easier to make the healthy choice.

The Modern Way of Life—*or Death*?

Let's say that today at lunch you ate a greasy cheeseburger, onion rings, and supersized soda—and then had a near-fatal heart attack. Would you wake up tomorrow and order the same thing? Of course not!

Yet every day, millions of us are eating foods again and again that are destroying our health. It may not happen right away, but after days, weeks, months, and years of poor choices, that heavy load of saturated animal fat, trans-fats, and high-fructose corn syrup—along with a lack of healthy vegetables—leads to an insidious rise in insulin, cholesterol, triglycerides, and a sinister state of inflammation. These substances, aided by our own immune system, lead to the formation of an atherosclerotic plaque, causing the artery wall to weaken.

What happens then? One Monday morning, the executive grips his chest in excruciating pain, and all those poor daily choices that didn't seem to matter much at the time begin to matter a lot. The coronary artery ruptures its endothelial lining and platelets quickly gather around the tear, forming a clot and cutting off the heart's blood supply. He collapses as a result of a massive heart attack at age fifty—and everyone's surprised. He seemed so healthy!

Here's the thing: eating that one cheeseburger didn't kill him. The body has an amazing ability to handle a few bad choices. What killed him was making similar bad choices day in and day out over the course of all those business lunches, year after year. It's ironic, isn't it? Our health is our most precious asset, yet the daily choices most of us make directly conflict with our ability to preserve it. Why? Because the negative results aren't obvious right away. Eating a cheeseburger today or bypassing the treadmill on your way to the couch won't cause a noticeable downturn in your health right away. By the same token, choosing a healthy vegetable for lunch today or going to the gym once or twice in January won't create a noticeable improvement. *What will make a difference is choosing actions on a daily basis that support your journey to optimal health.* Over time, those choices make all the difference in the world—the difference between death and radiant health.

Changing Our Focus

In our instant-gratification society, we tend to think of weight loss as a destination. In fact, it's really just a first step. Optimal health is a journey based on lifestyle change—a re-orientation from merely hoping to lose weight (all the while succumbing to daily stress and making poor choices) to creating health by allowing our minds and bodies to work together. That's very different than focusing on losing weight alone!

The Art of Compounding

Let's think about those choices as if they were money in the bank. Despite whatever get-rich-quick spin the latest financial gurus are touting, building wealth is really all about compounding. Here's a little exercise to try as an example.

Say you have to make a choice. I'll write you a check today for a million dollars or I'll give you a penny today and double it every day for thirty-one days. Two choices—a million dollars today or the sum of a penny doubled for one month.

What would you do?

It may surprise you to find out that by waiting patiently for thirty-one days instead of grabbing the instant million, you'll end up with $10,737,418! Yet, without thinking, most of us would put out our hand and take the check in a second. It's ingrained in our behavior. In today's instant society, we want gratification and we want it now! We're always looking for the next breakthrough, the next cure, the next pill that will help us lose weight fast. That's why people rush out and have gastric bypass surgery, or buy the latest prescription—often with no regard to long-term health risks or side effects. And take my word for it, *there are always side effects.*

True, drugs may lower your weight for a short time, but without changing your Habits of Disease—the cheeseburger, the salt, the lack of exercise, the six-pack—medications are nothing but a band-aid. In fact, I will be so bold as to say that *no breakthrough drug is on its way that can cure obesity.*

However, there is a powerful solution available to you right now—and it starts with the compounding effect of choice. It's about making small, doable choices that support health every day. When you make those choices today, and tomorrow, and the next day, day in and day out, the benefits compound much like the penny doubling over time. And in the end, you gain a treasure far more valuable than weight loss alone—you gain permanent optimal health.

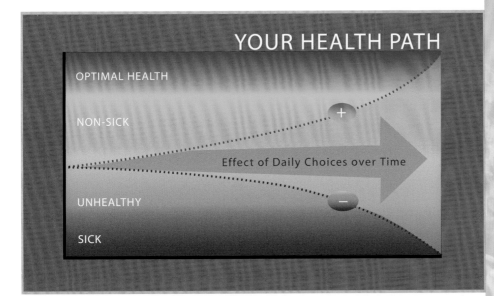

YOUR HEALTH PATH

OPTIMAL HEALTH

NON-SICK

Effect of Daily Choices over Time

UNHEALTHY

SICK

Your Health Path: The Effect of Daily Choices over Time. Making a positive choice (+) or a negative one (-) may not seem to make much difference at the moment. But as you can see from the chart, each of those little choices adds up over time, taking you in the direction of sickness or optimal health. Which direction are your choices taking you?

The Path to Optimal Health and Beyond

As I take you through the phases of your journey to optimal health, a number of improvements will begin to occur throughout your body. If your health is like most of ours, your body is probably in fat-storage mode right now, with progressive weight gain and an associated high insulin level. These unhealthy physical conditions create an inflammatory state that's a major contributor to heart disease, cancer, and premature aging.

As you start down your new path, we'll focus on your energy intake and the foods you're eating—things we can change immediately. Beginning in Phase I, we'll transform you from a fat factory to a fat-burning machine, stabilize your insulin, douse the inflammatory fires, and start building habits that support health. Here's a snapshot of some of those improvements as you journey through the phases toward optimal health:

THE PATH TO OPTIMAL HEALTH AND BEYOND					
	Your Current State of Health	PHASE I Beginning the Weight-Loss Phase	PHASE II Incorporating the Habits of Health	PHASE III Optimizing Your Health	PHASE IV Longevity
Fat vs. Muscle	Fat Storage	Fat Burning	Muscle Building	Muscle Optimization	Extreme Lean Muscle
Body Mass Index (BMI)	BMI High	BMI Decreasing	BMI <25	BMI <25	BMI 20–24
Habits of Health	Habits of Disease	Healthy Eating and Activity Habits	Habits of Health	Habits of Health Automated	Specific Longevity Strategy

*C-reactive protein, a common measure of inflammation

But before we begin, we're going to spend some time really looking at this choice you're making: the choice to be healthy. Because in order to reach and maintain your goals—for weight loss, for better health, for a more fulfilled life—it's essential to first understand where you are right now, where you need to be, and just what's standing in your way.

Chapter 3

Motivation for Change

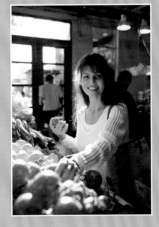

Much of the material in this chapter originates from the work of my friend and colleague Robert Fritz, best-selling author of The Path of Least Resistance *and many other important works that have changed the way we understand human motivation and the structure of change.*

The Motivation Factor

Why do you want to change?

The answer might seem obvious—so obvious in fact that we don't often think to ask the question, or to consider our answer. After all, if you're over-weight, have health problems, feel tired, and lack energy, the obvious answer is that you want to change in order to solve those problems. That's true of most changes we try to adopt—they're based on solving a problem or trying to get rid of an unwanted situation.

This type of motivation almost never leads to lasting change. Typically, you make some changes at first, but later you fall back into your old ways of behaving. Why? Because whenever you experience emotional conflict—that is, feelings of negativity—you want it to stop. Who wants to feel uncomfortable? You think about your health problems, or about how much you hate the way you look, and your natural response is to feel terrible. In order to end that discomfort, you take actions that make you feel better about yourself—maybe you go on a diet, or vow to change your couch potato ways and start exercising. But those actions aren't motivated by what you *want*—an outcome you desire—and so they lead you into a predictable cycle:

1. Emotional conflict leads you to act.
2. Because you've acted, you feel better—even if the situation hasn't changed much.
3. Feeling better takes the pressure off, lessening the emotional conflict.
4. Less emotional conflict means there's less reason to continue doing the things that reduced the conflict in the first place.
5. Since you feel better, you no longer feel a pressing need to follow through on your actions.
6. And the original behavior returns.

When you try to change in order to get rid of negative feelings or situations, you slip up once things get a little better. It just doesn't work long term.

A Habit of Health: Focusing on what you *want,* not what you *don't* want

Here's another way of looking at this cycle. Your bad feelings (intense emotional conflict) motivate you to take action, which reduces your emotional conflict:

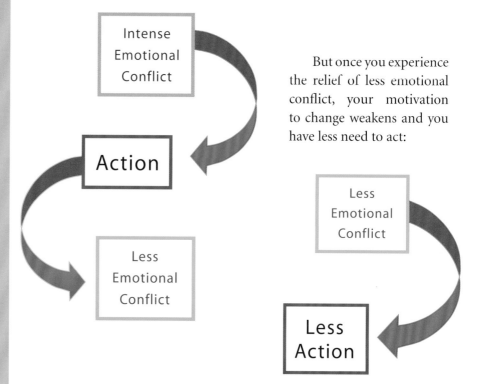

But once you experience the relief of less emotional conflict, your motivation to change weakens and you have less need to act:

It's a typical yo-yo pattern! And the most natural thing in the world is to fall back into your previous habits: eating, smoking, whatever it is you're trying to change. In fact, it's more than natural—it's inevitable. Here's a tip that's worth committing to memory:

Conflict-driven motivation is one of the major reasons people yo-yo.

And what's reinforcing this pattern? Look at our doctors, warning patients about the ill-effects of eating the wrong foods, of not exercising, of smoking, or of not taking care of themselves in myriad other ways. You leave their office ready to do anything to avoid the terrible things that could happen to you if you don't change your ways. Now, these doctors mean well. But, unbeknownst to them, they're setting a yo-yo pattern in motion by using *threat* to force a change in their patients. Their intentions are golden—their approach floats like a lead balloon.

Yet, despite the fact that relying on self-control is nearly impossible and unlikely to lead to long-term success, most of us regularly use this sort of conflict manipulation to try to lose weight. It just doesn't work long term, especially if you're an "emotional eater" (see box, page 25). That's why we're going to change the way you motivate yourself—and in the process create a fundamental new Habit of Health.

*You're going to motivate yourself by focusing on what you want—
not what you don't want!*

Problem Solving vs. Desired Outcome

Let's say you have two choices. You can:

1. Think in terms of trying to fix your bad health (a *problem* orientation)
   or
2. Shift your focus to creating health (an *outcome* orientation)

Most diet books fail to understand the difference between a *problem*-oriented motivation and an *outcome*-oriented motivation. Gosh, is it really that hard? The first has to do with trying to solve a problem, like being unhealthily overweight; the second has to do with creating a desired state, like being optimally healthy. In the first, you're motivated to take action to get rid of a problem; in the second, you're motivated to take action to bring what you truly want into being.

Changing our emphasis from *what we're against* to *what we're for* has a dramatic impact. Are we merely against something, or do we want to create an important result? And let me be clear here, I'm not talking about "positive thinking," but rather about the fundamental reason we act—with no spin on it, positive or otherwise.

Researchers regularly report the success of certain diets, all the while warning people that the subjects on these "successful" diets couldn't sustain weight loss for more than two years on average. And they always blame the diet itself for this long-term failing, because they don't know any better. The one factor that's never named—that's almost universally ignored—is that the dieter's motivation is usually a problem-solving, conflict-driven reaction to emotional anxiety.

You could try to adopt the healthiest diet that ever existed, but if your motivation is to fix a health problem you have or might have in the future, you'll be back to your old tricks in two years, with your weight back on and in worse shape than ever. No wonder so many people feel helpless after trying time and again to lose weight. They don't know why they can't pull it off. They're sincere about wanting to lose weight. They know the stakes are high.

As you'll learn in Phase I, choosing the right way to eat is one of the most critical factors in creating health. But how do you go about making this new approach a true lifestyle change—one that lasts beyond the two-year life span of most diets? As vitally important as the right approach to eating may be, that alone isn't going to do it. *And that's why reaching your healthy weight is only the beginning of our journey.* The motivation factor is what makes all the difference between yo-yoing—losing weight only to gain it back—and creating optimal health by adopting health habits you can live with.

What does that mean for you? That if you're adopting a new eating approach because you're reacting to the conflict you're feeling at the moment, you

The right eating approach is vitally important, but it's just the first step. For long-term success you need the right motivation.

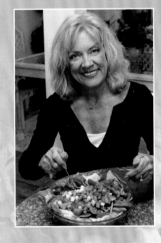

Why Modern Medicine Has Failed to Stop the Obesity Crisis

Most of our medical system's energy goes toward reacting to and preventing illness. Creating health—as obvious a goal as that may seem—just hasn't been part of the picture. Only recently are some of my colleagues beginning to shift their focus to exploring why people need help in the first place. They're beginning to realize that healing the sick, while a noble cause, just isn't as smart as making sure people don't get sick in the first place.

What have they learned? That it's not enough to simply react to illness. It's not enough to settle for a state of non-sickness. We need to teach people how to actively create health by building a healthy body, mind, and long-term Habits of Health.

ON FIXERS AND HEALERS

By Mark Nelson, MD, FACC, MPH

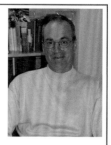

How are we to understand the predicament we now find ourselves in as health care providers? A health care system that provides neither health nor care, and is certainly not a system but rather a patchwork quilt of "fix-it" medicine and technology—a bureaucratic albatross sustained by enormous financial cost and surviving at the expense of untold human lives and suffering. How has it come to pass that we physicians have been taught, incentivized, and paid to fix but not to heal, to treat but not to prevent, to compartmentalize and fragment but not to create health?

I have taught my patient Frank to make his choices around the principles Dr. Andersen outlines in this book. He feels renewed and invigorated, and he says he has more hope and energy than he's experienced in many years. Thanks to the resulting weight loss, his doctor has been able to reduce his diabetic and anti-hypertensive medications because his conditions have improved. He's succeeded in creating health for himself and has integrated healthy habits into his life—eating small, frequent, healthy low-fat meals; having breakfast every day; exercising regularly; and weighing himself weekly. He's internalized my support as a coach and has incorporated that into his daily routine as well.

On a recent visit to his primary care physician, Frank's doctor told him, "Well, Frank, I guess you don't need me anymore." I wondered at this doctor's dilemma, of feeling helpless and perhaps even worthless in the face of his patient's health. How strange that he could envision no role for himself in his patient's quest for health, for a life without disease, labels, medications, and an endless litany of tests and procedures. And I wondered, couldn't his physician imagine himself as both fixer and healer? As doing more than simply reacting to disease? Could he envision preventing illness and creating health? Have we physicians become so tired of the bureaucratic entanglements, so inured to medication upon medication and test upon test, that we've forgotten (or perhaps never realized) our untapped potential to teach our patients Habits of Health, to work with them to create health and conquer disease?

Perhaps the ultimate test of our relevance and compassion as physicians is to have the courage to let go of the familiar and learn to walk with our patients, who yearn to learn and practice Habits of Health so that they may be not just free of disease, but free to create lives of unsurpassed health. ∎

won't be able to maintain your initial success. Or, in simple English: Friend, you're going to fail miserably. Sorry, but that's just how it is.

Think back to the last time you tried unsuccessfully to lose weight. Remember how you reverted to your old eating habits once the pressure to change diminished? Notice how easy it was to sink into your old behaviors. You know, it's not unusual for someone who's spent months losing weight to celebrate their accomplishment by chowing down at McDonald's or Burger King. Welcome to human nature! Soon you're back to where you were before, or worse. Study after study shows the negative impact of dieting once the diet's over. As you yo-yo from one diet to the next, you put yourself at higher risk for cardiovascular disease, more weight gain, and myriad other problems. It's not your fault. You simply didn't know that your problem-solving motivation was your downfall all along.

A Teachable Moment

So what do you do if you bought this book with problem solving in mind? Don't worry—you're not doomed! Your starting point is just your starting point—not your end point. You can recalibrate your motivation right now.

This is a teachable moment! And here's why it's possible:

1. *You're about to take a step forward.* You've made the decision to begin losing weight. And even if that first step is a reaction to the emotional conflict you feel. . . hey, at least you're committed and on the move to getting healthier. We just need to keep you going in the right direction on the path to optimal health.
2. *You're open to allowing the change process to succeed.* Until now, you didn't know how important motivation was. But now you can see the profound difference between avoiding bad stuff and supporting good stuff. With this new insight, you're able to make a major shift in your motivation, and as a result dramatically improve your chance of success.
3. *You truly want a positive outcome.* Sure, there are problems you'd like to solve, and future problems you want to avoid. But even more, there's a life you want to build. Think of it this way: even if those problems disappeared tomorrow, you'd still want to have the life you desire, right?

Imagine how your life will look once you've created optimal health for yourself. *Optimal*—the most desirable or favorable possible, the highest possibility there is. It's the perfect word for us. After all, we're all different. One person's optimal health might mean running a four-minute mile or breaking the record for weight lifting. For someone else, optimal might mean being able to play tennis or run a few miles every day. And for yet another person, it might mean they can play with their grandchildren and live a healthy, normal life.

Your optimal health profile—your personal best—is our goal. Not our only goal, but certainly one of our most important ones. And it all begins by shifting your motivation from being against bad things to being in favor of good ones.

Structuring Your Success

Having goals is a good first step, but goals alone aren't enough. We need to position those goals within a structure that supports them. With the right structure, our chance of success goes up. With the wrong structure, our chance of success goes down—and even with the best intentions we probably won't accomplish our goals in the long term.

Let's say optimal health is our goal. What do we need to know in order to put this goal into a useful structure? Well, look at it this way: if our goal were to go to Chicago, the first thing we'd need to know would be where we're starting from.

We need to know our starting point. And if our goal is optimal health, our starting point is our current state of health. We need to have a realistic picture of where we actually are right now.

To figure out how to get to our destination (optimal health), we must first look realistically at where we are. The space between these two points creates the tension that motivates us to change.

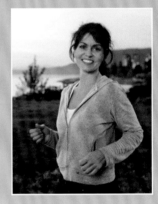

When where we are
is different from where
we want to be, we feel
tension—and
that tension is a
great motivator
for action.

A Habit of Health:
Being honest with
yourself

Honesty is crucial to
achieving our goals—
but what exactly do we
mean by honesty?

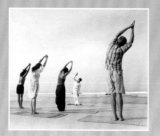

The Importance of Structural Tension

The difference between our *desired state* and our *actual state* creates a useful tension that author Robert Fritz calls structural tension. It is as if we've stretched a bow and aimed the arrow. The tension in the bow makes reaching the target possible—even probable. It's the type of tension that helps us take the actions we need in order to get the results we want.

In nature, all tension strives for resolution. So by establishing structural tension, we've created a powerful dynamic to help us achieve our goal. It's as if nature herself is on our side, and we find ourselves more able than ever to work on behalf of our goals.

Granted, our goals for optimal health aren't easy to accomplish. If they were, we'd have done it years ago. And the fact that we've tried to reach these goals in the past and failed makes them even more daunting. But with the right approach, within the right structure, we can change that pattern.

Tracking Your Progress

Where are you right now in relation to your goal? Remember, your current reality is constantly changing, so it needs regular updating.

The actions you're taking right now have impact you can measure. If one of your goals is to weigh 140 pounds, how much do you weigh now? Weigh yourself weekly to see. If your goal is to fit into that tight pair of sexy jeans, how close are you? Try them on every few days to find out.

You may have other health goals, each one with its own current status. Maybe it's a blood pressure, cholesterol, or blood sugar goal, or a goal for increased energy and stamina, measured by how far you can walk or jog or swim. Each of these is one part of your optimal health picture, and each one should be tracked and updated as you manage the relationship between your actual situation and your desired goal.

Being Honest with Yourself

Honesty is crucial to achieving our goals—but what exactly do we mean by honesty?

One aspect of honesty is being clear about our goals—*we shouldn't lie to ourselves about what we want.* Another is separating what we want from what we think is possible—*we need to describe our current reality honestly and objectively.*

Most of us aren't trained to be as honest with ourselves as we need to be. But being honest with yourself is an important Habit of Health. And like any new habit, it takes practice. The more you do it, the more it becomes part of who you are. This is one area where a health coach can come in handy, both to help you understand your current reality and to help you develop new habits.

The Power of Choice

Choice means it's your call—you can do it or not (whatever "it" is). Choice is the power to make a decision.

Now, if you just want one thing, making a choice is easy. But what happens when two things you want are in conflict with each other? Most of us never learn how to deal with this sort of conflict. In fact, most of the time we're not even aware that a conflict exists. But the reality is that we face situations like this all the time:

> *You want optimal health, and you also want to eat the banana split.*

Those two desires are mutually exclusive. You can't have both. You need to make a choice. But how? The overall principle is this: *Make the choice that supports your more important desire.* Of course, that means you need to sort out which of your desires are more important and which are less important.

Three Types of Choices

There are three distinct types of choice: *primary, secondary,* and *fundamental.* I'll discuss primary and secondary choice here, and leave fundamental choice for the next chapter.

Primary choice is a major choice—something we want more than other things that we may also want. When we think about optimal health versus a banana split, the question is, What's more important to us? The benefits of a long and healthy life, or the short-lived satisfaction of eating something that can harm our health? It's easy to see that the prospect of a long and healthy life is a far better proposition. But when confronted by a banana split, we sometimes forget our larger goal and succumb to temptation. Hey, we're only human. But it's also human to become a bit more savvy in distinguishing the things that support our health from the things that harm us.

Secondary choice concerns the actions we take to support our primary choice, even if we don't really want to. We're motivated to take these actions

> What should you do when two things you want conflict? Make the choice that supports the desire that's more important.

> Primary choice is about deciding that we want one thing—optimal health, for example—more than something else. Secondary choice is about taking the daily actions that support our primary choice—for example, choosing not to have a banana split.

Choice means we
can do it or not
(whatever "it" is).

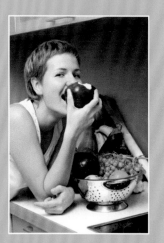

not because we like doing them, which we often don't, but because we like the result they bring. Dorothy Parker put it this way: "I like *having* written." In other words, she didn't like the process of writing, but she was willing to do it in order to produce the piece—which in the end she did like.

Once we know what our primary choice is, it's easy to figure out how to make our secondary choices. We make them in such a way as to support our primary choice. If optimal health is our primary choice, what secondary choices do we need to make to support that choice? Basically, these choices fall into two categories:

1. Doing some things we don't like doing
2. Not doing some things we like doing

Many secondary choices aren't things we would normally choose to do. In fact, if it weren't for the primary choice, we wouldn't do them at all. And yes, this may include exercise. Now, some people love to exercise. Aren't they lucky? But many more people don't like to exercise, and yet they do it anyway. Why? To support their higher, more important goal of creating health. So they adopt an exercise program—a secondary choice that falls into the category of doing things we don't like doing, but do anyway to support a higher goal. The same may be true for learning to eat in a new healthy way.

Now, that doesn't mean we can't try to find exercises that are as fun as possible, or make healthy eating easy and enjoyable. In fact, *making things easy and enjoyable increases our tendency to do them* and therefore supports our higher goals—in this case, optimal health. And, in fact, making things easy and enjoyable is a big part of my plan. But we must never lie to ourselves about our motivation. The reason we're doing this thing we may not want to do is because it supports something we *really* want—a lot. Because the real power of choice is not in doing things that are easy and enjoyable, but in doing things that are strategically critical to our goal.

That's important to keep in mind. We make secondary choices to support our goal—not because we particularly like the *actions*, but because we like the *outcome.*

To support our goal of optimal health, we may find that we no longer choose to do certain things—smoking, eating the wrong foods, being a couch potato, living in stressful situations, abusing alcohol and drugs, and other unhealthy habits that need to stop. But try to use conflict to make yourself stop, and the moment the pressure's off, you return to the unhealthy behavior. By understanding our primary choice, on the other hand, and making strategic secondary choices, we discover a whole new ability to support ourselves.

Now, what goes on in our heads when we're confronted by the need to make a secondary choice—in this case, let's say, that banana split. Here's our *internal* conversation:

I like the looks of that banana split.
Yes.
I could have it.
That's right, you could.
I want it.
Yes, you do.
But I also want to support my long-range goal of optimal health.
Sure.
I could eat the banana split or not.
That's true.
If I ate it, it would be harder to create my goal.
That's true too.
What do I want more: the banana split or optimal health?
Optimal health.
Therefore, while I could have the banana split, I choose not to have it to support my more important goal.
That's right!

And what goes on outside? Here's the *external* conversation:

"Would you like a banana split?"
"No thanks."

One thing's pretty clear: you are *very* aware of what you're doing when you make these choices. And that's part of the power of primary and secondary choice. You're not doing things unconsciously. Quite the opposite, in fact. You're becoming much more tuned in to what you're thinking and what you're doing. If you don't have that type of conversation with yourself when temptation rears its ugly head, you'll eat the banana split and regret it later when your senses return. *Mindlessness* is the enemy.

The Key to Discipline

Throughout your life, you're faced with situations that demand a choice. Even by not choosing, you've effectively made a choice. But this choice usually isn't in your own best interests. Knowing how to determine what's primary—and therefore, what's secondary—enables you to rise above any situation, however hard, to support your greater good.

So in fact it's in this relationship—between the primary and secondary choice—that the key to discipline is found. Once you know how to manage this relationship, you'll be able to accomplish more than you ever thought possible.

In the next chapter, we'll organize your life around what matters most— optimal health.

> To support our primary goal (optimal health), we do things we wouldn't otherwise choose to do, like exercising or eating right. We may not always like doing these things, but we like where they get us.

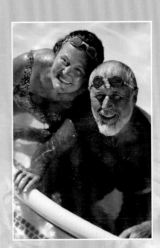

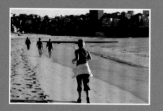

Life, liberty, and the
pursuit of happiness—
the inalienable rights
that our forefathers
determined to be a
fundamental choice.
To create optimal
health, you need to
make the *fundamental
choice* to be healthy.

Is anything in life more
important than health?
When people realize
that they're dangerously
ill, the answer to that
question becomes clear.

Chapter 4
Health Is All About Choice

In the previous chapter, we discussed primary choice (the creation of specific goals) and secondary choice (the actions we must take to support those goals). Both are key to successful change. But there's another type of choice that's equally important—*fundamental choice*. It's what organizational consultant Robert Fritz calls "the choice upon which all other choices rest."*

Fundamental Choice

Fundamental choice is what defines our state of being. It's where we stand.

It's our choice to be free and healthy. It's what we're willing to fight for!

Let's take an example: Say you try to quit smoking, but you've never really made the fundamental choice to be a nonsmoker. Nothing will work, even methods others have found successful. Soon you'll be back to your two-pack-a-day habit. If, on the other hand, you do make the fundamental choice to be a nonsmoker, just about any method will work—and in fact you'll find yourself attracted to those methods that work particularly well.

It's the same with any fundamental choice. Once you make the choice to be healthy, you've made it your business to act in accordance with your goal. You're taking full responsibility for your actions rather than letting circumstances drive your decisions. You become the author of your own life story.

It's important to accept the fact that no one can do it for you. Others can help with their advice, good wishes, guidance, experience, medical insight, and understanding of human patterns and motivation. But it will always come down to you. If you're thinking, "I'll do my best, but it's really someone else's job to see to it that it works," then you haven't made this fundamental choice.

Most of us have been raised to react to circumstances. We haven't been taught to believe that we can adopt a fundamental, self-generated resolve. But in fact this is how we take charge of our lives—by realizing that, no matter the circumstances, no matter the temptation, we can do what we know is right, because we've taken a stand for the choices we hold most important.

How to Make a Fundamental Choice

Right now, whatever your circumstances may be, you can make a profound, fundamental choice for optimal health. Begin by asking yourself this question: Do I want to be optimally healthy? (Notice that I didn't say, "Is it possible to be optimally healthy?") Most likely, the answer is a resounding *yes!*

*Robert Fritz, *The Path of Least Resistance,* Ballantine Books, 1984.

Let's think about it for a moment. Is there anything else in your life as important as optimal health? As you ponder that question, let me give you a little perspective. As you know, for twenty years I served as director of surgical intensive care at a large teaching hospital. The patients I managed would very likely have died without the intense, interventional care we provided—the full gamut of Star Wars medical technology, invasive monitoring, potent intravenous medications, and sophisticated nutritional intervention.

These vulnerable patients came from all walks of life, some young, some old. But they all knew that at any moment they could die. They shared a universal realization that changed them profoundly—that right now, surviving and getting healthy was all that mattered. It was more important to the millionaire than his portfolio. It was more important to the executive than his job promotion. It was more important to the teenager than the new car he'd just wrecked. Reality can be so enlightening!

In fact, health deserves to be right up there alongside freedom and the pursuit of happiness as our most prized possessions. It's certainly *my* most prized possession. I want to be healthy to go skiing with my young girls. I want to watch them graduate from college and be able to keep up with what they're doing. I want to see them get married and see my grandchildren go to school. I want to sail around the world with my wife, Lori, and I want her to be healthy too. I want these things more than anything I own. And they're all possible, as long as I make optimal health my top priority—my fundamental choice.

I hope that you too have decided that optimal health is your fundamental choice. Once you've made that choice, you simply need to arrange your primary and secondary choices to make it happen. Sound simple? It is! It really is!

Our task now is to:

- Organize the primary choices that will produce optimal health.
- Outline the secondary choices, or actions steps, that will support those primary goals.

By making these actions part of your daily life, step by step, you'll begin to embody Dr. A's Habits of Health.

Primary Choices for Optimal Health

Now that you've made health your fundamental choice, it's our job to bring it into being. I'll be your guide, but it's up to you to actually do the work to create optimal health, starting by focusing on the primary goals that will support your fundamental choice.

Optimal health is built on a foundation of behaviors that together create a lifestyle that restores your body and optimizes its ability to function. The basic components of a healthy lifestyle—what I call the foundations of health—are outlined in the box on page 30. You may already recognize and even practice some of these, such as a healthy weight or an active lifestyle, but our approach will help you solidify your grasp of *all* of these critical components by bringing them to life.

In the previous chapter, I described a new way of looking at health. Rather than thinking of issues such as your weight or your blood pressure as problems

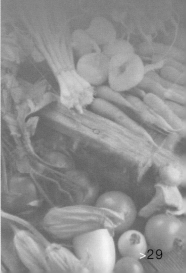

CHAPTER 4

HEALTH IS ALL
ABOUT CHOICE

Health Crisis and the Teachable Moment
According to a study by the National Weight Control Registry—a database of individuals who've lost thirty pounds or more and kept it off for at least one year—people who suffer a heart attack, stroke, or other serious medical crisis find themselves more committed to weight loss as a result. In addition, people with these sorts of medical triggers reported greater weight loss and less weight regain. The upshot? A medical event may provide a teachable moment for weight control.*

*Gorin, A. A., et al., "Medical Triggers Are Associated with Better Short- and Long-Term Weight Loss Outcomes," *Preventive Medicine* 39 (September 2004): 612–616.

Optimal health isn't
a destination, but a
state of being that you
achieve—a change in
orientation whereby
you create a new state
of being that revolves
around making the daily
choices that support
health.

Need some help and
guidance as you
identify your goals? It
might help to read the
chapters that cover the
primary health habit
you're targeting in your
chart. You'll also find
extra guidance and
assistance in *Living a
Longer, Healthier Life:
The Companion Guide
to Dr. A's Habits of
Health* (Habits of Health
Press, 2009) and in the
new DVD *Dr. A's Habits
of Health Video Series*
(forthcoming).

to solve, you learned to think about what you really want out of life, and to
use that motivation to adopt behaviors that support your health goals. Those
behaviors are the Habits of Health.

It's all about creating radiant health, whatever that means to you. Let's
begin by showing you how to identify your goals in each of the foundational
components that together form the basis of health and the Habits of Health.

The Foundations of Health

- Healthy eating, including vitanutrient support
- Healthy weight and a normal waist size
- An active lifestyle, including a daily activity program, a walking program, strength conditioning, flexibility, and agility
- Recuperative sleep
- Relaxation
- A microenvironment of health
- Well-being, including social activities, limited stress, a sense of purpose and meaning, spiritual health, and personal fulfillment
- A support system

Identifying Your Primary Choices

Take a look at the foundations of health in the box above and begin to think
about what each of them means to you. I want you to start becoming aware of
these fundamental determinants as we prepare you for your journey.

What's your goal in each category right now? I realize that at this point
you may not know how you'll reach these goals. That's OK—it's my job to
help teach you how to adopt the powerful Habits of Health that will help you
do just that. For now, just spend some time with a blank piece of paper and
write down what it would look like to be at your own optimal point in these
foundational areas. Since we're all at different stages of health, that's bound to
look different for each of us, and that's fine too. Remember, health is a journey,
not a destination. Where you are now is just a starting point.

As you're thinking about and writing down these goals, here are five simple
steps to help you hone your definition:

1. Form a mental picture of one of the foundational components (for
   example, an active lifestyle). Then ask yourself, "Is this the result I want to
   create?" If the answer is yes, that's great. If it's no, you'll need to refine your
   definition.
2. Quantify your goals. Be specific and include a time frame—for example, "I
   will have great aerobic stamina in twelve months."
3. Avoid comparative terms. For example, if you wrote, "I will have better
   health," rewrite your goal to say, "I will have very good health."
4. Make sure you're focusing on creating health, not on solving a problem.
   For example, if you wrote, "I will stop being so short of breath when I

walk," rewrite your goal to say, "I'm walking for half an hour every day and am able to talk to my dog the whole time."

5. Make sure you're describing an actual result, not a process. We'll talk about process—how we achieve something—when we discuss secondary choice. For now, focus on outcomes. For example, if you wrote, "I will lift weights three days a week," rewrite your goal to say, "I have a lean, toned body."

Describing Your Current Health Reality

In the next chapter, I'm going to ask you to answer a questionnaire I've created that will help you accurately assess your current health and behaviors in the foundational areas that determine your health. But for now, just take a moment to write down where you *think* you are currently in each of these areas, using some recent photos as your guide. Be objective. If you're not sure how to describe your current state, wait until after you've taken the questionnaire and come back to it.

Creating a Structural Tension Chart

A simple *structural tension chart* for each of the foundational components can be an important tool in your progress. These charts aren't difficult to make, and they give you a direct, visual way to compare your current reality to your desired goals. As we learned in the previous chapter, the relationship between where you are now and where you want to be creates a dynamic tension that serves as a powerful motivator as you work toward your goals.

Once you've taken the health assessment in the next chapter, you'll have a better sense of your current health reality and will be able to create a more refined structural tension chart for each goal that emerges on your journey. Right now, for example, your first goal may be to reach a healthy weight, and from doing the assessment you'll soon have a precise idea of your current weight, body mass index (BMI), and waist circumference. Those current realities will help you create a chart focusing on your healthy weight goal. Here's an example, on the right.

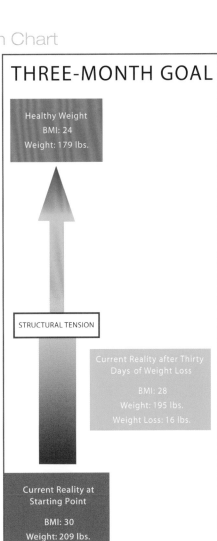

THREE-MONTH GOAL

Healthy Weight
BMI: 24
Weight: 179 lbs.

STRUCTURAL TENSION

Current Reality after Thirty Days of Weight Loss

BMI: 28
Weight: 195 lbs.
Weight Loss: 16 lbs.

Current Reality at Starting Point

BMI: 30
Weight: 209 lbs.

Visualize Your Goals
Find magazine pictures that represent radiant health and put them up on your walls. Or write out your goals and display them prominently on a wall, on the refrigerator, or as my wife does above her desk.

● ● ● ● ● ● ● ● ● ● ● ● ●

Sample Structural Tension Chart with Progress Report.
This chart identifies the person's current reality at the beginning of their program, their current reality at thirty days, and their three-month goal for healthy weight.

• • • • • • • • • • • • • • • • •

**Sample Structural
Tension Chart.**
This chart identifies
the person's
current reality and
their one-year goal
for optimal fitness.

For some extra help
drafting these charts,
check out the exercises
in *Living a Longer,
Healthier Life: the
Companion Guide to Dr.
A's Habits of Health.*

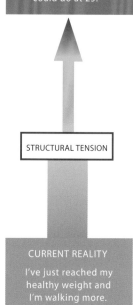

Now that you have a list of the foundational components for optimal health and a framework for creating goals, spend some time mapping out your future. Focus on what you're creating. Remember, this isn't "positive thinking," but rather simply a matter of writing and visualizing where you're going. By using where you are now as your starting point, you create the magical tension that begs resolution—the basis of action.

As you move forward, your current reality will change. You can use these charts as a road map to help you understand where you are in relation to your goal at any point, and to give you important feedback on your progress.

Now let's examine those important secondary choices—the action steps that make up your daily journey.

Secondary Health Choices: Daily Choices, Small Disciplines

Secondary choices—the action steps that support your primary choices—are the day-to-day behaviors that over time build your path to optimal health. They're not always fun, and we wouldn't necessarily choose to do these things if they weren't organized into our hierarchy of choice (in other words, if we didn't recognize them as actions that support our higher goal of thriving health).

Let's say you decided to become a world-class violinist. What would you do every day? You'd practice, of course! Even if you came home from work tired and would rather grab a drink, sit on the sofa, and kick off your shoes, you'd make the secondary choice to practice because it supports your primary choice—your goal of becoming a world-class violinist.

Pro golfer Jack Nicklaus taught me a valuable lesson about choice several years ago when I was playing golf with a friend at a course where Nicklaus practiced. As my friend and I warmed up by hitting a few balls, we had the privilege of witnessing Nicklaus and fellow pro golfer Greg Norman practicing hitting to a flag about eighty yards away. Although they were just getting started, the three dozen or so balls they'd hit so far were all within a couple feet of the pin. The tight grouping of balls on the rich carpet of the green was like an exclamation point showcasing the skill of these top professional golfers.

Mesmerized by their precision, I reluctantly left to tee off. As I hooked my drive into the sand trap and walked down the first fairway, I kept thinking how lucky these guys were to be so good.

We proceeded to play the first nine, and maybe I hit one shot (out of forty-five) that was as good as any of Jack's. The day was hot, and I was thirsty, so I headed back to the water fountain by the practice range. Imagine my astonishment when I discovered that Nicklaus and Norman were still there and still hitting the same shot! And every one of those now hundreds of golf balls were within a few feet of the pin. They'd just spent two and a half hours in the summer heat practicing a shot they had already performed to perfection. Talk about making secondary choices that support your primary choice to be the best golfer in history! These guys created perfection by spending years and years making the secondary choices that would enable them to perform even under intense pressure.

So much for luck!

Make no mistake—spending long hours practicing the violin or lobbing shots on a hot day isn't easy. But maybe, just maybe, it's a little easier when we know that we're supporting a goal we really want. And maybe that also applies to that thirty-minute walk, the healthy low-glycemic dinner, and going to bed at 10:00 p.m. instead of watching the late, late show. After all, being a great violinist or a great golfer are lofty primary choices—but they pale in comparison to your choice of optimal health. Without his health, I doubt even Nicklaus would have achieved his goals.

So let's get started pinpointing those secondary choices: the Habits of Health you'll be learning step by step in the next few chapters and practicing for life.

Identifying Your Secondary Choices

How do we determine whether our actions are likely to move us toward our goal? Here's a checklist of questions to ask yourself. Let's examine them in the context of the sample structural tension chart on page 32, with its goal of optimal fitness.

1. If you take these steps, will you achieve your foundational goal? For example, "If I lift weights once a month, will I reach my twelve-month goal of 14 percent body fat and lean muscle mass?"
2. Are your action steps accurate, brief, and concise? Picture the action step and then write it down in a couple of sentences—for example, "I will lift weights three days a week for thirty minutes."
3. Does every action step have a due date? For example, "I will walk ten minutes three days a week for the next two weeks."

The Habits of Health are behaviors that support your fundamental choice to be healthy.

Dr. A Says . . .

Make a list of the reasons you started your journey to optimal health and remember to pull it out when you need a little positive reinforcement!

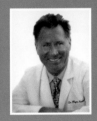

PART ONE

PREPARING FOR
YOUR JOURNEY

· · · · · · · · · · · · · · ·

**Sample Structural
Tension Chart
with Secondary
Choices.**
This chart identifies
the person's
current reality at
the beginning of
their program, their
secondary choices
(action steps), and
their one-year goal
for an active lifestyle.

Here's a sample structural tension chart that includes action steps to support the goal of an active lifestyle.

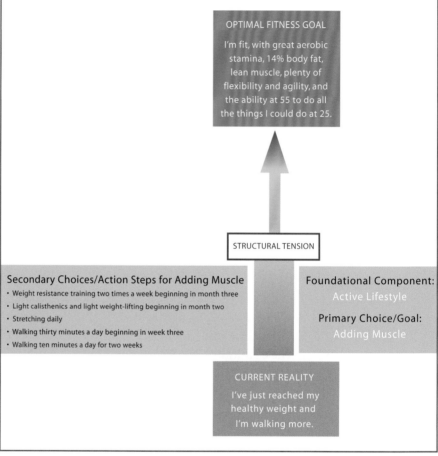

ONE-YEAR GOAL

OPTIMAL FITNESS GOAL

I'm fit, with great aerobic stamina, 14% body fat, lean muscle, plenty of flexibility and agility, and the ability at 55 to do all the things I could do at 25.

STRUCTURAL TENSION

Secondary Choices/Action Steps for Adding Muscle
• Weight resistance training two times a week beginning in month three
• Light calisthenics and light weight-lifting beginning in month two
• Stretching daily
• Walking thirty minutes a day beginning in week three
• Walking ten minutes a day for two weeks

Foundational Component:
Active Lifestyle

Primary Choice/Goal:
Adding Muscle

CURRENT REALITY

I've just reached my healthy weight and I'm walking more.

> The only way to keep your health is to eat what you don't want, drink what you don't like, and do what you'd rather not.
>
> Mark Twain

These secondary choices—daily, mundane activities—might seem insignificant in and of themselves. They might seem easy to do or not so easy to do. And as I mentioned before, given the choice we'd usually prefer not to do them. (Judging by his quote above, Mark Twain would surely have agreed!) It does seem, in this day and age of instant gratification, that most people are living in a world of impulse, with no regard to the effect their choices have over time. But in fact, time is the great equalizer. Time is either on your side, helping you build and maintain a thriving, vibrant life, or it's slowly but insidiously draining your health bank account.

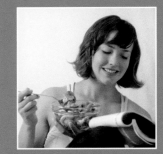

Remember the executive from chapter 2 who suffered a massive heart attack after years of eating the wrong foods? (That's what killed Mark Twain, by the way.) Today's cheeseburger doesn't make a difference today. And neither will substituting a salad. That's part of the problem.

We live in a society that's focused on instant results. Flip the light switch and, thanks to technology, we get results—now. That same mentality is what makes us believe that medicines will make us healthy or reduce our fat. After all, in the movies Rocky gets in shape in just two hours! A part of us expects the same. But that's just not how it works in the real world. The process of creating health takes time.

But in time, after taking those action steps day in and day out, you'll begin to enjoy optimal health, and through that feedback you'll know that your real work is already done. You'll have taken control of your daily choices and beaten the negative consequences of today's unhealthy lifestyle. A lifestyle affecting even our youth, resulting in ten-year-olds with *adult-onset* diabetes, or the ominous angiogram I saw at a recent medical conference of a patient with a "widow maker"—a lesion named for its ability to cause instant death by blocking the blood flow to the heart, which is seen often in men in their fifties. The conference hall let out a collective gasp when it was revealed that this patient was a seventeen-year-old boy!

It doesn't have to be this way. And it's never too late to start. But it's all up to you.

With the system I'm teaching you, making these small daily choices is doable. They won't make much difference today, but by practicing them patiently you can harness your most powerful ally—time. And if you do, you will get healthier. I promise.

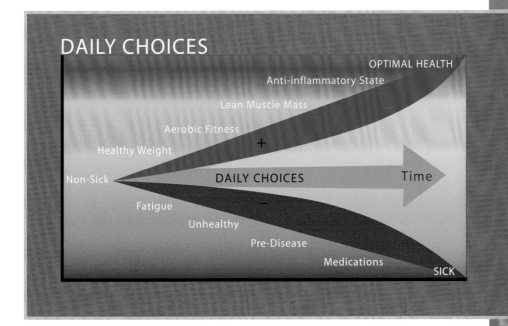

DAILY CHOICES

OPTIMAL HEALTH
Anti-inflammatory State
Lean Muscle Mass
Aerobic Fitness
Healthy Weight
+
Non-Sick
DAILY CHOICES   Time
–
Fatigue
Unhealthy
Pre-Disease
Medications
SICK

Daily Choices.
Will you take the green path to optimal health, or the red path to sickness? Over time, your daily choices can support your goals (a healthy weight, an active lifestyle) or lead you down the path to disease. It's up to you.

You've now learned a complete system to guide you in creating the life you want—a life of optimal health. That's your fundamental choice. You've outlined your primary choices—the foundational components of health that serve as your goals. You've begun to consider the day-to-day actions you need to take to reach those goals. And you've learned how important it is to look honestly at your current reality, using it as the basis for a structural tension chart for each of those foundational components.

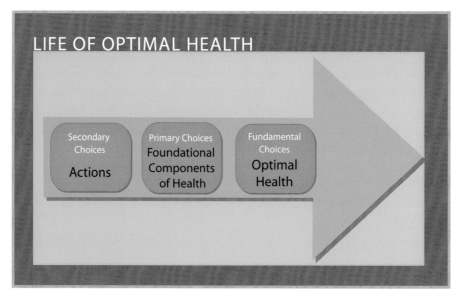

These critical factors can make all the difference between long-term success and reversal into previous patterns. In fact, they're the very framework of the path to optimal health.

You should now have a better understanding of where you want to go. But in order to get there, we first need a more precise idea of your starting point. Where are you *now* in relation to where you want to be? The next chapter consists of a health evaluation that will help us pinpoint your exact location on your health path, in much the same way that a GPS device helps you plot the most efficient path to your destination. Exploring current behaviors that affect your health—how you react to stress, how you spend your leisure time, even behaviors you may have ignored or considered unimportant—is our next step in putting *you* in charge of your own life's journey.

Chapter 5

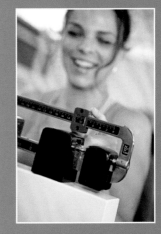

Where Are You Now?

Evaluating Your Current Health Status

Your answers to the following questions will give us valuable information on your current health status—something I believe is very important for you to know. That's why I urge you not to skip this step! In fact, many people have told me that this assessment has played a pivotal role in helping them understand how their daily choices have affected the reality of their health and their lives.

You and I are embarking on a journey—your journey toward optimal health. And as with any journey, to reach our destination we need to know our starting point. Understanding your health status as it is right now is an important part of building your personal health plan.

The following questionnaire is all about you. Be sure to give it your full focus, away from noise, interruptions, cell phones, and other distractions. Answer each question as truthfully as possible, basing your response on your most current and consistent behavior—what you're doing now, not what you did last week or last month.

Before you begin, take a look at the chart on the right. It depicts the health continuum, from sick, to non-sick, to optimal health. The higher the number, the healthier you are. Using a pencil, mark the spot that you think most accurately represents the state of your health right now. (Most people find themselves somewhere in the unhealthy range of scores, in the non-sick zone between sick and optimal health.)

Now let's get on with our evaluation and find out how well you guessed!

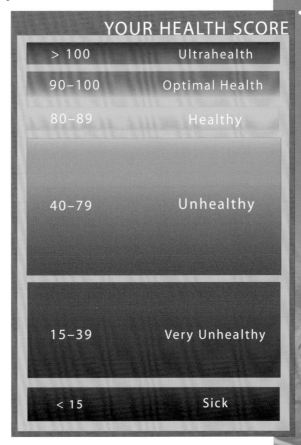

YOUR HEALTH SCORE

> 100	Ultrahealth
90–100	Optimal Health
80–89	Healthy
40–79	Unhealthy
15–39	Very Unhealthy
< 15	Sick

Your Predicted Health Score. Where do you fall on the health continuum: sick (red zone), healthy (green zone), or somewhere in between, in the unhealthy zone? Our goal is to move you toward the green zone and optimal health.

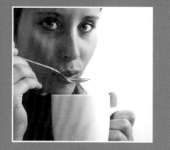

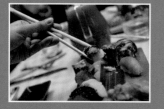

Note: Some questions may have multiple correct selections

1. You Are What You Eat

What you eat—and how much you eat—is critical to your health. Eating more calories than you use leads to weight gain; high-glycemic foods overwork your pancreas; and foods that stimulate inflammation such as saturated fats create chaos throughout your body. On the other hand, eating lots of fruits and vegetables turns off fat storage, satisfies hunger, stabilizes blood sugar, lowers insulin, and quells inflammatory fires.

In the previous twelve months, I have:

Lost more than 5 pounds	+5
Lost 2 to 5 pounds	+2
Stayed the same weight	0
Gained 2 to 5 pounds	-2
Gained more than 5 pounds	-5

I eat breakfast:

Every day	+3
Most days	+1
Occasionally	-1
Never	-2

I eat ___ small healthy meals or snacks a day.

6 or more	+3
4–5	+1
2–3	-1
1 huge meal a day	-3

In general, I eat ___ of my calories after 5:00 P.M.

Less than 35%	+3
35–50%	0
More than 50%	-2

I eat red meat:

Never	+3
2–3 times a week	-1
More than 3 times a week	-3

I eat fish that's high in omega-3, such as salmon, mackerel, or sardines:

More than 2–3 times a week	+3
1–2 times a week	+1
Less than once a week	-1
Never	-3
I take fish oil daily	+3

I eat dairy products that are:

Low-fat or skim	+2
Full fat (whole milk)	-1
I don't eat dairy (but get calcium from other sources)	+1

I prefer my poultry:

Skinless	+1
White meat only	+1
Dark and white meat	-1
Skin on	-2

I usually like my meat or fish:

Baked or steamed	+3
Broiled	+1
Grilled	-1
Charred	-3
Fried in unsaturated fats (olive oil or other vegetable oils)	-5
Fried in saturated or trans-fats (butter or solid shortening)	-8

I eat ____ servings of vegetables a day:

More than 5	+5
3–5	+3
1–3	+1
0	-3

I eat ____ servings of fresh fruit a day:

More than 3	+3
1–3	+1
0	- 2

I get my sugar primarily from:

Natural fruits	+3
Fructose	0
Table sugar	-1
High-fructose corn syrup	-3

I eat white starches such as white bread, white rice, tortillas, and pastas:

Never	+5
Less than 1–2 times a week	0
2–5 times a week	-2
1–2 times a day	-3
More than 2 times a day	- 5

I eat unprocessed, natural grains, cereals, and rice:

More than 2 times a day	+3
1–2 times a day	0
Never	-2

The type of fat or oil I use most often is:

Olive or canola oil	+3
Margarine spreads with no trans-fats (Smart Balance, Promise, Benecol, Enova)	+1
Margarine or vegetable oil	-1
Butter, lard, or vegetable shortening	-3

I drink alcohol:

Never	+5
1 glass of red wine with dinner	+3
Between 1 drink a week and 1 drink a month	+2
Less than 1 drink a day	+1
1–2 drinks a day	-1
3 or more drinks a day	-5

I salt my food:

Never	+3
Occasionally	0
Always	-2

I take vitamin and mineral supplements:

Daily	+3
When I remember	0
Never	-2

Total points for section 1: ____

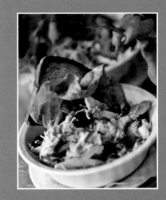

Dr. A Says. . .

Extra-virgin olive oil (olive oil that's unrefined) contains powerful antioxidants including vitamin E and is my first choice of oils. Just be careful, because it packs 119 calories per tablespoon!

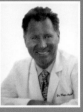

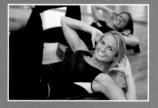

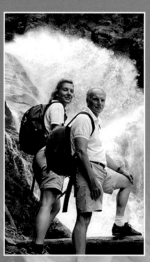

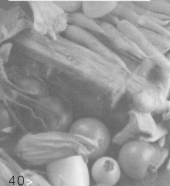

2. On the Move!

If you're like most of us, with our computer-driven, sedentary lifestyles, you're probably not very active at the moment. I understand! When you're tired and overweight, it takes a lot of effort to move your body. Just answer the following questions as best you can, and know that help is on the way. Once you've reached your healthy weight, we'll get you moving gradually through fun activities—including some cutting-edge calorie-burning methods you've probably never even heard of.

I walk:

At least 30 minutes a day	+5
Sometimes, but not every day	+1
To my car and my desk—that's it!	-3

I do aerobic activities (aerobics class, running, sports):

Daily	+5
Occasionally	+2
You kidding? I'd rather die!	-2

I do weight resistance training:

3 or more times a week	+5
Occasionally	+2
Does lifting a quarter-pounder with cheese count?	-2

On the weekend I usually:

Go for bike rides in the country	+3
Take a walk or walk my dog	+3
Sit on the sofa and watch TV	-3

When outdoor activity exposes me to the sun:

I always cover myself and use sunscreen of at least 30 SPF	+2
I avoid the sun at all times	-1
I put on sunscreen when I think of it	-1
I go out in the sun but never protect myself	-3

At my job, I'm:

Active and perform manual labor	+5
Usually walking and moving	+2
Sometimes walking, sometimes sitting	+1
In a chair seven hours a day	-5

During lunch and breaks:

I walk or take the stairs	+5
I go out to lunch or eat at the cafeteria	+2
I work at my desk, but get up and walk around whenever possible	0
I eat lunch at my desk—usually fast food that's brought in	-2

Total points for section 2: _____

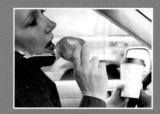

3. The Inner You

Today's chaotic schedules leave us with too much stress, too little free time, too little sleep, and not enough fun. We're just not enjoying ourselves like we used to! Many people shrug it off, but medical science is beginning to understand the impact of our emotional life on our health and our longevity.

My job:

Brings me lots of satisfaction	+5
Is OK, but I live for the weekends	0
Makes me really despise going to work	-5

At work, I find myself getting upset:

Never	+3
1–2 times a week	0
Most days	-5

My commute to work:

Isn't a factor—I work out of my house	+5
Is short, and I enjoy the drive	+2
Takes at least 30 minutes, and there's sometimes traffic	0
Is something I dread due to the length and traffic jams	-3

When I get home from work, I usually:

Relax in the garden or do something fun	+3
Read a good book and go for a walk	+3
Take a hot bath and play some music	+3
Chauffer kids to various activities	+2
Go home and get on the computer	0
Fight with my spouse and usually grab a drink	-3

I take part in some type of relaxation or spiritual endeavor:

Every day	+3
Occasionally, when I find time	0
Never	-3

The last time I had a really good laugh was:

This week	+2
A few weeks ago	+1
Last month	0
Can't remember	-3

I have ___ close personal friends.

More than 5	+3
2–5	+2
Fewer than 2	-2

I would describe my marriage or significant relationship as:

The best	+5
Happy	+3
Pretty good	+1
OK	-1
I'm unhappily married or recently separated	-5

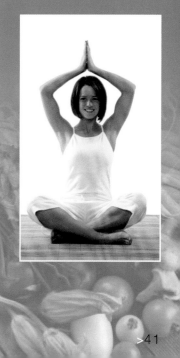

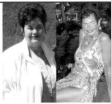

"Formerly flabulous. . .now fabulous!"

NANCY PETTIT *Over six years at optimal health*

At 5′ 6″ and 267 pounds, I was morbidly obese. I hated how I looked, hated how I felt; I hated myself. Ever since age twelve, I've been a weight watcher—watching as my weight steadily climbed northward. Six times, I lost more than 70 pounds. I joined gyms, signed up for weight-loss seminars, tried out the diet of the week from the supermarket magazine rack. I even considered gastric bypass surgery! But no matter what I did, I couldn't keep the pounds off. I wanted to, but I didn't know how.

Results vary. Typical weight loss is 2-5 lbs per week for the first 2 weeks and 1-2 lbs per week thereafter.

My prayers were answered when a man at our church told us about the program Take Shape for Life™, which had helped him lose 35 pounds. The program was so easy to follow! Soon I began to lose weight using the Medifast® meal replacements and more importantly, I felt great, better than I had for years. And because I kept losing weight steadily, I felt encouraged, and actually looked forward to jumping on the scale each day. My hunger went away, and I no longer craved food . . . and I lost 135 pounds!

It's been six years since I started the journey to optimal health, and now with Dr. A's Habits of Health I have all the tools necessary to stay healthy. It has made a radical difference in my health, self-esteem, marriage, and my relationships with others. ■

I get together with a group of friends for fun and companionship:

Two or more times a week	+3
Occasionally	0
Hardly ever	-2

My experience with pets is best described as:

I have a dog or cat that loves me	+3
I've had a pet in the past, but not currently	0
I don't like animals	-3

I sleep:

More than 7 hours a night	+5
6–7 hours a night	0
Less than 6 hours a night	-2
Less than 5 hours a night	-5

When I go to bed:

I fall asleep almost immediately	+3
It takes me a while to fall asleep	0
I toss and turn until I'm exhausted	-3

Once I fall asleep:

I sleep soundly through the night	+5
I wake up too early in the morning and can't always get back to sleep	-2
I wake up after a few hours and can't get back to sleep	-5

I wake up:

Totally refreshed and ready to attack the day	+5
Rested	+3
Feeling OK	0
Only if the alarm wakes me up	-1
Tired	-3
Exhausted	-5

Total points for section 3: _____

4. Breathe Deep!

You probably don't need to be told that smoking is devastating to your health. In fact, it's the single most important *controllable* health determinant—even more so than diet and physical activity. If you're a smoker, I recommend you make quitting your very first step, even before learning the other Habits of Health. Chapters 3 and 4 on motivation and choice can help you make a fresh start.

I've smoked:

Never   +5

I'm currently a smoker or I smoked at one point but have quit:

1. **First, calculate the number of *pack/years* that you smoked:**
   Multiply the number of packs you smoked per day by the total number of years you smoked, and make the result a negative number.

   For example: If you smoked two packs a day for fifteen years, multiply 2 by 15 for a score of -30 pack/years

   Packs per day × years = _____ pack/years

2. **Now, if you're no longer smoking, modify your score using the following formula:**
   _____ pack/years × healing factor (HF) = recovery points

   If you quit more than 10 years ago, your HF is .75
   If you quit 2–10 years ago, your HF is .5
   If you quit less than 2 years ago, your HF is .25

   For example: If your score is -30 and you quit smoking eleven years ago, multiply 30 by .75 = 22.5

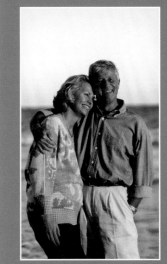

3. **Finally, calculate your total points using the following formula:**
   _____ pack/years (a negative number) + _____ recovery points (a positive number) = _____ total points (a negative number)

   For example: -30 + 22.5= -7.5 (final score)

I'm exposed to secondhand smoke:

Never	0
Occasionally	-1
Often	-5
Daily	-8

I live:

In the country	+3
In the suburbs	0
In a major city	-3

I work:

In the country	+3
In the suburbs	0
In a major city	-3

Total points for section 4: _____

5. Weighing You Down

Your current weight and the amount of abdominal fat you're carrying are key health predictors. Knowing your body mass index (BMI), waist circumference, and waist-to-hip ratio can tell you whether your current habits are on target or weighing you down.

Body mass index (BMI) is an important measure of disease risk and a helpful way to track your progress as you lose weight. Here are two alternative ways to find out your BMI.

1. **Use the following formula:**

$$\text{BMI} = \frac{\text{weight in pounds} \times 703}{(\text{height in inches}) \times (\text{height in inches})}$$

OR

2. **Find the correct number on this table:**

Body Mass Index Table

	Normal						Overweight					Obese										Extreme Obesity														
BMI	19	20	21	22	23	24	25	26	27	28	29	30	31	32	33	34	35	36	37	38	39	40	41	42	43	44	45	46	47	48	49	50	51	52	53	54
Height (inches)												Body Weight (pounds)																								
58	91	96	100	105	110	115	119	124	129	134	138	143	148	153	158	162	167	172	177	181	186	191	196	201	205	210	215	220	224	229	234	239	244	248	253	258
59	94	99	104	109	114	119	124	128	133	138	143	148	153	158	163	168	173	178	183	188	193	198	203	208	212	217	222	227	232	237	242	247	252	257	262	267
60	97	102	107	112	118	123	128	133	138	143	148	153	158	163	168	174	179	184	189	194	199	204	209	215	220	225	230	235	240	245	250	255	261	266	271	276
61	100	106	111	116	122	127	132	137	143	148	153	158	164	169	174	180	185	190	195	201	206	211	217	222	227	232	238	243	248	254	259	264	269	275	280	285
62	104	109	115	120	126	131	136	142	147	153	158	164	169	175	180	186	191	196	202	207	213	218	224	229	235	240	246	251	256	262	267	273	278	284	289	295
63	107	113	118	124	130	135	141	146	152	158	163	169	175	180	186	191	197	203	208	214	220	225	231	237	242	248	254	259	265	270	278	282	287	293	299	304
64	110	116	122	128	134	140	145	151	157	163	169	174	180	186	192	197	204	209	215	221	227	232	238	244	250	256	262	267	273	279	285	291	296	302	308	314
65	114	120	126	132	138	144	150	156	162	168	174	180	186	192	198	204	210	216	222	228	234	240	246	252	258	264	270	276	282	288	294	300	306	312	318	324
66	118	124	130	136	142	148	155	161	167	173	179	186	192	198	204	210	216	223	229	235	241	247	253	260	266	272	278	284	291	297	303	309	315	322	328	334
67	121	127	134	140	146	153	159	166	172	178	185	191	198	204	211	217	223	230	236	242	249	255	261	268	274	280	287	293	299	306	312	319	325	331	338	344
68	125	131	138	144	151	158	164	171	177	184	190	197	203	210	216	223	230	236	243	249	256	262	269	276	282	289	295	302	308	315	322	328	335	341	348	354
69	128	135	142	149	155	162	169	176	182	189	196	203	209	216	223	230	236	243	250	257	263	270	277	284	291	297	304	311	318	324	331	338	345	351	358	365
70	132	139	146	153	160	167	174	181	188	195	202	209	216	222	229	236	243	250	257	264	271	278	285	292	299	306	313	320	327	334	341	348	355	362	369	376
71	136	143	150	157	165	172	179	186	193	200	208	215	222	229	236	243	250	257	265	272	279	286	293	301	308	315	322	329	338	343	351	358	365	372	379	386
72	140	147	154	162	169	177	184	191	199	206	213	221	228	235	242	250	258	265	272	279	287	294	302	309	316	324	331	338	346	353	361	368	375	383	390	397
73	144	151	159	166	174	182	189	197	204	212	219	227	235	242	250	257	265	272	280	288	295	302	310	318	325	333	340	348	355	363	371	378	386	393	401	408
74	148	155	163	171	179	186	194	202	210	218	225	233	241	249	256	264	272	280	287	295	303	311	319	326	334	342	350	358	365	373	381	389	396	404	412	420
75	152	160	168	176	184	192	200	208	216	224	232	240	248	256	264	272	279	287	295	303	311	319	327	335	343	351	359	367	375	383	391	399	407	415	423	431
76	156	164	172	180	189	197	205	213	221	230	238	246	254	263	271	279	287	295	304	312	320	328	336	344	353	361	369	377	385	394	402	410	418	426	435	443

Source: Adapted from *Clinical Guidelines on the Identification, Evaluation, and Treatment of Overweight and Obesity in Adults: The Evidence Report.*

Now find your BMI on the chart below and enter the corresponding number of points here: _____

	BMI	Points
Ultrahealthy	20	+10
	21	+8
	22	+6
	23	+4
Healthy	24	+2
	24–24.9	+1
Overweight (pre-obese)	25	-1
	26	-2
	27	-3
	28	-4
	29	-5
Obese	30	-6
	31	-7
	32	-8
	33	-9
	34	-10
	35	-11
	36	-12
	37	-13
	38	-14
	39	-15
	Over 40	-20

Waist circumference measures your abdominal fat—both a predictor and a cause of poor health and disease. Use a tape measurer to determine your waist circumference in inches by placing it just on top of your hip—the blue line in the diagram.

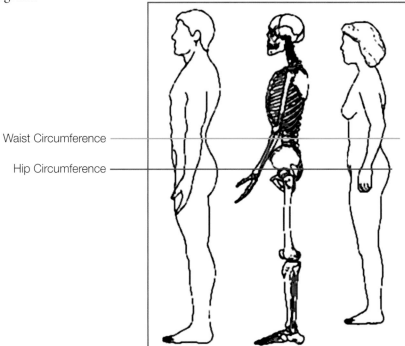

Waist Circumference

Hip Circumference

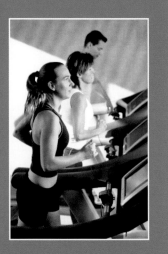

Now find your waist measurement in inches on the chart below and enter the corresponding number of points here: _____

Waist circumference (in inches)	Male	Female	Points
	<32	<29	+10
	32–34.9	29–31	+ 5
	35–37	31–32.5	0
	37.1–39.9	32.6–34.9	-3
	40+	35+	-10

Waist-to-hip ratio (WHR) compares the circumference of your waist to the circumference of your hips to see how much dangerous fat you're carrying. Carrying extra weight around your lower hips—sometimes called the pear shape—is much less harmful to your health than extra weight around your waist.

To find your waist-to-hip ratio:
1. Measure your hip circumference in inches.
2. Take your waist circumference from the previous question and divide it by your hip circumference. This is your WHR.
3. Now find your WHR on the chart below and enter the corresponding number of points here: _____

WHR	Male	Female	Points
	Over .90	Over .80	-2
	.90	.80	0
	Less than .90	Less than .80	+2

Total points for section 5: _____

6. Testing, testing

Had a check-up recently? If so, your doctor may have tested your blood for four types of fats that help assess your risk for heart disease: total cholesterol, high-density lipoprotein (HDL, the "good" cholesterol), low-density lipoprotein (LDL, the "bad" cholesterol), and triglycerides. He may have also checked your metabolic health by testing your fasting blood sugar and your hs-CRP, an important measure of your current health.

If you have these numbers, you can use them to answer the following questions. If not, just skip this section—but I highly recommend you have your doctor check these levels. Just ask to have a *lipid profile* done at your next visit, along with blood glucose and hs-CRP.

But if you don't have them, don't worry. Although these numbers give us a little more information, they almost always parallel your lifestyle scores, so we *can* get an accurate assessment even without them. And the Habits of Health you're about to learn are more powerful than the medications your doctor would use to treat you anyway! (Though it's fun to get the tests done so we can watch your scores improve!)

Total cholesterol helps the body form hormones, vitamin D, and other important substances—but too much of it can clog and damage blood vessels. Find your *total cholesterol* level on the chart below and enter the corresponding number of points here: _____

Total cholesterol	Points
Less than 100 (Ultra)	+10
100–149	+5
150–179	+2
199–180	0
200–239	- 3
240+	-5

Low-density lipoproteins (LDLs) build up in the blood and increase your risk of heart disease. Find your *LDL* level on the chart below and enter the corresponding number of points here: _____

	LDL	Points
Ultra:	Less than 70 mg/dL	+10
Very good:	70–100 mg/dL	+5
Good:	100–129 mg/dL	+3
Borderline:	130–159 mg/dL	0
High:	160–189 mg/dL	-3
Very high:	190 mg/dL or higher	-5

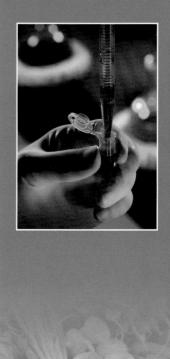

High-density lipoproteins (HDLs) carry cholesterol to the liver, where it is removed from the body. Find your *HDL* level on the chart below and enter the corresponding number of points here: _____

	HDL	Points
Low:	Less than 40 mg/dL	-5
Medium:	41–59 mg/dL	0
Very Good:	60–80 mg/dL or higher	+5
Ultra:	80 mg/dL or higher	+10

Triglycerides store energy for your body to use when needed. Too many triglycerides can block blood vessels and cause other health problems, such as abdominal pain and pancreatitis. Find your *triglyceride* level on the following chart and enter the corresponding number of points here: _____

"We have our life back!"

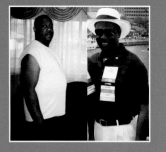

GARY SHAW
*Over five years at
optimal health*

My wife and I both lost over 55 pounds each on our journey to optimal health—and best of all, Dr. Andersen, as our personal coach, has given us the education, tools, and support to keep it off.

Adopting this healthy new lifestyle has been an incredible blessing in our lives! ∎

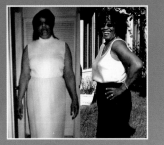

Josephine Shaw

Results vary. Typical weight loss is 2-5 lbs per week for the first 2 weeks and 1-2 lbs per week thereafter.

continued on next page . . .

	Triglycerides	Points
Ultra:	Less than 100 mg/dL	+10
Good:	100–150 mg/dL	+5
Borderline:	150–199 mg/dL	0
High:	200–499 mg/dL	-3
Very high:	500 mg/dl or higher	-10

Fasting blood glucose (sugar) measures the ability of your body to regulate your blood sugar and is an indicator of your metabolic health, as well as whether you're at risk for diabetes. Find your *blood glucose* level on the chart below and enter the corresponding number of points here: _____

	Blood glucose	Points
Ultra:	Less than 80 mg/dL	+10
Very good:	80–100 mg/dL	+5
Normal	100–110 mg/dL	+1
Borderline:	111–126 mg/dL	-1
High (diabetic):	126–150 mg/dL	-5
Very high:	150 mg/dl or higher	-10

High-sensitivity C-reactive protein (hs-CRP) evaluates the inflammatory state of your blood and body. This important test is a common measurement of your risk for a number of diseases, especially heart disease—but it also lets us know how healthy you are. If you haven't had this test, you'll want to once you read this book! Make sure you get the *high-sensitivity* version (*hs-CRP*). Find your *hs-CRP* level on the chart below and enter the corresponding number of points here: ____

	hs-CRP	Points
Ultra	Less than .5 mg/L	+10
Very good	.5–1.0 mg/L	+5
Normal	1.0–1.9 mg/L	0
Borderline (inflammation)	2.0–2.9 mg/L	-1
High	3.0–4.9	-5
Very high	5.0 mg/L or higher	-10

Total points for section 6: _____

7. Start Where You Are

Any medical conditions you have at the moment are, naturally, a major factor in your current health status. But don't be discouraged! *Remember, your health status isn't fixed—it's only the starting point of your journey*. By changing your health habits, we can neutralize and even eliminate many health problems and in some cases reduce or completely phase out your need for medication.

I've been to my primary care physician for my Periodic Health Examination (i.e., check-up):

At least once a year	+2
Sometime in the past	-1
Never	-2

I've been diagnosed with:

Pre-diabetes	-3
Gestational diabetes	-3
Pre-hypertension	-3

I currently take:

Over-the-counter medications for allergy, sinus, headache, etc.	-1 per medication
Birth control pills	-2
Birth control pills (and I smoke)	-5
No medications	0

I take a daily, low-dose aspirin of around 162 mg and:

I'm a male over 35	+2
I'm a female over 40	+2
I have metabolic syndrome	+2
I don't take daily aspirin	0

I have the following health conditions (*Choose as many as apply. Add -5 if you need medication to control these conditions, for a maximum of -15 per condition*):

High blood pressure	mild -5	moderate -8	severe -10
Metabolic syndrome	mild -5	moderate -8	severe -10
Polycystic ovarian syndrome	mild -5	moderate -8	severe -10
Diabetes	mild -5	moderate -8	severe -10
Thyroid condition	mild -5	moderate -8	severe -10

I have the following advanced health conditions (*Choose as many as apply. Add -5 for each condition that requires medication, for a maximum of -15 per condition*):

Heart disease (e.g., heart attack, CHF, stroke)	-10
Lung disease (e.g., COPD, severe asthma)	-10
Kidney disease (e.g., renal failure)	-10
Immune disease (e.g., lupus)	-10
Gastrointestinal disease (e.g., Crohn's disease)	-10
Other significant disease	-10

Total points for section 7: _____

"The difference between life and death."

JOSEPHINE SHAW

Over five years at optimal health

I was always an energetic person, but in my forties, my health began to deteriorate. I was overweight, and I couldn't even walk across the room without effort. I had incurable lung disease, diabetes, depression, fibromyalgia, and chronic fatigue. I remember thinking, "I'll probably just die this way."

It was then that Dr. A and his wife, Lori, told me about a way to regain my health. Thanks to my weight loss, my energy level began to climb and my blood sugar improved. Thanks to my weight loss, my doctor lowered my medications for cholesterol and high blood pressure.

Today, I can run upstairs if I want to! I haven't felt like this in years. I'm no longer watching life go by from inside my bedroom window… and in the process of getting better, I lost 55 pounds!

I didn't even realize how sick I really was until I started learning how to eat right and adopted a whole new set of healthy habits. But now, thanks to Dr. A, my grandchildren will have their grandma for many more years to come! This has been a miracle in my life. ■

Results vary. Typical weight loss is 2-5 lbs per week for the first 2 weeks and 1-2 lbs per week thereafter.

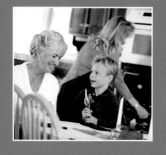

8. All in the Family

Your family's medical history reflects your genetic programming and is a big influence on your current health status and future risk. It can even affect your ability to control your weight. To find out your *genetic factor* (GF), add the points in the chart below for each condition that any of your parents or grandparents developed *before age 60*. Your GF is 1 minus that total.

For example: Your mother and grandmother had diabetes (.04 + .04) and your father had heart disease (.04), all diagnosed before age 60. Add .04 + .04 + .04, for a total of .12. Your GF is .88 (1 − .12 = .88).

ALL IN THE FAMILY

	Mother	Maternal Grandfather	Maternal Grandmother	Father	Paternal Grandfather	Paternal Grandmother
Heart Disease	.04	.04	.04	.04	.04	.04
Stroke	.04	.04	.04	.04	.04	.04
Diabetes	.04	.04	.04	.04	.04	.04
Colon Cancer	.04	.04	.04	.04	.04	.04
Breast Cancer	.04	.04	.04	.04	.04	.04
Ovarian Cancer	.04	.04	.04	.04	.04	.04
Alzheimer's	.04	.02	.02	.04	.02	.02
Obesity	.04	.04	.04	.04	.04	.04

Total from chart = _____

Genetic Factor = 1 − total from chart = _____

Genetic Factor (GF) from section 8: _____

To Total Your Score

1. Add your points from sections 1–7: _____
2. Multiply your result by your GF from section 8 for your Actual Health Score: _____

For example, if your total points from section 1–7 are 78, to calculate your Actual Health Score, multiply your total points by your genetic factor: 78 x .88 = 68.

As you can see from this example, your genetic history can move you from the healthy zone into the unhealthy zone—emphasizing the importance of optimizing your behaviors and environment in order to offset genetic risk!

Now that you've completed the questionnaire, place a mark on the following chart on the spot that corresponds to your Actual Health Score. Compare this chart to the one on page 37. How close was your prediction?

Your Current Health Score Status

So what does your health score mean and what can you do about it? Let's find out.

Less than 15

Health Status: Sick

You probably already have significant medical conditions that are affecting your health, or are on the verge of becoming ill. But we can help change all that.

I don't view sickness as a progressive and inevitable decay in quality and length of life, nor as a condition that should be "fixed" simply by dialing up more medications. Those beliefs are for practitioners in the world of "sick care" not health care. Rather, I believe that if you're willing to take control of your health and learn new habits, we can get you out of this sick state, despite any underlying disease. By making a fundamental decision to become healthy you'll fuel a whole new array of choices that can quickly improve your health, and you may soon be able to reduce or eliminate your medications and free yourself from their daily side effects—just by applying the Habits of Health to your life!

15–39

Health Status: Very Unhealthy

If you're not already suffering from significant disease, you're on track to develop it in the near future. But you can create dramatic changes in your health and in your life by adopting the Habits of Health—change that can alter your current health path and even save your life.

40–79

Health Status: Unhealthy

You may not suffer from disease at the moment, but your current condition is no recipe for optimal health. Over time, your poor daily choices and lack of discipline are sure to lead you down the path to disease. The good news is that your body will respond quickly to the changes we're going to help you make in your life!

YOUR HEALTH SCORE

> 100	Ultrahealth
90–100	Optimal Health
80–89	Healthy
40–79	Unhealthy
15–39	Very Unhealthy
< 15	Sick

Your Actual Health Score. Now that you've completed the health assessment, compare your actual health score to your prediction on page 37. How close were you?

Dr. A Says. . .

Remember that making healthy choices—the kinds of behaviors you'll be learning with the Habits of Health—can help you overcome your genetic history and raise your health score.

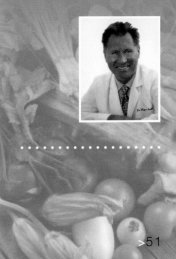

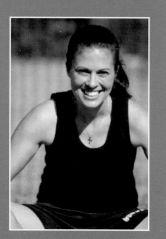

80–89

Health Status: Healthy

Congratulations! You have a number of positive habits that have helped keep you free from disease and within the healthy range. But don't get too comfortable—without constant vigilance and improvement, it's all too easy to slip. And working to make even better choices can put you firmly on the path toward the best possible health you can achieve.

90–100

Health Status: Optimal Health

You're in the small group of individuals who have made a conscious effort to create health for yourself . . . or you're still eighteen! But remember, optimal health is a journey that continues throughout your life. So there are still some areas where you can improve your health status, even within this optimal range. The techniques in this book will help you in areas you've mastered as well as in areas that need improvement, and will teach you ways to organize the Habits of Health into a system for continual growth.

In fact, our ultimate goal is to continue your optimal health growth into a state of Ultrahealth.

More than 100

Health Status: Ultrahealth

You naturally subscribe to a lifestyle that supports Ultrahealth—a state of health and behaviors that prevents disease, helps your body slow down aging, and has the potential to extend your lifetime.

In Part Three, we'll discuss ways to improve your Ultrahealth status and help you remain there indefinitely. Together, we can work on not just reaching and maintaining optimal health but actually extending this thriving life much longer than you ever thought possible!

Where Do We Go from Here?

As you can probably tell from the questions you've just answered, I'm interested in much more than just your medical history—I'm interested in the dynamics of your life. That's because in order to create health, *you* need to take an active role. Your daily choices can support or undermine your health. And that's good news—because it means that in each and every question where you scored zero or lower, you can improve immediately. But your ability to completely reverse the effects of your current choices weakens with age. It's critical that you examine the choices you're making right away—in fact, there will never be a better time.

How many of the healthy choices above are you incapable of making? What's stopping you? Maybe making healthy choices didn't seem to make much difference in the past. Not today, perhaps, and not tomorrow. But over time those choices add up—and together they've given you the health score you have today. But we can change all that.

Did you know that your body today is made up of entirely new cells than were there twelve months ago? Change your nutrient intake, add a little physical activity—and imagine where you could be twelve months from now! We can't pick our parents and our genetic background, but we *can* take control over the state of our health. If you're a spectator in your own life, you leave yourself open to sickness and disease. But if you're ready to play, we have all the equipment you need to get in the game. We have the Habits of Health.

The First Step

I've prepared you for your journey. Now it's time to take the first step. As with any new adventure, this is a time of excitement and perhaps some anxiety. Will this plan work? Can I do it? Will I end up back where I started?

It's not unusual to be afraid as you move out of your comfort zone. Our current habits are secure, familiar, and efficient—they've been part of us for so long that we do them automatically, every day, without thinking. When they're mostly healthy habits, they make us stronger. Unfortunately, for most people that's just not the case.

The Habits of Health will give you those healthy habits—if you're willing to change. Let me start by helping to allay any concerns or fears you might have.

First and foremost, let me assure you that all the principles and techniques I'm teaching you to improve your health are safe. They're based on clinically proven methods, with sound scientific research to validate their effectiveness.

Second, everything in my plan is doable. I've paid particular attention to making sure these new habits are convenient and can be incorporated into our time-starved lives.

And third, I've chosen the first step very carefully—because I know that if I can help you succeed right off the bat, you can use that success to build a lifetime of health. That first step changes everything.

Shall we begin?

Dr. A Says . . .

The Habits of Health will give you healthy habits if you're willing to change. I'm here to help allay any concerns or fears you might have.

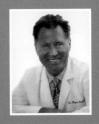

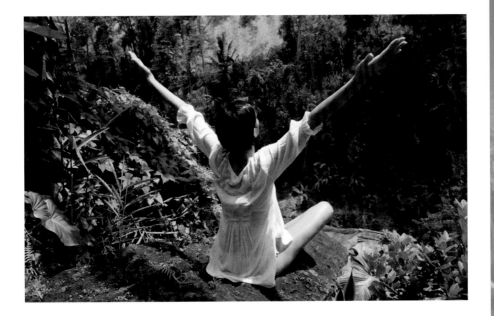

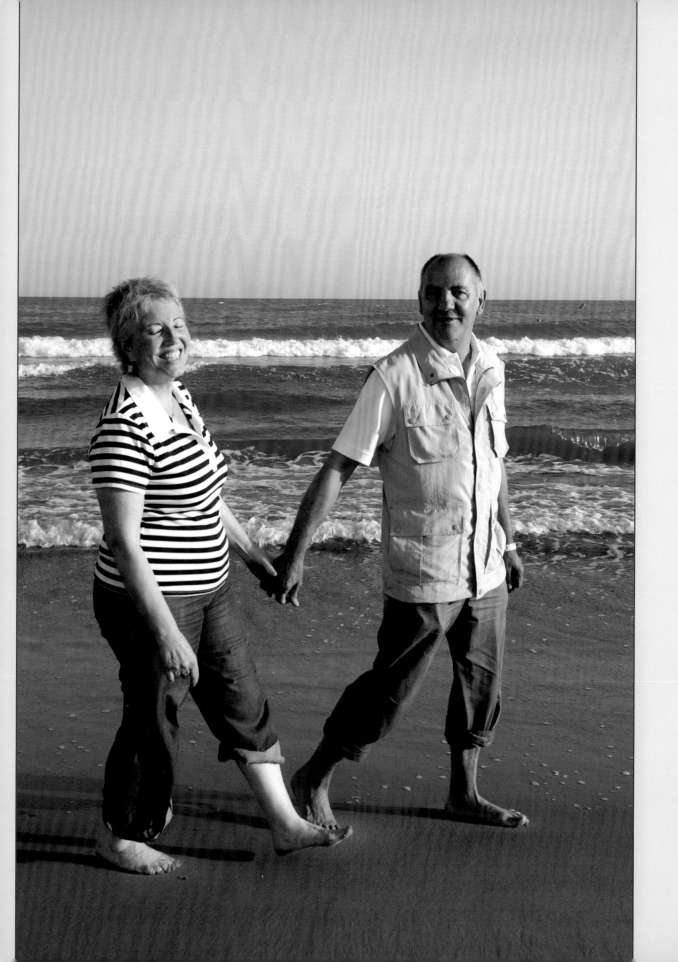

Part Two

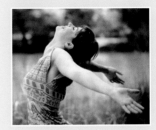

....>

Your Journey to Optimal Health

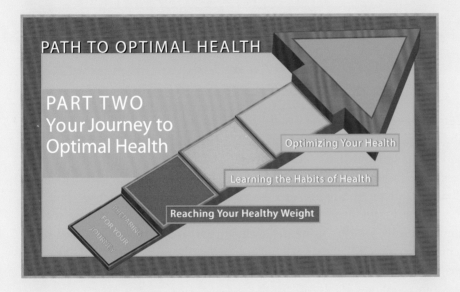

In Part One, Preparing for Your Journey, we explained how our basic biological design clashes with our environment, making it hard to maintain a healthy weight. We concluded by evaluating your physical health and lifestyle and determining your current health status as a starting point on your path to optimal health.

In Part Two, Your Journey to Optimal Health, we will begin the series of phases that make up your journey. In each phase, you'll build the knowledge, skills, and techniques you need to take control of your life and develop behaviors for lasting health. These Habits of Health—designed to be digested in bite-sized pieces at your own pace—are the structure that supports this new world.

Each phase on the journey follows the next in a logical fashion. All are based on one unifying principle: using energy management—the relationship between the energy you consume and the energy you use—as a catalyst for health.

As you learn and practice the Habits of Health, the daily choices you make will begin to help you master your energy balance. These new behaviors will quickly become automatic—and by the time you complete Phase III, the world of nutritional pollution will have lost its influence over you.

Let's review this energy management system.

· · · · · · · · · · · · · · ·

Your New Energy Path to Optimal Health and Longevity. In the Before stage, you were taking in more energy (energy in, red line) than you were expending (energy out, green line), resulting in weight gain. In Phase I, we'll shift that balance by changing the quantity and quality of your energy intake until you reach a healthy weight. In Phase II, you reach a new healthy state of equilibrium, and ultimately optimal health in Phase III. Phase IV takes you beyond optimal health, to Ultrahealth—a state where you can actually increase your longevity.

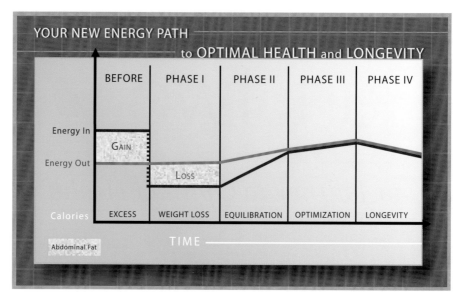

Before refers to the point at which most of us start our journey—with excess abdominal fat as a result of too many calories from foods loaded with sugar and fat combined with too little activity.

Phase I is all about tapping into the excess energy stored in fat by changing the quantity and quality of your energy intake. I'll provide you with a comprehensive strategy using medically formulated portion-controlled meal replacements (PCMRs) that will put you in a fat-burning state so you can lose weight safely and quickly. As your health improves, you'll find it easier and easier to adopt new Habits of Health.

Phase II puts you into a new state of energy equilibrium. Once you've reached your healthy weight, we'll start increasing your energy intake in relation to your energy output. My diversified eating plan makes healthy eating a pleasure for life, while my progressive activity plan increases your energy expenditure— without requiring a gym pass. The Habits of Health introduced in this phase will make it easier for you to make choices that support and solidify your health and increase your ability to control your lifestyle. From improving your sleep to providing you with plenty of support, this phase will help you regain control over your life.

Phase III adds the final pieces to create optimal health and life. We'll look at external and internal factors to eliminate the health-robbing forces of inflammation, and will examine your state of well-being in order to align your life with what really matters to you. As your body gets leaner and more efficient and your energy requirements increase, we'll fine-tune your cellular health by exploring nutritional supplementation. These final refinements will help you use the Habits of Health—which are now deeply engrained—to make your new lifestyle one that supports optimal health.

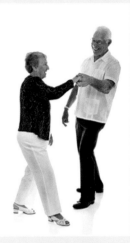

Phase IV takes you beyond optimal health, in a process that we'll discuss in Part Three, The Path to Longevity. You'll discover how further reducing your intake of processed food and substituting nutrient-dense food enables you to decrease your total calories and can actually extend your life. It's all part of an exciting, cutting-edge movement, backed by an increasing body of scientific and medical evidence and based on the principle of *calorie restriction*. By lowering your daily caloric intake 15 percent below our optimal health recommendations, you can actually put your body into a state of ultra-efficiency. Preliminary studies suggest that this state may extend your life by as much as 30 percent—and increase its quality.

Thrive alive! That's how I want to spend my 80s and 90s and—who knows—100s!

Phase I
Reaching Your Healthy Weight
The First Step

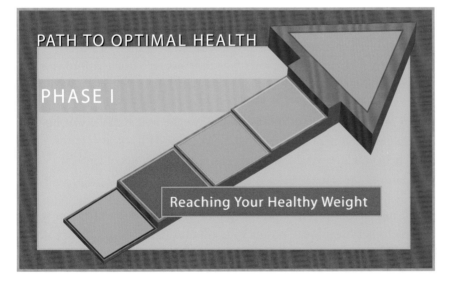

PATH TO OPTIMAL HEALTH

PHASE I

Reaching Your Healthy Weight

Why is reaching a healthy weight so important, anyway? Well, for starters, it can:

- Help you live longer
- Improve the quality of your life
- Slow down the aging process
- Give you more energy and vitality
- Improve your mental outlook and increase your happiness
- Improve your work performance
- Improve your sleep
- Lower your blood pressure, cholesterol (especially bad cholesterol), and triglycerides

Just a 10 percent
reduction in your
weight lowers your
risk of disease by
over 50 percent.

- Lower your risk for heart attack or stroke
- Lower your blood sugar
- Eliminate insulin resistance
- Reverse and possibly eliminate metabolic syndrome
- Dramatically lower your risk of developing diabetes or, if you have diabetes, arrest and even reverse its progression
- Lower your risk for liver and gall bladder disease
- Lower your risk for varicose veins, deep vein thrombosis, and blood clots
- Help you breathe better
- Eliminate sleep apnea
- Lessen or eliminate asthma, bronchitis, and other lung problems
- Lower your risk of getting arthritis or, if you have arthritis, relieve your pain
- Reduce or eliminate the amount of medication you use
- Increase your chances of becoming pregnant (if you don't want to get pregnant this is your warning—be careful!)
- Improve the health of you and your baby during pregnancy
- Markedly lower your risk for many types of cancers

Just a 10 percent reduction in your weight lowers your risk of disease by over 50 percent—and that risk continues to drop as you reduce your BMI (body mass index) below 25. In fact, the only drawback to weight loss that I've ever encountered is that you'll have to spend money on a new wardrobe!

Let's take a look at how the next few chapters will teach you to reach a healthy weight and set the stage for optimal health:

Dr. A Says. . .

In Phase I, we're going to give you a jumpstart to help you reach a healthy weight.

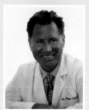

Chapter 6 outlines our plan for rapid, safe weight loss. You'll learn how to prepare your environment and kitchen for success, and I'll reveal a very effective system to help you lose weight and start learning the Habits of Healthy Eating for Life.

Chapter 7 introduces you to a powerful tool that provides a safe, consistent way for me to help you break out of your rut and launch you on the path to optimal health. This tool will be our catalyst to helping you reach a healthy weight.

Chapters 8, 9, and 10 show you practical ways to use my low-glycemic portion-control approach for optimal health and teach you the Habits of Health that support healthy eating—including a complete, long-term eating system to help you stay healthy for the rest of your life.

Chapter 11 gives a detailed explanation of the science behind weight loss, healthy eating, and how we'll use your body's design to help you reach and maintain a healthy weight.

But first, let's help you reach a healthy weight!

Chapter 6

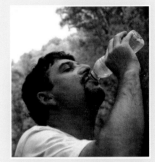

Your Blueprint for Safe, Rapid Weight Loss

If you've been through more than a few weight-loss plans, you've probably figured out that there are a multitude of recommendations on how to lose weight.

Many plans view weight loss as an end in itself. Through any number of methods—low-carb or low-fat diets, medication, colonics, exercise boot camps—they get you to your destination (sometimes), at which point they basically drop you off. The problem with plans like these is that even if you do get through the deprivation involved and manage to lose weight, you almost immediately start meandering back to your old ways—kind of like when a golf course tries to get rid of a flock of Canada geese by moving them down the way a few miles. Sooner or later, they're back.

Other plans take a more conservative approach, advising you to eat sensibly and be more active. Well, that's great advice if you're already healthy and in shape. But the problem here is that the sort of subtle changes these programs recommend just don't make enough of a difference in the short term to give you the positive reinforcement you need to continue with them. The lure of fast food and a weekend on the couch are just too strong!

I've spent six years studying why most diets don't work on their own, and why most people never change. And as a result, I ask a very different question than most people do—not just "What is the most effective way to reach a healthy weight?" but "How can I go beyond weight loss to achieve optimal health and stay healthy for the rest of my life?"

I believe that the answer lies within our own bodies. After thirty years of medical practice, I still marvel at the human body's incredible ability to adapt to a wide range of physical, mental, and social conditions. Unfortunately, today's world is challenging these adaptations—overwhelming our defenses, eroding our health, and moving us down the path toward non-sickness or worse. But one amazing human attribute can help us change direction—resiliency! No matter how much we abuse our bodies, if we stop the assault of unhealthy habits and put ourselves back into position to function as we were designed, we can tap into the body's inherent capacity to heal itself. And what's the best tool we have for doing that? *The food we eat!* Why, all the medicines and treatments in the world pale in comparison to the impact of a healthy eating strategy!

The healthy eating system you're about to learn is built around Habits of Health that give you the ability to control the quantity and quality of your energy intake. Most people aren't able to master this most fundamental principle even after a lifetime of struggle. You see, they're relying on their internal programming to select their food choices. But as we've discussed, that programming—which was optimal for a different time, when we needed to grab onto and hoard every calorie we consumed—is no longer helping us. Today, unlike 10,000 years ago, we lack the activity we need to dispose of all that excess energy. So if we consume more than we need to run our body, the extra calories get stored away—as fat. That fat around your middle is a symptom of an imbalance between your energy intake and energy output, with your intake set higher than it should be.

In this chapter, you will learn the fundamentals behind our healthy eating system—a system that was strategically developed to change your health *rapidly*, but with *long-term health* as the goal. And we're going to start by focusing on the central principles of energy management.

Creating a New Energy Management System

As your body's boss, you need to fire your old energy management system. It's not working!

Eating a little healthier or walking a little more isn't going to get you to your healthy weight. The evil forces out there—tempting you with calories and offering you a nice, cushy ride in place of exercise—are just too powerful. We live in an instant-gratification society. If our pizza's not here in thirty minutes, it's free! If we have to wait more than five minutes for anything, we go crazy!

Nope, the steady-as-you-go approach just isn't going to work for most of us. It's certainly never worked for me. So instead, let's use your biological design to our advantage and revamp your energy management system. We'll start by giving you a new eating strategy.

Look at it this way: If I can help you lose two to five pounds of weight per week for the first two weeks and one to two pounds of weight per week thereafter while keeping you from being hungry and eliminating your cravings for carbohydrates, and if a little later (after you have lost some weight) all I ask of you is thirty minutes of your time for a nice walk. . . will you do it?

I hope your answer is yes! Let's see exactly how we're going to go about changing your energy management system to help you lose weight in Phase I.

Energy Management in Phase I: Weight Loss.
In Phase I, we'll lower your energy intake (red line) while keeping your energy use (green line) fairly steady. As a result of this decreased intake, you'll see your body mass index (white line) go down.

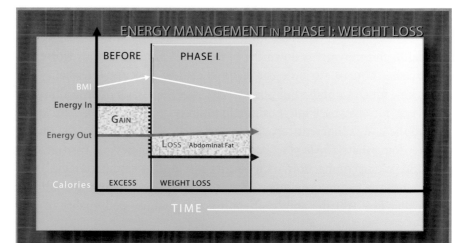

ENERGY MANAGEMENT IN PHASE I: WEIGHT LOSS

BEFORE   PHASE I.

BMI

Energy In

GAIN

Energy Out

LOSS   Abdominal Fat

Calories   EXCESS   WEIGHT LOSS

TIME

Our goal in this first phase is to get you to a healthy weight and a body mass index (BMI) of 24.9. We'll do that by lowering your caloric intake below your energy expenditure.

But don't worry—based on my experience of helping thousands of people through this process, you'll still have plenty of energy, and you won't be hungry. How is that possible? We're going to use the abundant stores of energy in that extra fat around your belly to turn you into a fat-burning facility!

To do that, we're going to alter your food intake in order to create a stable energy source, a process that taps into two core principles of energy management:

- Controlling your energy intake
- Managing your insulin pump

These principles form the basis of the healthy eating strategies we'll be learning in this weight-loss phase, and mastering them is, quite simply, the key to long-term success!

Let's take a look at the typical Western eating pattern and see what happens when these core principles are ignored.

Want to know more about the science behind our healthy eating plan for weight loss and optimal health? You'll find a detailed discussion in chapter 11, *The Science of Healthy Eating and Weight Loss.*

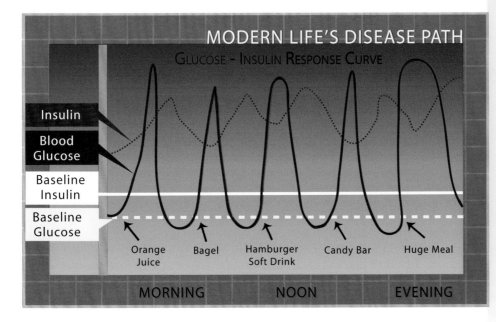

MODERN LIFE'S DISEASE PATH
GLUCOSE - INSULIN RESPONSE CURVE

Insulin
Blood Glucose
Baseline Insulin
Baseline Glucose

Orange Juice · Bagel · Hamburger Soft Drink · Candy Bar · Huge Meal

MORNING · NOON · EVENING

Modern Life's Disease Path: Glucose-Insulin Response Curve. The typical Western diet of highly processed, energy-dense, high-glycemic foods causes blood sugar (blood glucose) to rise dramatically, which then causes insulin levels to rise. But that in turn causes blood sugar to plummet, resulting in cravings and a cycle of poor eating patterns that lead to obesity and disease.

As you can see above, the typical Western diet of highly processed, high-glycemic foods—soft drinks, candy bars, bagels—causes blood sugar (also called *blood glucose*) to rise dramatically. And that makes the level of insulin rise. What happens next is interesting—this elevated insulin level actually causes blood sugar to plummet, creating the rapid rise and fall you see in the chart.

As blood sugar falls below normal, the brain sets off a series of messages that cause cravings—and soon you're scrambling for something sweet and full of calories. And so the cycle of high and low blood sugar levels continues, reinforcing eating patterns that lead to poor health and obesity.

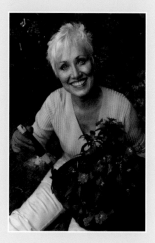

When insulin levels stay elevated this way, the body continuously uses glucose for fuel, rather than both glucose and fat. And when it's not used as energy, all that ingested fat—along with excess glucose and high-fructose corn syrup—is laid down in fat cells. In short, you become a fat-storage factory. On top of which, that huge meal right before bed keeps your body in fat-storage mode through the night and disrupts your sleep, leading to even poorer eating habits and even more weight gain.

Ask yourself these questions to see if your body is currently getting its energy by burning fat or by using quick carbohydrates.

1. Do you eat a lot of refined, processed foods and drinks?
2. Do you have a hard time concentrating or staying focused?
3. Do you skip meals and end up eating only one or two a day?
4. Do you struggle with cravings and low blood sugar?
5. Are you irritable if meals are missed or delayed?
6. Do you struggle with midmorning or afternoon slumps?
7. Do you have difficulty staying asleep?

If you answered yes to more than a couple, you probably have a high level of insulin that's keeping you in fat-storage mode and creating weight gain.

How can you break that cycle? Let's look at a study that offers some clues to a new, better way of eating that also happens to be a core Habit of Health!

The Myth of Three Squares

A study by David Jenkins, MD, PhD—the University of Toronto pioneer in low-glycemic eating—demonstrates that eating small portions at frequent intervals is good for your health in a number of important, even remarkable, ways.*

The researchers divided their subjects into two groups. Both ate the exact same food with the exact same number of calories. But one group ate their food divided into the usual three meals a day. The other ate more often, consuming lots of little meals.

Surprisingly, the group that ate small meals throughout the day lost more weight. It wasn't that they were less hungry (although, in fact, they *were* less hungry). They lost weight because their blood sugar didn't continually spike and then dip down to an even lower level, the way it does after a big meal. Their glycemic levels—the amount of sugar in their blood—remained steady . . . and their craving for sweet foods went down.

That's not all. After only two weeks, they found that the people who ate every three hours reduced their blood cholesterol by over 15 percent and their blood insulin by almost 28 percent. That's key—because, in addition to regulating your blood sugar level, insulin plays a pivotal role in fat metabolism, inflammation, and the progression to metabolic syndrome. When your body produces less insulin, you're much less likely to convert dietary calories into

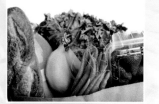

*Jenkins, D. J., et al., "Nibbling versus Gorging: Metabolic Advantages of Increased Meal Frequency," *New England Journal of Medicine* 321 (1989): 929–34.

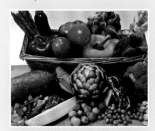

body fat. Your body begins to work differently, and you're no longer the fat factory you once were.

So what does this study tell us? That it's not just *what* you eat, it's *when* you eat it. Small amounts of nourishment throughout the day are better than the same amount of food concentrated in three big hits. If we feed the body at regular intervals, we send a signal to the body that it doesn't have to store calories. Conversely, when we skip meals we send just the opposite signal for the body to *store* calories, creating a negative effect on the metabolism.

Eating regularly satisfies our ancient programming, prevents activating the alarms of starvation, and turns off fat storage. It's our modern-day version of hunting and gathering! And by adding low-glycemic foods to those meals, making them more like our ancient diet, we do even more to control blood sugar and turn off the insulin pump that leads to dreaded fat storage—fat that's crippling our health and leading directly to disease.

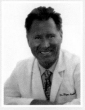

The Science of Six Fuelings

What are the benefits of eating a small amount of food more often? Preliminary research supports the idea that when the typical "three squares" diet is replaced by smaller, more frequent meals, it can:

- Help you lose weight
- Control hunger
- Reduce blood insulin (a factor in fat storage and inflammation)
- Lower total cholesterol levels
- Reduce LDL ("bad") cholesterol
- Reduce levels of apolipoprotein b (the "very bad" stuff!)
- Depress glucose levels
- Increase bile acid secretion
- Suppress free fatty acids levels
- Reduce serum uric acid levels, a common risk factor for coronary heart disease
- Increase uric acid excretion
- Reduce adipose tissue enzyme levels
- Reduce fluctuations in satiety (fullness)

So now we know that eating smaller, low-glycemic meals is a great way to turn off insulin and provide healthier fuel for our body. What else can help us achieve long-term weight loss?

Patterns of Success

In the introduction, you learned that over 85 percent of those who go on a diet without other behavioral supports fail. But on the flipside, that means that just under 15 percent succeed. What can we learn from them? Studies provide some intriguing answers. In one of the most impressive, led by Dr. James Hill and Dr. Rena Wing from the National Weight Control Registry, researchers gathered data from over 10,000 individuals, many of whom lost over 65 pounds and kept the weight off for at least five years. The weight-loss methods varied, but what these individuals had in common were certain core practices that have proven critical to successfully and safely maintaining a healthy weight. Here's what they did:

- They ate breakfast.
- They ate a balanced diet, paying close attention to the amount of dietary fat.
- They increased their physical activity quite a bit.
- They monitored their weight regularly.

So we want to add breakfast, lower fat content, make sure our food is nutrient dense, become more physically active, and monitor ourselves for early warnings of weight regain. And in fact, these scientifically proven fundamentals are crucial components of our weight-loss and long-term maintenance eating strategy. Let's put these healthy behaviors all together and see just how that strategy is going to look.

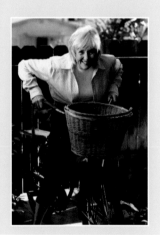

Why Exercise Alone Won't Help You Lose Weight

Trying to fight fat with exercise? You may want to rethink your strategy.

When you take in more calories than you expend, the excess gets stored as fat—3,500 calories in one pound. Eating just 100 extra calories a day—a bagel, a candy bar, a soda—translates to 36,500 calories of excess energy over the course of a year. Even if your body stores only half of that, the result is over five extra pounds of fat a year!

You could try burning those excess calories through exercise alone. But in order to burn just one pound, you'd have to run 33.8 miles. Just for one pound! And nearly one-third of us have an extra thirty pounds of fat. To burn that much, you'd have to run 1,040 miles—the equivalent of forty marathons.

The Key to Healthy Weight Loss

What's the key to successful mastery of both weight loss and long-term health? There are really two main components:

1. The ability to master the amount of fuel you take in
2. The quality of that fuel

So if we can devise a plan that delivers lower-calorie, nutrient-dense foods in the proper proportions, we have a recipe for success.

How does it work? Portion size is key. When you eat healthy foods—that is, low-glycemic carbohydrates, healthy fats, and high-quality protein—in smaller portions than your body is used to, a magical transformation occurs. Your body turns to Plan B and begins to utilize the unhealthy fat around your middle to make up the deficit. Remember that 10,000-year-old programming we discussed? That storage system of fat begins to be used *as it was intended*, providing your body with a constant source of calories while signaling it to turn off insulin, hunger, and cravings for carbohydrates.

And there's another great benefit. By providing your body with these nutrient-dense, protein-rich feedings in small portions throughout the day, you protect your muscles from being cannibalized, unlike in some low-calorie weight-loss programs. But that doesn't mean you won't see results. In fact, you can expect to lose two to five pounds per week for the first two weeks and one to two pounds per week thereafter.

But this efficient, safe platform not only carries you through your initial weight-loss phase, it also sets the stage for a whole new pattern of healthy eating—for life. Let's see how your body's going to respond to this new healthy fueling strategy.

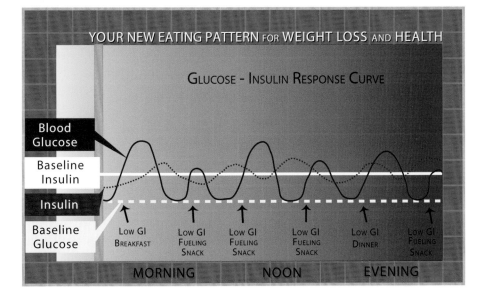

That's a whole different picture than before (see Modern Life's Disease Path, page 61). First, we've reduced your total energy intake by introducing smaller, portion-controlled meals and snacks. Second, we've switched to low-glycemic meals that keep your blood sugar and insulin levels from spiking. This constant, stable energy source means no more wide swings in blood sugar. You've turned off your insulin pump and taken control of cravings!

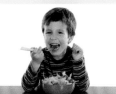

Your New Healthy Eating Pattern for Weight Loss and Health: Glucose-Insulin Response Curve. In your new eating plan, you'll have small, frequent, low-glycemic meals and snacks in order to prevent blood sugar and insulin levels from spiking.

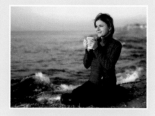

Eating this way—every three hours, starting with a healthy breakfast—helps you build a whole new energy management system, one that disperses energy throughout the day in accord with your body's natural design. And once you begin to use energy more efficiently this way, your body quickly starts to offload excess calories, producing the perfect internal environment for hunger control and weight loss.

That's the science behind our plan. Now how is that going to translate to your daily life?

The Logistics of Healthy Eating

Can you eat every three hours? If so, you can change your life. Let me help you figure out how to make this sort of meal schedule fit easily into your day. Here's the schedule you'll use during Phase I, the weight-loss phase.

First, eat a healthy breakfast within thirty minutes of rising, say at 7:00 in the morning. Three hours later, eat a little something else. And so on, through the day:

> 7:00 breakfast
> 10:00 nourishment
> 1:00 nourishment (or small lunch)
> 4:00 nourishment
> 7:00 dinner
> 9:30–10:00 small nourishment

You'll see that our plan includes a healthy evening meal. It may be smaller than the standard American dinner of enough meat and potatoes to feed an army. But the good news is that your body won't want a big meal. You'll be satisfied with a modest amount of healthy food, because your body's desires will have changed.

Like many of my new patients, you may be thinking: *I don't have time. It takes too much effort to prepare meals. It's inconvenient. It doesn't fit my lifestyle.* Don't worry—I've got you covered. In the next chapter, you'll learn about an amazing technology that's going to help. In my many years of practice, I have yet to encounter a single person who wasn't able to make this plan work once I showed them how. By planning your meals in advance and making sure to have healthy fuelings with you wherever you go, the program is actually quite easy to manage logistically. More importantly, it's easy to manage *biologically*—and that's the point. You want your body to cooperate with you, which won't happen if it's starving.

In our plan, you won't feel hunger pangs. You won't feel the lack of anything. You'll feel satisfied. You'll feel in control again! And as a bonus you'll begin to restore your sense of taste and learn to experience the flavors of food in new and exciting ways. All while losing weight!

Creating a Microenvironment of Health

In chapters 3 and 4, you learned how to develop an internal framework focused on the motivation and choices that support your goal of optimal health. Now

There's always something tempting us to eat. That's why it's so important to create a microenvironment of health in our own homes by filling them with healthy foods and other things that inspire positive behaviors.

we're going to begin supplementing that healthy *internal* environment with a healthy *external* environment. This brave new world—what I call a *leptogenic* world—supports optimally healthy, fit individuals. Here's how we're going to start building it.

From the moment we get up in the morning until the time we hit the pillow at night, somebody or something is tempting us to eat. This world of nutritional pollution is hard to ignore.

It all goes back to our development as a species. Over the course of many thousands of years, our brains perfected a system that rewards behavior it deems essential to our survival. Food gives us sensations of pleasure, which we've learned to anticipate and seek out. In fact, food—especially high-calorie junk food filled with fat and sugar—affects our brain receptors in just the same way that drugs and alcohol do. Back in our ancestors' day, this was an important survival mechanism. High-density foods were rare, and it was always in our best interest to eat as much of them as possible. But even today, this conditioning is so strong that we're stimulated by the mere hint of food—just by being in certain environments or around smells that we associate with eating.

So, what's the take-home message? In your kitchen, you have a 100 percent chance of finding food. But today, unlike in the past, it's not helping you survive. In fact, it's harming you.

You need to change the inventory, bring in the Hazmat team, detoxify, and outwit your ancient hard-wiring, especially in the beginning when your new Habits of Health aren't yet automatic. In essence, you need to build a microenvironment that gives you the best chance of success—a protective bubble of health.

As we proceed, I'll teach you additional techniques to support your new healthy world. By the time you've reached your target weight, you'll be armed inside and out with the motivation, structure, and daily choices you need to maintain optimal health.

But for now, let's set you up for success by giving your house a health makeover.

Reduce Your Refrigerator

Begin by bringing a trash can over to the refrigerator. Get ready to dump the following foods, take them to the local food bank, or give them to your neighbors—depending how much you like those neighbors!

Here's what needs to go:

- whole-fat dairy products such as milk, cheese, yogurt, butter, cottage cheese, and mayonnaise
- processed deli meats and bacon
- sugary sodas
- beer and wine
- foods high in calories, fat, or sugar, including peanut butter, jellies, and salad dressings (except low fat and low calorie)

***Leptogenic:* Your Brave New World**
Leptogenic comes from the Latin word *lepto*, meaning thin or slender. It's the polar opposite of the *obesigenic* world we've been living in!

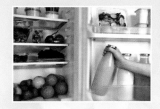

Note: This list of healthy
foods is a general
guideline for long-term
healthy eating. Your
actual shopping list
for Phase I will be
outlined in the following
chapters!

Now fill your fridge back up with these:

- fat-free or low-fat dairy products such as skim or soy milk, low-fat cottage cheese, and low-fat yogurt
- low-fat protein sources such as lean chicken and meats, tofu, hummus, and eggs
- fresh fruits and vegetables (and frozen fruits and vegetables for the freezer)
- condiments such as mustards, pickles, and vinegars

Perk Up Your Pantry

Get rid of any of these tempting foods that could sabotage your healthy eating choices. Please do not use this time to finish off the bag of cookies you find! It's better to just throw them away; a bigger waist will result from putting that unhealthy food into your body! (If you have children or teenagers, this is a great chance to help them eat healthier too. But if you must keep foods for them in the house that don't fit your plan, put them in a low, out-of-the-way cupboard and don't go near them!)

Start by getting rid of these:

- white rice, white flour, and white bread
- hydrogenated vegetable oils, including hard or semi-soft margarine and shortenings such as Crisco
- refined cereals (whole grain is OK) and flavored oatmeal
- cookies, candy, cakes, and muffins
- chips, crackers, pretzels, and peanuts

Now fill your pantry back up with these:

- brown rice
- canola and olive oil
- natural, non-flavored oatmeal
- whole grain, high-fiber breads and pitas
- whole wheat flour
- walnuts and beans
- a variety of spices and herbs

Clean Up Your Kitchen and Your Kitchen Behaviors

- Put away any cookie jars or food triggers that are sitting out on the counter.
- Smaller plates support smaller portions. Put your regular dinner plates in the back of your cupboard and bring out the 6- to 9-inch salad plates.
- Never stand or walk while you're eating. Take the time to sit down at the table.
- Buy some blue placemats and plates. The color blue has been proven to decrease appetite, while yellow and red increase it. Guess where the inspiration for the golden arches came from, and why the interiors of many fast food restaurants are yellow, gold, or red—to make you salivate, increase your appetite, and tempt you to buy their fat- and grease-laden food!

- Never use serving bowls on the table. Plate your meals in the kitchen (using 9-inch plates).
- Turn up the wattage! Bright lights have been shown to make us eat less.

Ready Your Bedroom

Creating an environment that optimizes sleep quality is critical to good health. In fact, several studies confirm that poor sleep directly contributes to poor eating habits. We'll spend considerable time in Phase II giving you some tips to improve your sleep, but for right now here are a few simple steps to make your bedroom more conducive to healthy sleeping:

- Organize your bedroom and put away clutter.
- Don't watch TV in bed. If you have a TV in your bedroom, remove or un-plug it.
- Choose a bedtime that allows you to get eight hours of sleep and stick with it.
- Keep your room cool while you sleep.
- Never eat in bed.

Create a Journal

Keeping a journal of everything you put into your mouth can give you further insight into your current behaviors and eating habits. I recommend you get one when you're out buying your new groceries! You'll find some great journal ideas in *Living a Longer, Healthier Life: the Companion Guide to Dr. A's Habits of Health* and at the Web site, www.habitsofhealth.net.

Your Weight-Loss Strategy

My years of experience as a physician helping people who have previously strug-gled with losing and maintaining a healthy weight have taught me what works in the real world. I'm not going to teach you theory based on some laboratory findings in rats, or hype created in some company's marketing department. The specific eating strategy I'm about to describe works because it's practical, cost-effective, and it provides consistent weight loss. It delivers the simplicity of a turnkey system that helps you get results quickly, and it's easy to learn. It allows you to lose weight while I teach you a practical plan to eat healthy for life.

The two components I'm about to describe differ in the time, effort, and skills they require to master. Combining them into an overall strategy allows you the time necessary to learn the Habits of Health while you reach your healthy weight. I want to bring you along at a pace that relates to your level of cooking experience and your understanding of healthy food choices. Learning both of these strategies will arm you with the best possible preparation to create the outcome we want—long-term success. You'll be able to pick and choose from a compendium of tools that provide you with several options based on your current weight, time availability, and even personality. You'll finally have the ability to reach a healthy weight quickly while you learn the habits of healthy eating for life.

The color blue has been shown to decrease appetite, while red and yellow increase it. Guess where the inspiration for the golden arches came from?

Dr. A Says. . .

Now that you're cleaning out the pantry and stocking up on healthy snacks, it's a great time to teach your kids to eat healthy too!

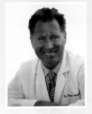

Both components of our overall eating strategy work in synergy and share these important features:

- They're based on my two core principles of energy management for safe weight loss.
- They both set the stage for all the other Habits of Health.
- They contain important techniques you can incorporate into your daily habits as you build the tools, skills, and techniques for long-term success.
- Both approaches have been studied extensively at major universities around the world and have extensive research to support their efficacy and safety.
- They offer simple, straightforward ways to fuel your body efficiently, lower your energy intake, turn off your insulin pump, and put you in fat-burning mode.
- Both allow you to choose from diverse, satisfying, and balanced foods for sustainable weight loss.
- Both focus on foods that are low glycemic, low fat, and contain high-quality protein.
- With each method, you'll eat breakfast every morning and continue to eat every three hours through the day.
- They provide the versatility to customize a plan that fits your lifestyle.

Let's spend a little time discussing both of these components to our overall strategy and see how they apply directly to you.

The Catalyst to Reaching a Healthy Weight: Medically Formulated Portion-Controlled Meal Replacements

For quick, effective weight loss without a lot of preparation, medically formulated, low-calorie portion-controlled meal replacements (PCMRs) offer a convenient, ready-to-use food system in the form of pre-packaged, low-glycemic meals. In fact, the success of these systems is well documented in the medical literature.

As I mentioned previously, I have considerable experience using meal replacements to help people lose weight. I've found them to be a powerful tool that consistently delivers predictable weight loss. Because they're so easy to use and fit so nicely into a busy lifestyle, I highly recommend them. In fact, for people who need to lose more than a few pounds, this is the tool I use to assure that they get a strong start as they begin their journey on the road to optimal health.

How does it work? Medically formulated, low-calorie portion-controlled meal replacements provide a low-glycemic, healthy-protein mixture that enables you to safely and comfortably lower your caloric intake when you eat them in place of meals. They're also fortified with vitamins and minerals. Once each day, at a time that works for you, you'll supplement the meal replacements with a healthy portion of lean meat, poultry, or fish, along with a salad or choice of vegetable. This combination allows your body to rapidly enter a reliable fat-burning state that produces safe, effective weight loss.

Medically formulated, low-calorie, balanced meal replacements are easy and convenient and can help you lose weight quickly. And once you've met your initial weight-loss goal, you can continue to use PCMRs while learning the basics of eating healthy for long-term success.

In short: Meal replacements are convenient, varied, and effective. As you're learning to eat healthy for the first time, the ease and fast results of this ready-to-go approach are very appealing. As you learn the fundamentals of healthy eating, meal replacements enable you to grasp the principles of low-glycemic eating and menu choice gradually, in bite-sized pieces. We'll also use them as a convenient, high-quality portable fuel as part of our long-term healthy eating system.

Dr. A's Healthy Eating System: A Low-Glycemic Portion-Control Approach to Support Optimal Health

This simple, straightforward approach to shopping, preparing, and cooking healthy meals makes nourishing your body every three hours easy and convenient. It will teach you everything you need to develop an eating strategy that will last a lifetime. If you have only a few pounds to lose or are already at a healthy weight, this easy system will help you maintain your weight and can be used with the medically formulated, low-calorie PCMRs to give you the best of both worlds.

How does it work? You'll utilize the principle of low-glycemic eating to shut off excess insulin secretion and turn off fat storage.

This plan gives you everything you need to control portion size and lower your intake of calories, including a unique color-coded system to make shopping for healthy foods stress free. You'll find information on selecting acceptable carbohydrates, proper fats, and proteins that work together to promote weight loss, as well as flexible menu choices that make meals fun. I'll even teach you to use a portable cooker to prepare delicious, easy meals wherever your busy day takes you!

In short: This healthy eating system teaches you how to make good choices and prepare healthy meals from day one. It's going to take a little practice, but once you have it mastered you'll have a complete eating strategy for life. If you take the time to learn this system while you're losing weight on the medically formulated PCMRs, you'll be in perfect position to transition into my permanent healthy eating strategy once you reach a healthy weight. If you're already close to your goal weight, you can simply adopt my healthy eating system, which includes medically formulated PCMRs, right out of the gate.

The Teachable Moment

Now that we've described your weight-loss strategy, I encourage you to jump right in! In just a week or so, as you start to lose weight, you'll see substantial improvement in your physical and mental health. You'll feel better, have more energy, sleep better, and quite likely begin to reduce medications for certain weight-related health conditions. Soon you'll notice an improvement in your thinking, your memory, and your desire to learn more.

It's the period I call the teachable moment, and it's the best building block I've found for long-term success. It's the moment when the Habits of Health truly begin to take root!

Dr. A Says. . .

This system sets you up for a lifetime of healthy eating, with all the knowledge and strategies you need for success.

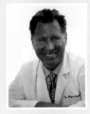

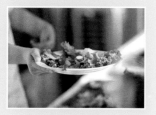

Medically formulated
PCMRs are a
powerful tool as part
of a comprehensive
approach to healthy
eating.

Chapter 7

The Catalyst to Reaching a Healthy Weight

In this chapter, I am going to outline the system I have found most effective in helping people who need to lose a lot of weight. This plan will get you results right out of the gate and allow me time to teach you my healthy eating system.

We'll use this incredible tool to help you lose weight and begin your journey toward optimal health. Then, in chapters 8 through 10, I'll outline my healthy eating plan, which will empower you to have complete command over your eating environment. You will learn a comprehensive approach that provides the techniques, shopping methods, and a meal plan that will deliver your body a full array of healthy food. But first, let me describe this tool that I use daily to help people start their journey to optimal health. If you're still a little skeptical, keep reading and you'll learn how easy it is to get going.

Medically Formulated Portion-Controlled Meal Replacements: Catalyst to Success

A lot has changed since portion-controlled meal replacements (PCMRs) were first developed in the 1970s. Originally created to spur weight loss in extremely obese, high-risk patients, PCMRs provide specific combinations of nutrients in small dose-controlled portions that protect lean muscle while burning fat.

Patients in those days received all their nutrients from these packets, often taking in as few as 300 calories a day. PCMRs were extremely efficient at helping patients lose weight, but they came under a lot of criticism, particularly when used long term. Medical experts complained that those early PCMRs didn't teach people healthy eating habits, and patients found them expensive and restrictive.

Fast forward to today. Medically proven low-calorie portion-controlled meal replacements have undergone significant improvement in the last few decades. In fact, I truly believe that they're on the verge of becoming an overnight sensation, or at least an integral part of many of our lives. Why? Because they're a powerful tool—not as a complete diet in and of themselves, but as part of a comprehensive approach to healthy eating. And one that's coming in the nick of time.

Our fast-paced society puts tremendous demands on us. As a result, we're facing a deterioration of our health that's just not sustainable. We need a breakthrough!

Now, I realize that meal replacements alone can't do the trick. As I've already discussed, isolated weight-control strategies that don't address the whole person and his or her unhealthy lifestyle are universally unsuccessful. In fact, there's not one documented case of a stand-alone diet, drug, or dietary supplement that has brought about consistent, sustained weight control over the long term by itself. A comprehensive approach that includes lifestyle change and proper support, on the other hand, when orchestrated correctly, is extremely effective in sustaining long-term health.

The Habits of Health is such an approach. One of the most critical components of the Habits of Health is eating small, healthy meals throughout the day that are portion-controlled and low glycemic. But for many of us, finding the time and energy to prepare these meals can be daunting. And then there's the learning curve. While teaching you to fix healthy, low-glycemic meals is one of my most important goals, I'm also a realist. I know, for example, that most of you have never programmed your DVD player, and that the LED clock is probably still blinking. We just have too much on our plates—no pun intended!

Today, more than ever, we need an easy, straightforward approach to healthy eating and energy management—a catalyst to get the ball rolling. Or to use another metaphor, just think of yourself as a jet on the runway. Takeoff requires a huge amount of energy, but once you've reached your cruising altitude you can settle down into a comfortable rhythm. Meal replacements will help you get past those first bumpy patches by minimizing the effort of planning meals and making a lot of choices at the beginning. And before you know it, you'll be cruising down the runway toward health.

I know—because I myself could never seem to find the time to eat healthy. I was standing still, getting heavier and heavier, until one day I started looking for answers and found the technology of meal replacements. And that made all the difference!

My Own Journey with PCMRs

As a critical care physician working as many as 110 hours some weeks, I was eating and living the Habits of Disease. Up at 5:00 a.m., grab a glass of high-glycemic orange juice (like many of you, I thought that was a healthy start to my day!), and off to the hospital. By 10:00 a.m., I was ravenous from hypoglycemia as a result of my sugar-laden OJ, so I'd satisfy those cravings by sneaking a piece of candy from a patient's nightstand. What with all those well-meaning relatives, I was never short on high-glycemic ways to elevate my blood sugar enough to get through the next surgery. Add in long hours, 10:00 p.m. dinners, poor sleep, not enough exercise, and soon enough I started gaining weight— twenty-seven pounds, nicely concealed by my drawstring scrubs. I was heading down the path to disease. Finally, I decided to do something about it. But I realized that I had no idea how to change my bad habits to healthy ones. I didn't really understand how to eat healthy, and besides, I had no time to cook. That's when I discovered PCMRs. And thankfully, they helped me lose those extra twenty-seven pounds.

Warning: For safety and effectiveness, choose only medically formulated, low-calorie PCMRs.

Results vary. Typical weight loss is 2-5 lbs per week for the first 2 weeks and 1-2 lbs per week thereafter.

Today's PCMRs are a whole new ballgame. Here are just some of the benefits:

- **They're cost effective.** Because you'll be replacing most of your groceries and snacks with PCMRs, you'll be spending the same or even less than you are now on food.

- **They offer plenty of variety.** Today's PCMRs help you fight taste fatigue with lots of great-tasting flavor options.

- **They help you control calories.** New technologies have developed advanced medically formulated PCMRs with the nutritional footprint to keep you in a fat-burning state while protecting muscle.

For more information on the medical science backing low-calorie PCMRs, see the following:

- Crowell, M. D., and Cheskin, L. J., Johns Hopkins University School of Medicine, "Multicenter Evaluation of Health Benefits and Weight Loss on the Medifast Weight Management Program."
- Cheskin, L. J., et al., Johns Hopkins University Bloomberg School of Public Health, "Efficacy of Two Diet Plans Designed for People with Type 2 Diabetes on Weight and Health Measures."

Now I've enjoyed six years at a healthy weight, I get eight hours of sleep a night, and I have plenty of time to spend with family and friends. Whether in the format of medically formulated PCMRs or whole foods, I eat a low-glycemic menu every day. I've gotten pretty good at picking healthy foods both at home and when I'm out to eat. PCMRs are especially helpful when I'm busy, on the road, or just feeling lazy. Grabbing a meal replacement helps me ensure that I eat a little something every three hours.

Best of all, my professional focus has gone from keeping unhealthy people alive to creating healthy lives. I spend my days finding better ways to help people reach a healthy weight and learn habits that support great health.

The PCMR that I used so successfully, and that I've helped others experience with success, is made by Medifast®, the company I now serve as medical director. Medifast's products and programs set the gold standard, with more than thirty years of efficacy and safety, backed by studies conducted by researchers from prestigious institutions such as Johns Hopkins Bloomberg School of Public Health and recommended by over 20,000 doctors since 1980. And to top it off, we've gathered a medical and research team committed to keeping these meal replacements at the forefront of science and technology.

PCMRs: Healthy Fast Food for the Twenty-first Century

In our chaotic lives, we rarely find time to plan meals. In fact, most of us don't even think about fueling our bodies until we're hungry and hypoglycemic. That's the mentality that's given rise to the fast food phenomenon, now a $129 billion a year business.

If you were driving across the desert, you'd definitely fuel your car before you started, and you'd probably give at least some thought to where the next gas station was located. But I'll bet you start your day in a hurry by skipping breakfast or, worse, grabbing a doughnut and coffee. Then, just at the moment your body's screaming for food, the fast food industry steps in with the sights, smells, and convenience that lead to bad decisions.

Sadly, those unhealthy fast food fueling stations aren't going away any time soon, so it's all the more important to find healthy alternatives that are convenient, readily available, and support the Habits of Health. So I'd like you to think of PCMRs like Medifast's as high-quality fast food—a "safety net" to protect you from nutritional pollution.

PCMRs give you what you need to fuel your body when hunger strikes and you don't have time for a sit-down, prepared meal. They're completely portable for convenience. They're sealed for safety. They're individually packaged for reliable portion control. And they taste good! Today's medically formulated PCMRs come in abundant variety with an array of flavors and textures tailored to breakfast, lunch, or dinner.

Most important, medically formulated PCMRs provide a balance of high-quality protein and complex carbohydrates, along with twenty-four vitamins and minerals, to protect your body and help you feel full and satisfied. And because they give you a scientifically determined dose of energy—between 90 and 160 calories per dose—you'll find it much easier to control your energy intake. Soon you'll be turning on your fat-burning machine and safely losing two to five pounds per week for the first two weeks and one to two pounds per week thereafter.

I believe that PCMRs are the easiest way to enter the path to optimal health. In time, I'll help you develop a complete healthy eating strategy to support you for the rest of your life, including advice on how to choose groceries, select from a restaurant menu, and cook a quick, low-glycemic meal. PCMRs can give you just the boost you need to get started on your journey to permanent weight loss and optimal health—just as I did.

The PCMR System

Remember in the last chapter, when I asked if you could eat every three hours? If you answered yes, you're going to find using PCMRs a breeze.

I can't overemphasize, however, that your success depends on choosing a high-quality brand of PCMR. Let me tell you a brief story about early generic pharmaceuticals. In the 1970s and '80s, a lot of companies started getting into the pharmaceutical business, many of which didn't use the rigid testing and dose standardization of the big companies that had set the gold standard. As a result, patients were injured, some seriously, or worse. The only way that we as physicians could assure our patients' safety was to specify medication *by brand name*.

I truly believe that, just as with these specific medications, in order to be assured of using a safe, effective PCMR, you must use only those backed by a medical research team and clinically tested. Please don't try to save a few pennies

It's important to choose low-calorie, medically formulated PCMRs that contain a high-quality protein, and soy is an excellent choice. A highly digestible primary protein, soy is a rich source of calcium, zinc, iron, phosphorous, magnesium, B vitamins, omega-3, and fiber. I recommend you use only products in which the soy is water-washed to maintain all the health-giving benefits of the phytonutrients. (For more information on the role of phytonutrients in optimal health, see chapter 20.) High-quality whey is a good substitute for those who are allergic to soy or who choose not to use it for other reasons.*

*Lycan, T. W., Davis, L. M., Andersen, W. S., Cheskin, L. J., "The Health Effects of Soy: Benefits and Risks for Women," forthcoming.

Important: Before You Begin

Before you start your journey, I suggest you schedule a visit to see your primary care provider, usually your family doctor. No doubt your doctor will be excited that you've decided to lose weight and create health in your life. After all, it makes their job easier! In the appendix, you'll find a sheet of information to give your physician that explains this "health makeover" you're doing. It's also available for download at my Web site at www.habitsofhealth.net.

A special note for those with type 2 diabetes: Checking in with your doctor before you change your diet is particularly important if you have type 2 diabetes. As you switch to my low-calorie, low-glycemic diet, your blood sugar will lower immediately, and your level of medication will need to be reduced accordingly. The great news is that this is a signal of your body's initial step toward health. Your disease progression is being arrested! But do remember to watch your blood sugar closely in the beginning to make sure your medications are properly adjusted.

by using some cheap product that turns out to be ineffective. It doesn't serve your best interests, and it certainly doesn't serve your health.

Of course, I have a bias toward the system I use, Medifast, because I've helped influence its development into the extremely versatile, clinically effective tool it is today. On top of that, we've worked to keep these high-quality meal replacements affordable and obtainable to you without the additional costs associated with obligatory office and lab visits or program fees. That means that unlike other PCMR systems out there, you can use Medifast products in conjunction with your health clinic, a private health coach, or just by purchasing them directly, as you would any other food.

Your Phase I Eating Pattern

Remember our old friend, the Glucose-Insulin Response Curve? Let's take another look to see your Phase I eating plan using PCMRs.

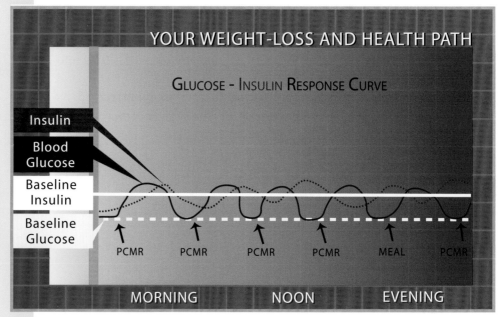

Your Weight-Loss and Health Path: Glucose-Insulin Response Curve. A steady dose of low-glycemic PCMRs helps stabilize blood sugar and keep your insulin level in control. With the PCMR system, you'll fuel your body throughout the day with one PCMR every three hours, a healthy meal in the evening, and a late evening PCMR.

You'll note from the graph above that a steady dose of low-glycemic PCMRs helps you stabilize your blood sugar and keep your insulin level in control. With the PCMR system, you'll fuel your body throughout the day— one PCMR every three hours, supplemented by a healthy meal in the evening, or whenever it fits best into your schedule. As you lower your energy intake and enter a fat-burning state—one of our core principles—you'll start losing weight almost immediately. On average you'll lose between 2.5 and 3.5 pounds each week (women) or between 3.5 and 4.5 pounds each week (men).* Your weight-loss results may be a little slower if you have hypothyroidism or are on medications such as hormone replacement therapy.

The low-calorie state you'll enter during Phase I—somewhere around a thousand calories a day—may seem low compared to what you're eating now,

*Crowell, M. D., and Cheskin, L. J., Johns Hopkins University School of Medicine, "Multicenter Evaluation of Health Benefits and Weight Loss on the Medifast Weight Management Program."

but within three days you'll turn on your fat stores as your energy source. Soon you'll feel great and have plenty of energy, and you won't be tired or hungry.

Getting Started

Before you start using your PCMRs for Phase I, there are a few things you should think about. Remember, you'll need five meal replacements on hand each day. I highly suggest you purchase a month's supply of PCMRs right off the bat for the sake of variety, economy, and to ensure you don't run out.

Choosing a system designed like Medifast's has a number of benefits, including the diversity of menu choices it offers. Choosing from fifty different varieties of PCMRs helps minimize "taste fatigue," a condition that occurs when an individual tires of the same monotonous tastes, textures, and flavors. But because all of those varieties are part of a carefully designed system, they work together using the same building blocks to support your health and burn fat. So while you're enjoying your cappuccino, scrambled eggs, or oatmeal PCMRs for breakfast, you have the backing of ingenious food technologists who've kept the nutritional footprint of all these various PCMRs nearly identical.

Best of all, with a medical-based system such as this, you can choose your shakes, chili, soups, bars, and whatever else appeals to you without having to think about calories, nutritional content, or glycemic index. It's an intelligent system that provides the nutritional footprint, portion control, low-glycemic ingredients, and reduced calories you need to optimize your body, creating a safe, healthy environment for fat burning while protecting precious muscle mass.

As medical director of Medifast, I've been part of a team that developed and uses an effective system of meal replacements. In the following pages, with permission from Medifast, I will use our sample menus, charts, and plan to demonstrate an efficient system of rapid, safe weight loss using PCMRs.*

Your Phase I Eating Strategy

Your Phase I eating strategy is simple: just select any five medically formulated meal replacements and one healthy, low-glycemic meal each day.

Ideally, you'll have your first PCMR within thirty minutes of rising, and then choose another every three hours. You'll also eat one healthy, low-glycemic meal a day, at whatever three-hour interval you prefer. Most people choose to have this healthy meal—what we call the "lean and green"—in the evening, to coincide with family dinner. It's designed to give you your necessary fats, natural enzymes, and phytonutrients, while maintaining the low-calorie, low-glycemic requirements that keep you in a fat-burning state. During Phase I, your lean and green meal includes *lean* meat, fish, or poultry (white meat only) and a *green* vegetable or salad. So, depending what time you wake up, your day should look something like this.

*Used with permission from Medifast, Inc. with all rights reserved. Lean and Green™; for more information on this specific system, see *The Secret Is Out: Medifast, What Physicians Have Always Known about Weight Loss,* by Brad MacDonald and Lisa M. Davis, PhD, PA-C (Medifast, Inc., 2006).

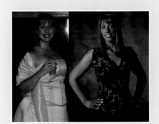

"I have a whole new life!"

JENNIFER DILLON
Over two years at optimal health

Through the techniques Dr. Andersen outlines in the Habits of Health, I lost 110 pounds using the Take Shape for Life™ program—and best of all I've maintained my weight and health goals ever since.

I can't possibly describe what this has done for me and my family. I now have a whole new life! I never imagined that I'd be able to run a 5K, which I did to celebrate one year at my healthy weight. And not only have I regained my own health, I get to help others change their lives, too. What an amazing feeling! Thanks, Dr. A, for giving me back my health and showing me what I need to do to stay that way. ■

Results vary. Typical weight loss is 2-5 lbs per week for the first 2 weeks and 1-2 lbs per week thereafter.

Sample Meal Plan

7:00 a.m.	**Breakfast**	*Choose one PCMR:* oatmeal, scrambled eggs, or cappuccino
10:00 a.m.	**Fueling**	*Choose one PCMR:* chocolate shake, hot cocoa, or chai latte
1:00 p.m.	**Lunch**	*Choose one PCMR:* chili, beef stew, or chicken and wild rice soup
4:00 p.m.	**Fueling**	*Choose one PCMR:* oatmeal raisin bar or vanilla pudding
7:00 p.m.	**Dinner**	*Lean and Green™ meal*

For example:

- 5-ounce steak; green salad with low-fat dressing
- 6-ounce grilled chicken breast; 1½ cups cooked asparagus with one teaspoon olive oil
- 5-ounce portion grilled salmon; salad (two cups mixed salad greens, ½ cup total of diced tomatoes, cucumbers, and celery with two tablespoons low-carb salad dressing)

10:00 p.m.	**Fueling**	*Choose one PCMR:* banana pudding or strawberry crème shake

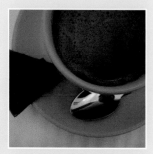

Shopping for Your Lean and Green

One thing that's great about this eating strategy is that there's actually very little you need to do in terms of preparation. The PCMR system you choose will include simple instructions on preparing and using their products, and getting ready for your lean and green meal involves little more than clearing out your pantry (as detailed in chapter 6) and making a quick trip to the market.

If you haven't had much experience selecting healthy protein and vegetables, you may want to take a bit of time to ask the butcher or produce department for help. I learned a great amount simply by asking store employees which items were fresh, healthy, and locally produced. Once you have it down, you should be able to get your weekly shopping done in no more than fifteen minutes.

Your shopping list should include selections from these four major groups:

1. Lean protein
2. Healthy fats and oils
3. Green vegetables and salad
4. Healthy snacks and condiments

Let's take a closer look at each.

1. Lean Protein

Shopping for protein is a great opportunity to try out new food sources, flavors, and recipes, and to learn a very specific Habit of Health. By choosing the leanest meats, experimenting with meat alternatives, and increasing your variety of fish and seafood, you're lowering and even eliminating unhealthy fats, while

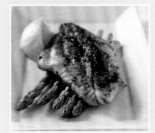

adding healthy omegas to create a powerful, nutritious meal. To keep that fat content low, you'll be grilling, baking, broiling, or poaching your selections. And to make it easier for you to choose the leanest options, I've devised a color-coded system that takes you from *lean* (light green) to *leanest* (dark green). Here's a rundown of your lean and green protein sources.

Seafood

When you eat fish, you're not only choosing a great protein source—you're also significantly reducing your risk of disease. Eating fish one to three times a week is an important Habit of Health and can have a profound impact on your well-being over time. In fact, one serving of fish a week may reduce your risk of fatal heart attack by 40 percent!

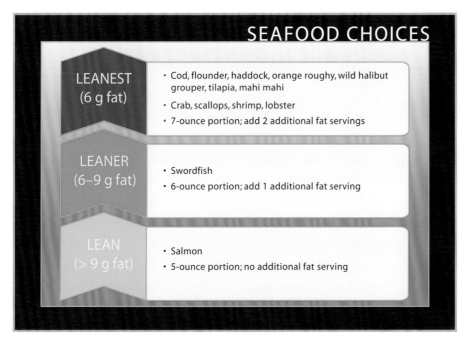

SEAFOOD CHOICES

LEANEST (6 g fat)	• Cod, flounder, haddock, orange roughy, wild halibut grouper, tilapia, mahi mahi • Crab, scallops, shrimp, lobster • 7-ounce portion; add 2 additional fat servings
LEANER (6–9 g fat)	• Swordfish • 6-ounce portion; add 1 additional fat serving
LEAN (> 9 g fat)	• Salmon • 5-ounce portion; no additional fat serving

Dr. A Says. . .

One serving of fish a week can reduce your risk of fatal heart attack by 40 percent.

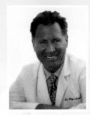

Meat and Poultry

I was brought up in a family where meat was part of daily life, and although I eat much less now, I still enjoy an occasional steak for dinner. It's important to lower your consumption of meat and eat more fish, white-meat poultry (skinless), legumes such as beans, and low-fat or nonfat dairy. But if you're like me, and once in a while need that savory taste of meat, just minimize the amount of saturated fat so you can enjoy this great protein source and still stay healthy.

Did you know that wild meat—the kind our ancestors ate 10,000 years ago—contains much less saturated fat than farm-raised meat? Our cattle are fed on high-glycemic foods and as a result contain an unhealthy amount of fat. By eating them, we concentrate our ingestion of fat and calories. Wild meats, on the other hand, such as buffalo and elk, contain very little fat. I've found both of these very enjoyable, as well as venison (deer), which although a bit strong-tasting can be quite good if prepared properly. Many of these wild meats are

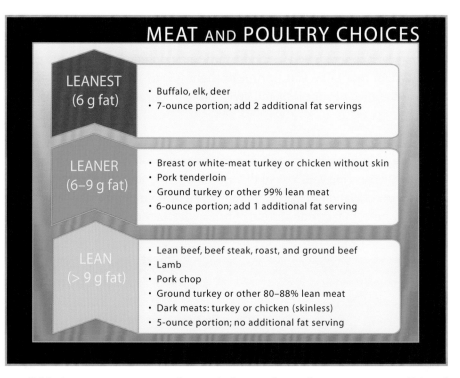

MEAT AND POULTRY CHOICES

LEANEST (6 g fat)
- Buffalo, elk, deer
- 7-ounce portion; add 2 additional fat servings

LEANER (6–9 g fat)
- Breast or white-meat turkey or chicken without skin
- Pork tenderloin
- Ground turkey or other 99% lean meat
- 6-ounce portion; add 1 additional fat serving

LEAN (> 9 g fat)
- Lean beef, beef steak, roast, and ground beef
- Lamb
- Pork chop
- Ground turkey or other 80–88% lean meat
- Dark meats: turkey or chicken (skinless)
- 5-ounce portion; no additional fat serving

available in grocery stores such as Whole Foods Market. But even traditional American beef can be a fine choice if you select cuts such as filets and sirloins rather than those that contain excess marbling from fat.

Meat Alternatives

If you'd like to eliminate meat from your diet, or just reduce the amount you eat, there are some great meatless selections available. I recommend that you stick with just the choices on the list, but if you do find an additional alternative you'd like to try, please make sure it contains no added sugar.

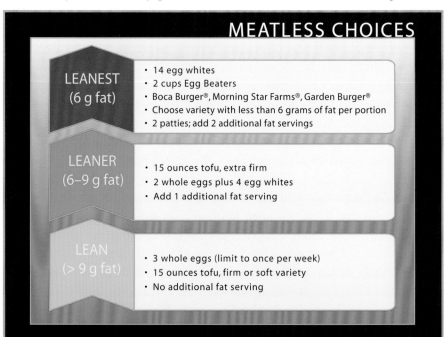

MEATLESS CHOICES

LEANEST (6 g fat)
- 14 egg whites
- 2 cups Egg Beaters
- Boca Burger®, Morning Star Farms®, Garden Burger®
- Choose variety with less than 6 grams of fat per portion
- 2 patties; add 2 additional fat servings

LEANER (6–9 g fat)
- 15 ounces tofu, extra firm
- 2 whole eggs plus 4 egg whites
- Add 1 additional fat serving

LEAN (> 9 g fat)
- 3 whole eggs (limit to once per week)
- 15 ounces tofu, firm or soft variety
- No additional fat serving

2. Healthy Fats and Oils

One of the important modern improvements in today's meal replacement systems is that they now ensure that users get the right amount of healthy fats. An adequate supply of fat helps your body absorb fat-soluble vitamins such as A, D, E, and K, and contributes to gall bladder health. Fats also help you lose weight by giving you a sense of fullness and adding texture to your meals.

Our focus in Phase I will be on eliminating unhealthy fats while supplementing your diet with healthy omegas that can accelerate your journey toward optimal health. Having a good supply of omega-rich antioxidants is particularly smart now during the weight-loss phase, when your body is unloading fat cells and unhealthy fat-soluble substances.

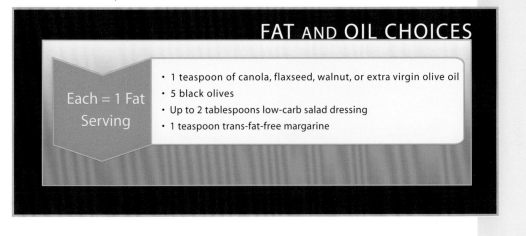

FAT AND OIL CHOICES

Each = 1 Fat Serving

- 1 teaspoon of canola, flaxseed, walnut, or extra virgin olive oil
- 5 black olives
- Up to 2 tablespoons low-carb salad dressing
- 1 teaspoon trans-fat-free margarine

3. Green Vegetables and Salad

I love vegetables and salads. As you'll discover in the following chapters, I believe you just can't eat too many healthy fruits and vegetables (with very few exceptions) once you reach your healthy weight. During Phase I, however, I'm going to ask that you avoid fruit, which can be extremely high in carbohydrates, and really focus on selecting moderate amounts of vegetables.

When we talk about vegetables during this phase, we're referring to nutrient-dense, low-glycemic carbohydrates that support your health while you lose weight. Some popular diets reduce carbohydrates to such a low level that they bring about a profound state of ketosis, accompanied by dehydration and juicy-fruit breath. I don't advocate that. Rather, this plan will create an efficient physiologic state of mild dietary ketosis. This allows you to burn fat while providing enough carbohydrates to maintain muscle and brain health—around 80 to 85 grams per day. The list on page 82 is designed to create this ideal state for optimal weight loss.

As you'll see, your choices are again color-coded, this time based on the amount of carbohydrates they contain. Darker green selections give you fewer carbohydrate calories. So if you're having trouble getting into a fat-burning state or if your weight loss slows down, it's probably a good idea to confine your choices to the dark green group, while also reducing or eliminating condiments and making sure your salad dressings are low fat and very low carb.

Medically formulated meal replacements are designed to place your body in an optimal state of fat burning.

From the list below, select any combination of three servings each day.
(One serving = 1 cup raw salad greens or ½ cup cooked or raw vegetables.)

GREEN VEGETABLES AND SALAD

Lowest Carbohydrate

Serving size = ½ cup unless otherwise specified

- Mustard greens (1 cup)
- Collards, fresh/raw (1 cup)
- Romaine lettuce (1 cup)
- Endive (1 cup)
- Lettuce, butter head (1 cup)
- Celery
- Cucumber
- Mushrooms, white
- Radishes
- Sprouts, alfalfa or mung bean
- Turnip greens

Moderate Carbohydrate

Serving size = ½ cup unless otherwise specified

- Asparagus
- Cabbage
- Cauliflower
- Eggplant
- Fennel
- Kale
- Mushrooms, portabella
- Spinach, cooked
- Summer squash, zucchini and scallop

Highest Carbohydrate

Serving size = ½ cup unless otherwise specified

- Broccoli
- Cabbage, red
- Collards or mustard greens, cooked
- Green or wax beans
- Kohlrabi
- Okra
- Peppers, green/red/yellow
- Scallions
- Summer squash, crookneck/straightneck
- Tomato, red ripe/canned
- Turnips
- Winter squash (spaghetti squash only)

4. Snacks and Condiments

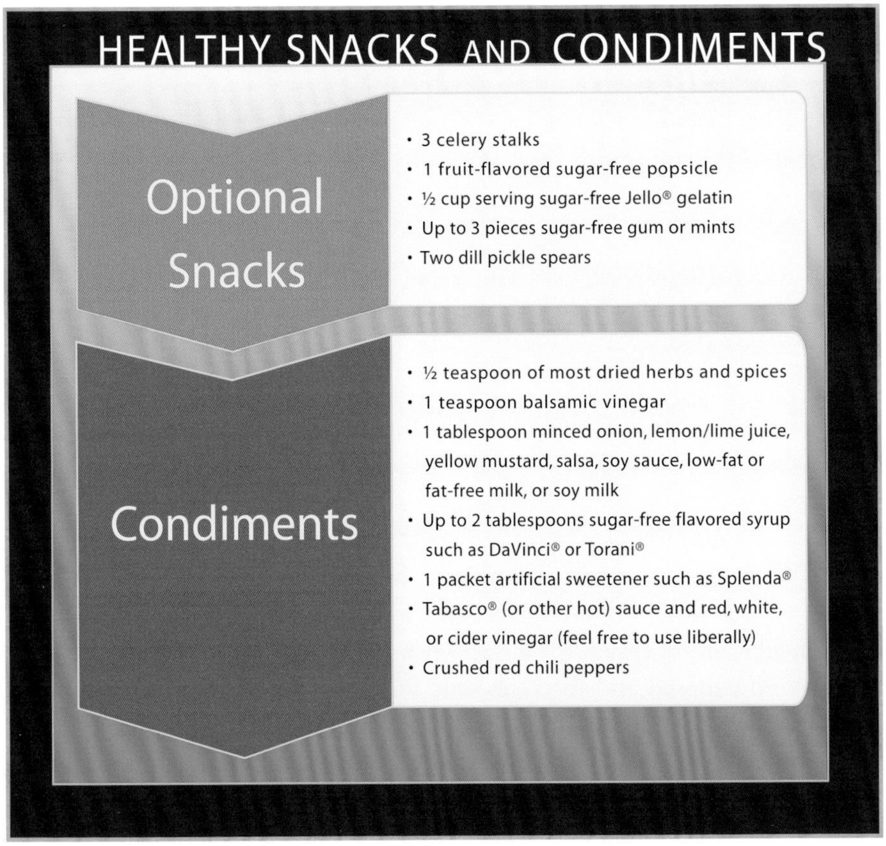
HEALTHY SNACKS AND CONDIMENTS
Optional Snacks
• 3 celery stalks
• 1 fruit-flavored sugar-free popsicle
• ½ cup serving sugar-free Jello® gelatin
• Up to 3 pieces sugar-free gum or mints
• Two dill pickle spears
Condiments
• ½ teaspoon of most dried herbs and spices
• 1 teaspoon balsamic vinegar
• 1 tablespoon minced onion, lemon/lime juice, yellow mustard, salsa, soy sauce, low-fat or fat-free milk, or soy milk
• Up to 2 tablespoons sugar-free flavored syrup such as DaVinci® or Torani®
• 1 packet artificial sweetener such as Splenda®
• Tabasco® (or other hot) sauce and red, white, or cider vinegar (feel free to use liberally)
• Crushed red chili peppers

So now you have your four-part grocery list and the entire inventory you need to restock your kitchen for Phase I using PCMRs. It couldn't be simpler—but remember, it's a precise eating strategy that works best exactly as outlined. That means that *for best results, you must confine yourself to only the foods on these lists.*

Now let's spend a moment looking at a typical meal schedule.

Your Daily Meal Plan

Begin each day by having your first PCMR within one hour—or better yet, thirty minutes—after you wake up. Your day should look like this:

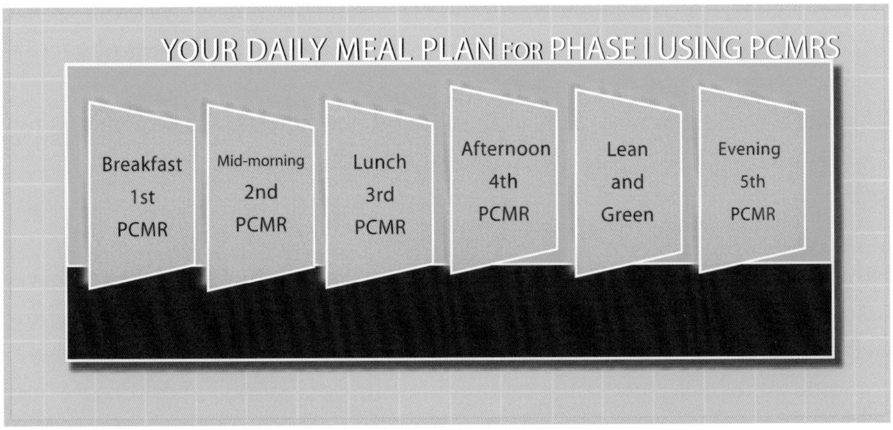
YOUR DAILY MEAL PLAN FOR PHASE I USING PCMRS
Breakfast 1st PCMR
Mid-morning 2nd PCMR
Lunch 3rd PCMR
Afternoon 4th PCMR
Lean and Green
Evening 5th PCMR

Your Daily Meal Plan for Phase I Using PCMRs. With the PCMR system, you'll have one PCMR every three hours throughout the day and a healthy "lean and green" meal in the evening, followed by one more late evening PCMR.

What, No Exercise?
No exercise for the first three weeks? I know it sounds crazy, but getting your body into a fat-burning state requires certain conditions. If you increase your energy demands now, you'll just add stress, slow down your weight loss, and sap your energy. That's why I'm asking that you reduce or eliminate exercise during this early stage of weight loss.

That being said, exercise is an important part of long-term health, and in chapters 13–16, you'll find an entire progressive plan that gradually increases your flexibility, activity, and strength. But for now I'd rather you focus on getting into a solid, consistent fat-burning state, without having to worry about damaging your knees or back. Trust me, once you're on track with weight loss, you'll be in a much better place physically and mentally to make physical activity a part of your long and healthy life.

So there you have it—a very simple method to help you lose weight quickly and safely while introducing you to crucial dietary habits, including:

- fueling every three hours
- eating breakfast
- making healthy food choices
- eating low-glycemic foods
- planning your meals

Once you have a handle on these habits, you'll have the framework for success—not only for weight loss, but for a lifetime of maintaining your healthy weight and optimal health.

Checklists for Change

Before you begin your weight-loss plan, make sure you've taken these important first steps:

✓ You've created a microenvironment of health.
✓ You've gone shopping and replaced your pantry and refrigerator with foods from all four groups on the grocery list.
✓ You've purchased and received your PCMRs. (For more information on ordering your PCMRs, see the resource list on page 370.)
✓ You've taken the health assessment and if possible are using the workbook, *Living a Longer, Healthier Life: The Companion Guide to Dr. A's Habits of Health,* to plot your health path.
✓ You've created a structural tension chart for your first goal of reaching a healthy weight. (For more information, see chapter 4.)
✓ You've bought a journal and are regularly recording your daily eating habits. (See *Living a Longer, Healthier Life: The Companion Guide to Dr. A's Habits of Health* for more information on using a journal as a tool for tracking choices that support optimal weight and health.)

Once you're on the move, here are some tips:

✓ Get through your first three days successfully.
✓ If you need some extra motivation, review chapters 3 and 4 on motivation for change, fundamental choice, and the discipline of daily choices.
✓ By day four you'll enter a fat-burning state, characterized by lots of energy and the beginning of weight loss.
✓ After a week, if you're ready and feel good enough, start slowly increasing your daily activity. Avoid active exertion for the first three weeks.

How Long Will I Be in Phase I?

How long you stay in Phase I depends primarily on how much weight you have to lose and how long you take to lose it, as well as your target BMI. While your weight-loss goal can be whatever you've determined is healthy for you, there are some guidelines concerning body composition. Generally speaking, if your

Secrets to Success

- Eat one PCMR every three hours. Don't skip meals even if you're not hungry. It's absolutely critical to fuel as scheduled—in fact, your weight loss may be slower if you don't.
- Get some extra rest. You may feel a little tired during the first three days as your body switches on its fat-burning mechanism and gears up to use its stores of fat.
- Drink at least eight 8-ounce glasses of water every day.
- Eat slowly.
- Stay busy and avoid sights and smells that remind you of food, especially during the first few days. Soon enough, your own energy stores will kick in and you'll feel more in control.
- Use your support system. If you have a coach, call them. (See chapter 18 for more information on building a support system.)
- Limit caffeine to no more than three servings a day. You may find that your body is more sensitive to the effects of caffeine, making this a great time to cut back on your daily consumption.
- Avoid alcohol. It causes dehydration, throws you out of the fat-burning state you've worked so hard to achieve, and it's a powerful appetite stimulant.
- If you slip up, just get right back on track. But remember, it will take about two to three days after a slip-up to get back into a fat-burning state. (For some extra motivation, review chapters 3 and 4 on making good choices.)
- Keep a journal. This is a great way to monitor your progress and help you focus.
- Avoid exercise for the first three weeks. Or, if you do choose to exercise, reduce your usual amount by half.

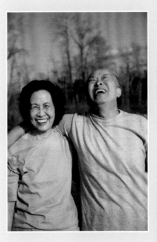

waist circumference is less than 37 inches (for men) or 32.5 inches (for women) and your BMI is less than 25, you're ready to transition to Phase II. In general, you should count on being in Phase I until you meet your goals and are able to maintain them for at least two weeks. Here's what to expect:

- *If you have just a small amount of weight to lose,* you'll transition to Phase II fairly quickly. You should read the chapters on my healthy, low-glycemic portion-control system (chapters 8–10) before you begin transitioning in chapter 12, because you'll be using much of that information as you learn to eat healthy for life. After that, you'll begin the progressive movement plan outlined in chapters 13–16.

- *If you have a lot of weight to lose,** you'll be in Phase I for a while. When the time comes, and you've reached your healthy weight, chapter 12 will teach you about transitioning to Phase II. In the meantime, you should read the chapters on my healthy low-glycemic portion-control system (chapters 8–10) because you'll be using much of that information as you learn to eat healthy for life. *In addition, once you've settled into a fat-burning state (after the first three weeks), you should start the progressive movement plan outlined in chapters 13–16.*

*You can expect to lose two to five pounds per week for the first two weeks and one to two pounds per week thereafter. So dividing the total weight you plan to lose by 12 will give you a rough idea of how many months you'll be in Phase I. However, this figure can vary greatly depending on your gender and certain medical conditions that may slow down your weight loss, such as hypothyroidism and PCOS (polycystic ovarian syndrome).

What's Next? Transitioning to Phase II

Our first goal—reaching your healthy weight—is the underlying dynamic that unlocks all the possibilities to follow. It's also our signal that you're ready to begin transitioning into Phase II.

In Phase I, we've laid the foundation for a more efficient energy management system. As you transition to Phase II, we'll boost both your energy intake and your energy expenditure. The thread that connects the phases is the relationship between energy in and energy out. Let's take another look at the energy diagram. Notice that the colored boxes in Phase II highlight our three key focal areas: a healthy body mass index, or BMI (white), increased activity and exercise (green), and increased caloric intake (red).

Energy Management in Phase I: Moving into Transition. Before you transition to Phase II, you'll have decreased your daily energy intake (red line) as well as your body mass index, or BMI (white line). Once you've reached a healthy weight and BMI, have begun to develop the fundamental Habits of Health, and have read the chapters on healthy eating (and started your movement program if you've been in Phase I for more than three weeks), you're ready to begin transitioning to Phase II.

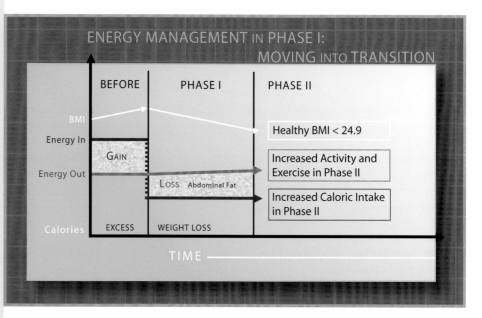

Before you move on to Phase II and learn how to maintain your new healthy weight, consider the following:

- Have you identified and started to develop the fundamental Habits of Health that will help you keep weight off, including proper motivation and choice?
- Have you reached your goal weight and BMI?
- Have you read and studied the healthy eating habits in chapters 8–10?
- If you've been in Phase I for more than three weeks, have you read chapters 13–16 and started your movement program?

If you can answer yes to these questions, you're ready to transition to Phase II!

Chapter 8

Dr. A's Healthy Eating System

*A Low-Glycemic, Portion-Control Approach
to Support Optimal Health*

"Tell me what you eat, and I will tell you what you are."
–Jean Anthelme Brillat-Savarin

In the last chapter I described meal replacements, the technology I've found most reliable in helping people lose weight while keeping up with today's busy, chaotic lifestyles. While this packaged system provides an effective tool for weight loss and maintenance, it's critical to master eating healthy using a traditional food approach as well. We're now going to give you the additional Habits of Health you will need to complete a comprehensive eating strategy and help reinforce long-term success.

If you're close to or at a healthy weight, this will be your entry point to the path to optimal health. Taking the healthy food approach to weight loss doesn't just tell you how to lose a few pounds; it teaches you how to build a permanent eating strategy for health.

The next three chapters are designed to give you an in-depth understanding of how to make healthy selections with all your food choices. I designed this system to make habits of healthy eating easy to learn, and over time they will become automatic. You'll discover new ways to think about food, including whole new ways to shop, prepare food, and eat. Our goal is to make healthy eating so easy, so portable, and so satisfying that you'll no longer be tempted by food industry tricks—like those flashing yellow and red signs that stimulate appetite. Those all-too-familiar golden arches will just seem to disappear!

You'll also set the foundation for new eating habits that will support your new healthy weight for the rest of your life. And as a bonus, as you learn to eat healthy, you'll awaken sensations of taste, smell, sight, and texture that have been dulled by the illusionary satisfaction the food industry creates by way of bulk, salt, fat, and high-fructose corn syrup.

The USDA Pyramid: An Outdated Model?

In the early 1980s, the U.S. Department of Agriculture (USDA) began developing guidelines for healthy eating, eventually adding information on serving size and what's needed to maintain a healthy weight. You probably recognize the USDA pyramid, which divides foods into six major groups. The size of each section represents the portion of your daily diet that the USDA believes should come from that group.

**Important Note:
The information presented here contains key Habits of Health that will prepare you for the permanent eating strategy you'll need for long-term success. However, if you have significant weight to lose, the PCMRs provide the most consistent results and are the method I recommend. You will then add this whole food eating system once you've reached a healthy weight and have gone through transition as outlined in chapter 12.**

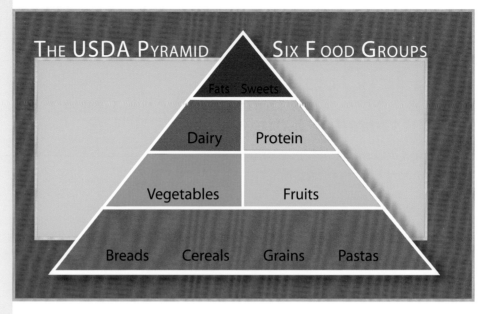

Fats   Sweets

Dairy   Protein

Vegetables   Fruits

Breads   Cereals   Grains   Pastas

The USDA Pyramid: Six Food Groups. You may be familiar with the USDA pyramid, which divides foods into six major food groups based on the portion of your daily diet that the USDA believes should come from each group. Unfortunately, this effort hasn't helped bring down obesity rates, because this model doesn't distinguish between healthy and unhealthy foods within each group and doesn't fit today's habits and lifestyle.

A Habit of Health: Learning to control your portions

While I applaud the USDA for its efforts, our rates of pre-obesity and obesity have continued to rise despite the guidelines. So why aren't they working? Because they don't fit today's habits and lifestyle. The cereal group, for example, doesn't distinguish between whole wheat bread and a doughnut, despite the fact that eating these two products leads to very different outcomes over time—one promotes a Habit of Health, the other a Habit of Disease.

Our goal is to take all the information that's available—including pieces of the USDA guidelines—and build a practical eating strategy that supports both weight loss and optimal health.

My healthy eating system helps you monitor and manage your energy intake while ensuring that you get a healthy, balanced diet. It's a simple visual system that teaches you the basics of portion size and the correct proportion of foods from our three designated major food groups: vegetables and fruits, proteins, and starches. And you'll be assured of getting the correct vitamins, minerals, and phytonutrients you need to support health without having to count calories. It's so easy you can even use it in restaurants.

With my system, you'll use a nine-inch plate to help you judge proper portion size and proportion. If you don't already have a nine-inch plate in your kitchen, now is as good a time as any to go out and buy a few. Ideally, the plate should be shallow with just a small lip to prevent you from heaping it with too much food.

Now take a look at the following diagram. I've simplified the USDA pyramid's six food groups into a three-component system that mirrors the way most people eat. Our typical meal is made up of:

• healthy vegetables or fruits
• healthy protein (meat, chicken, fish, dairy, nuts)
• healthy starch (rice, potato, pasta)

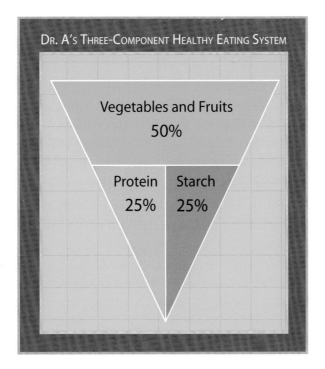

DR. A'S THREE-COMPONENT HEALTHY EATING SYSTEM

Vegetables and Fruits
50%

Protein
25%

Starch
25%

This breakdown gives you a healthy balance of nutrients in the right amount to satisfy your hunger and burn fat. All you need to do is visualize this chart on your nine-inch plate, and plan your meals accordingly.

As long as you maintain this ratio of starch, protein, and fruit or vegetable, you can be sure that you're getting a healthy, balanced diet. In fact, we'll be using these proportions to build your long-term health plan—so you're already learning an important Habit of Health!

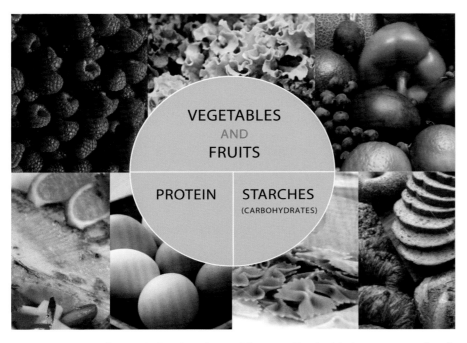

VEGETABLES
AND
FRUITS

PROTEIN

STARCHES
(CARBOHYDRATES)

Dr. A's Low-Glycemic Portion-Control System. For the ideal percentage of each food component and proper portion control, divide your nine-inch plate into these three sections: (1) fruits and vegetables 50%; (2) protein 25%; and (3) starch 25%.

Serving Size? Portion Size? What's the Difference?
A fruit drink may seem like a reasonable, healthy choice at 125 calories. That is, until you read the label more closely and find out that there are three servings in the bottle—a fifth of your daily calorie allowance. Unlike *portion size*, which basically means whatever's on your plate, *serving size* is a measured amount that's used by nutrition scientists on food labels as well as by the USDA in their food pyramid. Learning to understand serving sizes when you're shopping is an important skill— particularly when processed foods are involved.

For an even stronger visual cue, use a food-safe marker to draw these proportions right on your plate.

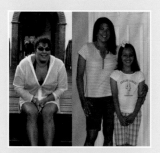

"I'm once again loving life!"

BECKY HORA
Over three years at optimal health

Before I met Dr. A, I was truly miserable. I even had trouble keeping up with my daughter! All that has changed now. I'm down to a healthy weight, and once again loving life and having fun with my family. I've maintained my healthy weight and I am using the Habits of Health to help reach and maintain optimal health. ■

Results vary. Typical weight loss is 2-5 pounds per week for the first two weeks and 1-2 pounds per week thereafter.

If you're at a healthy weight and are using this system to start eating healthier, or if you just want to get a little leaner by using Phase I, you'll be preparing two meals a day until you have reached your goal. You'll have four more opportunities for smaller fueling breaks each day, using foods from the list in chapter 10 or PCMRs. Altogether, this customized meal plan will provide you with an average of 1,200 to 1,300 calories per day, through two 400-calorie meals (breakfast and dinner) and four 100-calorie fueling breaks. Here's a breakdown.

Breakfast	Mid-morning Fueling	Lunch Fueling	Mid-afternoon Fueling	Dinner	Evening Fueling
300 – 400 calories	100 calories	100 – 200* calories	100 calories	400 calories	100 calories

*Although it's best to treat lunch like any other 100-calorie fueling break, I've included an option for extra calories at lunchtime to accommodate business lunches or the demands of a high-energy job. If you opt to make lunch a 200-calorie meal rather than a fueling break, you can either choose two fueling-break options or remove the starch from your nine-inch-plate meal selection. In other words:
• Choice A: Two 100-calorie fuelings combined (for example, cottage cheese with olives and apple slices with walnuts).
• Choice B: The protein and vegetable/fruit components of your nine-inch-plate meal (no starch).

I've found that this plan works well for people with a wide variety of lifestyles and metabolisms. It will put you well on your way to learning two important Habits of Health—*portion control* and the *proper proportion of the three major food groups*. Both are essential habits that will help you reach and maintain an optimal sustainable weight.

If you're already at a healthy BMI, you can graduate to my permanent healthy eating schedule outlined in chapter 12 and use the energy formula to calculate how many calories you should be consuming per day to fill out your eating schedule.

Dr. A's Low-Glycemic Portion-Control System

The practical system you're about to learn has three important benefits.

It's automatic. Any system that teaches new habits needs to be simple, easy, and doable. My goal is to make your life so simple that when you go to a store or prepare a meal, your choices will naturally support optimal health. This needs to be as automatic as driving up to the window at Burger King and ordering a number 3!

It supports weight loss. Weight loss is a critical first step to creating optimal health. What most people don't realize is that the USDA pyramid is designed to maintain a healthy weight, not to help you lose weight in the first place.

Learning this system of healthy foods will support your goal of an optimal weight and help you remain that way. You can use the two-meals approach of my system to actually knock off a few pounds.

It teaches you to eat healthy for life. The principles, skills, and strategies you'll begin learning on day one of my system will become part of your permanent eating strategy—so you can be assured that every moment of your time is well spent!

This simple, effective strategy has its own basic guidelines. These are the most critical ones to understand at the beginning:

- You'll incorporate my two core principles of energy and insulin pump control.
- You'll eat breakfast within an hour of awakening (thirty minutes is ideal).
- You'll eat something every three hours.
- You'll have a healthy dinner.
- You'll eat only lower-glycemic carbohydrates during Phase I (more information on this in chapter 9).
- You'll gradually begin increasing your daily activity.
- You'll learn the key habits necessary to maintain a healthy weight, including support, monitoring, and reinforcement.

If you're not already familiar with the basics of healthy eating, don't worry! The next few chapters will explain in detail exactly how to choose and prepare foods that support optimal health. I'll show you how to shop for and plan great-tasting meals on your own, or you can simply follow my preplanned menus in chapter 10 using the recipes in the appendix. I'll even make it easy for you to prepare foods at work or while traveling. Soon, with my guidance, you'll be able to:

- Shop for and prepare healthy low-glycemic meals that will turn off your insulin pump and use your excess fat as an energy source.
- Read food labels to distinguish healthy from unhealthy foods.
- Choose high-quality proteins and health-supporting fats.
- Understand portion size as a critical factor in energy consumption.
- Fill your plate the healthy way with my easy visual portion-control system.
- Master the logistics of eating healthy every three hours.
- Redesign your pantry, refrigerator, and freezer to support low-glycemic and healthy eating.
- Understand the importance of water.

Your New Fueling Pattern

Remember the chart on page 61, Modern Life's Disease Path? It showed you the dramatic spikes in blood sugar and insulin that result from the chaotic way most people eat. For most Americans, there's no pattern or rhythm to their meals. Throughout their busy days, eating becomes nothing more than a reaction to stress, hunger, boredom, and a million other problems. It brings instant relief, but leads to the overconsumption of high-calorie, nutritionally polluted foods that rob us of our health.

Overwhelmed by the idea of shopping and cooking for yourself? If so, go back to chapter 7 to learn more about using portion-controlled meal replacements (PCMRs). They'll make it easier to learn the basics of healthy eating at your own relaxed pace.

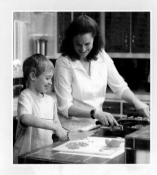

A Habit of Health:
Fueling your body every
three hours

What many people don't understand is that it's not just the type of food they eat and the excess calories that cause weight gain, but the erratic nature of the fueling pattern itself. Learning how to fuel your body efficiently—through small meals every three hours—is one of the most basic and critical Habits of Health. In fact, it's what humans were designed to do! Just making this simple adjustment will have a dramatic effect on your body, by:

• Turning on fat burning
• Increasing your metabolism
• Protecting muscle mass
• Suppressing appetite naturally
• Improving your energy level
• Lowering your cholesterol

And that's even before we start changing the quantity and quality of your fuel! Here's what your new healthy schedule might look like:

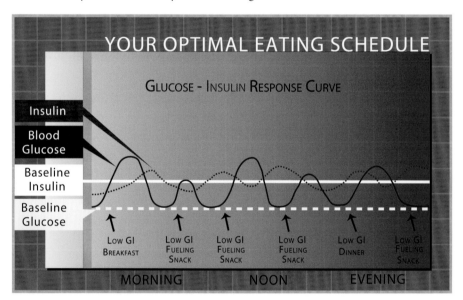

Your Optimal Eating Schedule: Glucose-Insulin Response Curve. Your new healthy daily eating schedule starts with a solid breakfast and continues fueling you every three hours while you're awake with low-glycemic choices, including a healthy dinner. This plan helps keep blood sugar and insulin levels steady.

This steady fueling schedule starts with a solid breakfast and continues every three hours while you're awake. My simple system, which we'll explore in the next few chapters, will help you design a menu of low-glycemic choices.

As you build on your new healthy eating habits, you'll be able to eat whatever you want—in moderation—because you'll have integrated the Habits of Health, and your body will begin operating at peak efficiency. Once your body has gained back its full recuperative powers, even the occasional hot fudge sundae or slice of pizza will have no overall effect on your health. In truth, though, I doubt you'll even want these types of foods once you're fully aware of their negative effects. You'll begin to understand how processed food has robbed you of the almost spiritual experience of nature's flavors, and you'll be amazed how wonderful real food can taste and smell. And speaking of great flavors, it's time to make this new healthy fueling pattern come alive.

Think of Phase I as not just a time to lose weight, but as the starting point of a new habit—healthy eating for life.

Chapter 9

Choosing Wisely

Dr. A's Color-Coded Shopping System

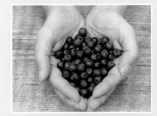

A Habit of Health:
Choosing low-glycemic
carbohydrates,
lean proteins, and
healthy fats.

Many experts in the medical establishment think that learning how to choose healthy, low-glycemic foods is just too difficult for most people to grasp, despite the proven health benefits. I disagree! Our simple color-coded charts make it easy for you to master shopping for healthy proteins, starches, and fruits and vegetables. When combined with our easy visual portion-control system, this color-coded shopping system puts you well on the way to creating meals that help you lose weight and build optimal health.

Low-Glycemic Foods for Optimal Health

The message couldn't be simpler: eating low-glycemic foods is the best way to lose weight and create health.

Many Western nations that, like the U.S., are experiencing obesity epidemics have embraced the glycemic index—a standard for measuring and communicating the glycemic content of food—as an important way to help people understand how to make healthy choices. Sadly, the U.S. medical community has been slow to endorse this powerful tool, claiming that it's just too hard for most people to understand.

That's why I've developed a system to make choosing and preparing low-glycemic foods a breeze. At the core is a series of color-coded charts highlighting choices from each food group. You can use these charts at home when you're preparing meals, while shopping, or when you're ordering food in a restaurant.

Here's your rule of thumb:

- Dark green = lowest glycemic (the best foods for weight loss and optimal health)
- Light green = moderate glycemic (foods to be eaten in moderation)
- Red = high glycemic (foods to be avoided)

As you begin your journey, your healthy eating selections should come from the dark green charts. These foods are highly effective at turning off your insulin and fat storage, and will facilitate reaching and maintaining an optimal weight. The light green charts list foods that are healthy but should be used sparingly in the first phase of our journey. Foods on the red chart should be used with care, only after you've reached optimal health.

And of course, the PCMRs are designed specifically to provide a high-quality, low-glycemic choice, and are always an excellent way to obtain a nutrient-dense, calorie-friendly fueling.

For your convenience, you can also download my color-coded shopping charts from www.habitsofhealth.net.

One reason people sometimes get confused about glycemic content and the glycemic index is that some foods that are *low glycemic* can be *high carbohydrate*. So how can you avoid picking the wrong foods? Just choose foods from the dark green charts, and be sure that your portion size fits in the right compartment on your nine-inch plate. As long as you stick with these two basic rules, you'll keep your insulin level stable and your fat-storage machinery turned off.

Nutritional intervention is a more powerful medicine than any pharmaceutical—and it's the very basis of health.

> ### Turn Down the Dial with These Easy Tips for Lowering the Glycemic Index!
>
> Take low-glycemic eating even further! Here are some simple ways to help keep your blood sugar under control by lowering the glycemic influence in the foods you eat each day.
>
> - Use vinegar and lemon juice, pickle your vegetables, and eat sourdough bread (not in Phase I, though!) to slow down starch digestion and the rate at which your stomach empties.
> - Undercook your spaghetti, oatmeal, and other pasta-like starches (in other words, cook them al dente) to slow digestion and prevent starch from gelatinizing.
> - Use stone-ground rather than finely milled flours. Larger-sized particles (less refined) have less glycemic content.
> - If you eat higher-glycemic foods (which should be avoided during weight loss), combine them with low-glycemic choices to lower the overall effect on blood sugar and the glycemic content of your meal.

The Power of Functional Foods

One criticism that's sometimes made about the traditional USDA food pyramid is that it doesn't help people distinguish between healthy and unhealthy choices. It doesn't discourage the consumption of red meats high in saturated fats, or encourage the use of health-enhancing oils. It gives equal classification to energy-giving whole grain products and the health-robbing refined grains found in many processed foods.

My plan, on the other hand, teaches you to replace the processed foods you're currently eating with healthy, life-giving foods—for a powerful healing effect on your body. By choosing healthy foods from my three designated major food groups, we're going to tap into the ability of nutrient-dense foods to actually improve the health of your cells, putting you in an ideal state to shed excess weight while moving you from non-sickness to optimal health.

In essence, we'll be using food to heal you instead of medicine. It's all part of an exciting new discipline called *nutritional intervention*—a much more powerful medicine than any pharmaceutical I've ever seen. And it's the very basis of optimal health.

So why would a critical care physician who spent over twenty years using pharmaceuticals utter such heresy? Because in those twenty years I never saw one of my medications create radiant health. Nutritional intervention, on the other hand, has the power not only to resolve pre-obesity, hyperinsulinism, and other unhealthy states without dangerous side effects, but also provides a platform for optimal health that traditional medicine doesn't.

I call the healthy foods we'll be selecting *functional foods*—a term first used in Japan in the 1980s to describe foods that provide particular health benefits. In my plan, I use the term to describe foods that add value to your body and move you up the path toward optimal health. It's one way of thinking of your nutritional intake as good medicine.

This new way of looking at food will unfold a whole new healthy world for you. Understanding how to select foods for optimal health is just as important as the total number of calories you consume—if not more so. In fact, the Habits of Health you're about to learn are among the most important daily decisions you can make.

Getting Ready to Shop

Today's supermarkets can be confusing places, with all too many choices. Before you head out to the store, here are a couple of guidelines to steer you toward foods that promote health and away from those that lead to disease.

- *Fresh* is better than frozen, canned, or in a jar.
- *Natural* is better than processed.

That's all well and good—but what do those terms really mean, and how can you know you're getting what you think you are?

So What Do We Mean by *Fresh*?

It's a tricky question! Too often what's advertised as *fresh* really isn't, as in the following examples:

Problem: Those greens may have been fresh at one time, but since then they've sat in a warehouse for weeks losing vitamins and nutrients. By the time you buy them at the store, the freshness is depleted.

Solution: When possible, buy locally grown produce. It was picked closer to the sale date and spent less time traveling.

Problem: Many commercially grown foods are "protected" with chemicals designed to preserve freshness. But do they? The veggies maintain their color and texture, but lose their flavor and much of their nutritional value.

Functional foods have particular health benefits that enhance your meals and move you toward optimal health. They're nutrient dense and calorie friendly, and contain healthy fiber.

Dysfunctional foods rob you of your health and promote disease. They're energy dense, nutrient poor, and usually over-processed.

Before You Shop

- Be sure you've created the microenvironment of health we discussed in chapter 6. For starters, that means clearing your house of all junk food. Have fun doing it! Imagine that you're getting rid of your bad food demons, and renewing your kitchen as a source of health, life, and energy.
- Arm yourself with a shopping list before you enter any sort of food shop to avoid impulse buying.
- Stay along the outer aisles of the store, where the produce, meat, fish, and other fresh, healthy items are found. Avoid the tempting processed foods on the inner aisles.
- Never go shopping when you're hungry!

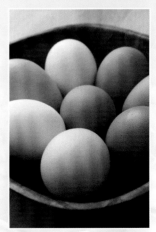

**What Is
Organic Food?**
Organic foods are produced according to certain production standards, meaning they're grown without the use of conventional pesticides, artificial fertilizers, human waste, or sewage sludge, and that they were processed without ionizing radiation or food additives. Livestock are reared without the routine use of antibiotics and without the use of growth hormones. In most countries, organic produce must not be genetically modified.

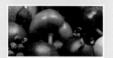

**Going Organic?
Look for the 9s!**
Discover whether the produce you're buying is organic or conventionally produced by checking the PLU (price look-up) code—the four- or five-digit number usually located on a small sticker affixed to fruits and vegetables. If the code has four digits, it's conventional. If it has five digits and begins with the number 9, it's organic.

Solution: A local green grocer may carry fruits and vegetables that haven't been treated. You'll get healthier, better-tasting food that's higher in nutritional value than the supermarket variety.

Natural, Processed, Organic: Is There Really a Difference?

The short answer is yes! Take peanut butter, for example. Natural peanut butter consists of peanuts and sometimes a bit of salt. That's it! Processed peanut butters, including most of the familiar national brands, contain peanuts and salt as well as sugar or high-fructose corn syrup, along with other ingredients that are completely unnecessary and can have a negative effect on your health—not to mention that once you've gotten used to the real thing, the processed stuff tastes like plastic.

Today's beef, lamb, pork, and poultry are all processed with antibiotics and even growth hormones—a practice that increases production for the food industry, but brings its own set of problems, including increasing resistance to antibiotics on the part of bacteria. If you can, try to buy meats that aren't processed—those labeled *natural* to indicate that the animal hasn't been given antibiotics or growth hormones. A wide assortment of these, as well as grass-fed meats, can usually be found at stores like Whole Foods Market.

And what about organic? Organic products are becoming more and more available, even in the large supermarket chains. For products to be labeled *certified organic* by the USDA, the producer needs to uphold a rigorous set of standards that go beyond *natural*. As demand for organics grows, so does the industry. In time, this could prove a tremendous counterforce to the big food industry, which all too often is more concerned with high production and profit than with quality. Yes, organic products usually cost 10 to 20 percent more, but the difference is worth it. You're better off eating less meat and dairy products, but going organic, than eating more of the processed stuff.

The Economics of Healthy Food

When your body's working well, it needs less food. Let's do the numbers. Say you spend $100 a week for food right now. Once your body wants less to eat, you can spend the same amount, but you'll be able to buy higher-quality food.

How Do I Know If It's Organic?

The term organic can mean different things on food labels, depending how it's used. Here's a quick guide to some common labeling terms.

- 100% certified organic: all the ingredients are certified organic
- Organic: contains at least 95 percent organic ingredients
- Made with organic ingredients: at least 75 percent of the ingredients are organic

In addition, some packages may not state organic on the label, but still list some ingredients that may be organic.

> ### *Keep in Mind!*
>
> Here are the main points about your healthy eating system to keep in mind as you plan your daily meals:
>
> - Choose all your carbohydrates (vegetable, fruit, and starch components) from the green lists, with the majority from the dark green sections.
> - Remember to serve your new, healthy food choices on a nine-inch plate.
> - Maintain the proper proportions for healthy eating and weight loss: 50% vegetable/fruit (mostly vegetables during the weight-loss phase), 25% starch, and 25% protein.
> - Select healthy fueling-break foods from the choices provided, choosing those that you enjoy and that fit your lifestyle. Remember to choose from the healthy periphery of the store, not the interior aisles that are full of unhealthy processed foods!
> - Keep with your Phase I meal schedule: two meals (400 calories each) and four fueling breaks (100 calories each).

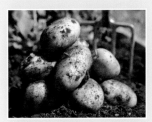

Fresh foods are critical for optimal health. If you're not sure which foods are fresh, ask your grocer.

Better food costs more, but you need less of it. When you eat bad processed food, your body is never really satisfied—so you eat more and more, even if you're stuffed to the gills. So much of our food is energy dense, but nutrient poor, leaving your body deficient in the nutrients it so desperately needs. With higher-quality food, your eating habits change—you're eating nutrient-dense food that fulfills the body's requirements. And when your sense of taste is satisfied, your body's satisfied, and as a result you're able to stop eating before you're stuffed. You'll find yourself leaving the table before you've eaten everything in sight, and you won't even want to make that midnight raid on the refrigerator!

Ready? Let's Go Shopping!

The charts that follow are designed to steer you toward foods that rev up your health. Think of them as the octane-disclosure sheets at the gas pumps. Watch your engine's performance improve as you switch from regular gas (the low-octane, nutrient-poor foods you're eating now) to premium (functional foods that are nutrient-dense, highly efficient fuels that turn down your insulin pump and turn on fat burning).

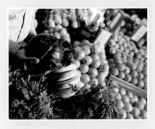

Don't forget to take these charts along with you while you shop. For your convenience, you can copy them from the companion workbook to this text or download them to your PDA, iPod, or printer at www.habitsofhealth.net. They'll also soon be available on your iPhone and iPad

As you shop, remember to visualize your nine-inch plate, with its divisions based on the proper proportion of foods for optimal health and weight loss. You'll need to have plenty of vegetables and fruits on hand, as well as lesser quantities of healthy, complex starches and lean proteins to create healthy, delicious meals.

Your Nine-Inch Plate, Divided into Food Types. When you're shopping, think about the meals you're planning. A meal on your nine-inch plate should be made up of 50% vegetables and fruits, 25% protein, and 25% starch from my healthy food choices.

Vegetables and Fruits

(50% of Your Plate)

Functional: Rich in vitamins, minerals, phytochemicals, and fiber, vegetables and fruit are at the core of your long-term plan to reach and maintain optimal health. And because they're low in calories and provide plenty of bulk to fill

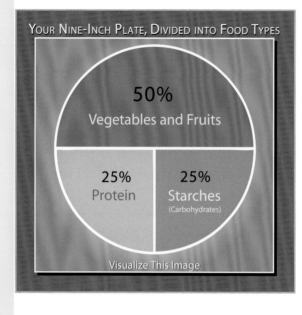

YOUR NINE-INCH PLATE, DIVIDED INTO FOOD TYPES

50%
Vegetables and Fruits

25%
Protein

25%
Starches
(Carbohydrates)

Visualize This Image

you up, they're a great tool to help you take charge of your energy intake.

Dysfunctional: The fried vegetables typical of fast food chains and other restaurants, as well as many common packaged fruit juices, have been stripped of their nutrients and are loaded with fat and sugar.

Vegetables and fruits represent half of your meal in our system. These essential foods provide nutrient-dense functional support to help you lose weight, as well as a wealth of antioxidants and anti-inflammatories for building optimal health. And you'll never tire of their abundant variety of flavors and textures: sweet to sour, crunchy to smooth, from the mild lettuces to power-packed blueberries.

Healthy vegetable and fruit choices: A wide variety of vibrant foods including salads, crunchy raw vegetables, and nutrient-packed berries.

Proportion of your meal: 50% of your nine-inch plate.

A healthy portion of vegetables and fruits is about the size of a small paperback book.

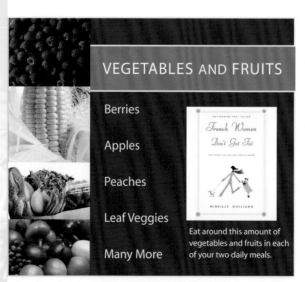

VEGETABLES AND FRUITS

Berries

Apples

Peaches

Leaf Veggies

Many More

French Women
Don't Get Fat

THE SECRET OF EATING FOR PLEASURE

MIREILLE GUILIANO

Eat around this amount of vegetables and fruits in each of your two daily meals.

Portion size: About the size of a small paperback book of about 100 pages. But green low-glycemic vegetables are so beneficial, you could probably even use a great big Tom Clancy book as your point of reference for judging the proper amount and still not overdo it!

Note: A small amount of low-glycemic fruit is permitted while optimizing your nutri-

tional intake in this phase. But because fruits are high glycemic and calorie dense, they should be the minor contributor to your vegetable/fruit group in this phase. Once you've reached a healthy weight and transition to Phase II, you'll be able to increase the amount of fruit in your diet.

Vegetable and Fruit Choices

Vegetables and fruits make up a whopping 50 percent of your meals—so it's especially important to select the lowest-glycemic varieties. Although a small amount of low-glycemic fruit is permitted while you're optimizing your weight, it's best to focus on vegetables for your vegetable/fruit component. The following charts are arranged from lowest glycemic (dark green) to low glycemic (light green) to high glycemic (red). Vegetables from the dark green charts have very little effect on blood sugar and insulin, and should be used freely. In fact, if you find that you absolutely need a little something extra as you're settling into your new eating strategy, you can always select from this component. Celery is a great crunchy choice!

VEGETABLES

VERY LOW GI ≤ 30

GI 15 or less

• Zucchini	• Alfalfa sprouts	• Brussels sprouts
• Spinach	• Artichokes	• Bell peppers
• Peppers	• Arugula	• Broccoli
• Onions	• Asparagus	• Chives
• Mushrooms	• Fennel	• Leeks
• Lettuce	• Cucumber	• Celery
	• Cabbage	• Cauliflower
	• Squash	• Chili peppers

GI 20 or more

• Eggplant	20	• Green beans	30
• Carrots, raw	30		

HIGH GI > 50

• Peas	50
• Taro	54
• Corn	65
• Red beets, canned	64
• Carrots, cooked	80

Unhealthy Vegetables and Fruits: A Habit of Disease

It's truly criminal what the processed and fast food industries do to once-healthy fruits and vegetables. Think of such "delights" as the Bloomin' Onion, tempura vegetables, and, sadly, the number-one selling vegetable in our country: french fries. In fact, I've had to put the poor potato—a healthy vegetable in some circumstances—in the starch category based on the high-glycemic, high-carbohydrate manner in which it's usually prepared and eaten.

A recent study found that most Americans eat fewer than two servings of vegetables and fruits a day—far below the recommended five to seven daily servings. Even more troubling, half of those respondents named french fries as one of their daily choices!

But what about fruit juices? Surely that's a healthy choice! The sad reality is that most packaged juices contain nothing more than high-fructose corn syrup with a little fruit "waved" over them. As such, they contain a high level of non-nutritive calories in a form that's so hard for the body to detect that it

FRUITS

VERY LOW GI ≤ 30

· Olives	15	· Blackberries	25
· Avocado	10	· Grapefruit	25
· Limes	20	· Cherries	25
· Lemons	20	· Tomatoes	30
· Raspberries	25		

LOW GI ≤ 50

· Apples	30	· Oranges	35
· Nectarines	30	· Apricots, dried	35
· Peaches	30	· Plums	35
· Pears	30	· Figs	40
· Strawberries	35		

HIGH GI > 50

· Apricots	57	· Grapes	53
· Bananas	60	· Mango	51
· Blueberries	53	· Melon	60
· Cantaloupe	67	· Pineapple	59
· Kiwi	50	· Watermelon	76

Unhealthy Vegetable and Fruit Choices.

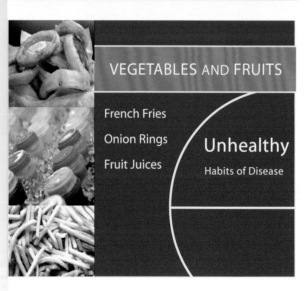

VEGETABLES AND FRUITS

French Fries
Onion Rings
Fruit Juices

Unhealthy

Habits of Disease

Fruit juices may seem like a healthy choice, but they're usually loaded with sweeteners and empty calories that don't fill you up, but rather lead to weight gain.

doesn't even sense it's being overloaded with calories. The result is excess weight and a whole host of diseases —including an epidemic increase in childhood obesity.

Protein

(25% of Your Plate)

Functional: Lean proteins form the building blocks of your vital tissues and organs. They contain amino acids that protect your muscle during weight loss and are the best macronutrient to help you feel full.

Dysfunctional: Many common forms of protein are high in unhealthy saturated fat.

Healthy protein choices: Very lean meats, eggs, fish, seafood, white-meat poultry, low-fat yogurt, low-fat milk and cheeses, legumes, nuts, seeds.

Proportion of your meal: 25% of your nine-inch plate.

Portion size: About the size of a deck of cards (after cooking).

Protein Choices

Proteins are a critical component of weight loss. Most protein sources, including fresh meats, poultry, and fish, contain no carbohydrates at all, so their glycemic level is negligible. And to top it off, calorie-for-calorie they're better than any other food at giving you a sense of fullness and satisfaction. To support weight loss and optimal health, choose lean protein that's low in saturated animal fats. Great sources include eggs, fish, and white-meat poultry, as well as vegetable sources such as soy and other legumes, which I'll discuss later. While dairy products are included in the protein category, bear in mind that they can contain considerable amounts of carbohydrates.

The charts below don't list glycemic levels for meat, fish, or poultry because the glycemic content for these foods is negligible. However, the charts do include total fat and saturated fat levels for meats. To guide your choices for optimal health, just choose any fish from the charts, or any meats that fall in the green area.

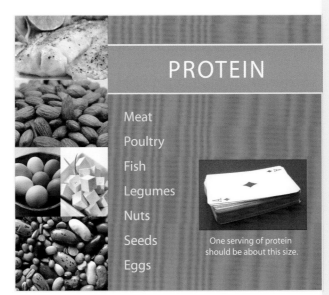

PROTEIN

Meat
Poultry
Fish
Legumes
Nuts
Seeds
Eggs

One serving of protein should be about this size.

A healthy portion of protein is about the size of a deck of cards. With their power to eliminate hunger and renew muscle for optimal health, healthy protein selections are highly supportive of weight loss.

Fish and Seafood

When you eat fish, you're not only choosing a great protein source—you're also significantly reducing your risk of disease. Eating fish one to three times a week is an important Habit of Health and can have a profound impact on your well-being over time. In fact, one serving of fish a week may reduce your risk of fatal heart attack by 40 percent!

Note: Pregnant women and young children should limit their intake of fish to once a week due to the potential for high mercury content in some fish.

A Habit of Health:
Eating fish one to three times a week

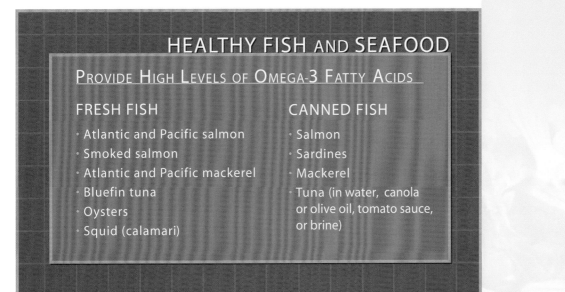

HEALTHY FISH AND SEAFOOD

PROVIDE HIGH LEVELS OF OMEGA-3 FATTY ACIDS

FRESH FISH
• Atlantic and Pacific salmon
• Smoked salmon
• Atlantic and Pacific mackerel
• Bluefin tuna
• Oysters
• Squid (calamari)

CANNED FISH
• Salmon
• Sardines
• Mackerel
• Tuna (in water, canola or olive oil, tomato sauce, or brine)

Meat

It's an important Habit of Health to lower your consumption of meat and eat more fish, white-meat poultry (skinless), legumes such as beans, and low-fat or nonfat dairy. But if you're like me and once in a while need that savory taste of meat, just minimize the amount of saturated fat so you can enjoy this great protein source and still stay healthy.

Did you know that wild meat—the kind our ancestors ate 10,000 years ago—contains much less saturated fat than farm-raised meat? Our cattle are fed on high-glycemic foods and as a result contain an unhealthy amount of fat. By eating them, we concentrate our ingestion of fat and calories. Wild meats, on the other hand, such as buffalo and elk, contain very little fat. I've found both of these very enjoyable, as well as venison (deer), which although a bit strong-tasting can be quite good if prepared properly. Many of these wild meats are available in grocery stores such as Whole Foods Market. But even traditional American beef can be a fine choice if you select cuts such as filets and sirloins rather than those that contain excess marbling from fat.

FAT CONTENT OF MEAT

	TOTAL FAT %	SATURATED FAT %
• Buffalo, elk, venison	17%	7%
• Pork loin	26%	9%
• Round steak	27%	10%
• Veal chop	39%	17%
• Canadian bacon	41%	14%
• Filet mignon	42%	16%
• Sirloin steak	44%	16%
• Flank steak	44%	19%
• Lamb ribs	48%	22%
• Spare ribs	52%	22%
• Ground beef (very lean)	58%	23%
• Sausage (beef)	80%	33%

Unhealthy Proteins: A Habit of Disease

With our processed lunch meats, hot dogs, and hamburgers, most of us eat far too much protein that's high in saturated fat. Foods like these stimulate inflammation and have a profoundly negative effect on your heart, your blood vessels, and your brain. They create oxygen free radicals that attack the lining of the vessels in all your organs and contribute to heart disease, high blood pressure, strokes, and cancers and accelerate aging.

To make matters worse, we stick these fatty meats on the "barbie" to char them. This forms extremely dangerous substances called *advanced glycation endproducts (AGEs)*, which can make these foods up to 200 times more immunoreactive, attacking your body with a vengeance. (For more information on the dangers of inflammation, see chapter 19.) As you can imagine, eliminating these foods can have a dramatic effect on your health!

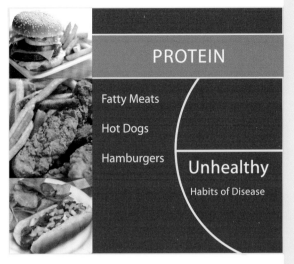

Unhealthy Protein Choices.

Poultry

Chicken, turkey, and other forms of poultry are healthier choices than red meat. But be careful! The health value and calorie content of poultry can vary significantly depending on the type of bird, which part you eat, and how it's prepared and cooked. For example, while a skinless turkey breast is 18 percent fat, the fat content of a skinless chicken breast is 24 percent. And manufactured products such as sausages, hot dogs, and burgers made from turkey and chicken aren't really much healthier than their meat counterparts.

As a general rule, avoid eating the dark meat (legs and thighs) and always remove the skin before eating—though it is a good idea to keep the skin on while you bake, grill, or broil your poultry to help lock in flavor and maintain moistness without adding significantly to the fat content of the finished

FAT CONTENT OF POULTRY

	SKIN?	FAT %	SATURATED FAT %
· Turkey breast		18%	6%
· Chicken breast		24%	7%
· Chicken breast	Yes	36%	10%
· Turkey breast	Yes	38%	5%
· Chicken dark meat		43%	12%
· Turkey dark meat	Yes	47%	14%
· Turkey sausage		50%	15%
Duck	Yes	50%	19%
· Chicken dark meat	Yes	56%	16%
· Cornish game hen	Yes	63%	28%
· Turkey hot dog		70%	19%

The amount of fat in poultry varies widely depending on type.

dish. As far as portion size, you want to end up with a piece that fits in the 25 percent protein portion of your plate (about the size of a deck of cards)—around 3.5 ounces of cooked poultry.

A final piece of advice: free-range or organic poultry can help you avoid the antibiotics and growth hormones that are given to many commercially raised birds.

Eggs

Eggs are an incredible source of protein that deliver all the amino acids, B_2, B_{12}, folate, and vitamins D and E. The whites are a wonderful digestible source of iron as well. While eggs are low in saturated fat, they're a major source of cholesterol, and even though we now know that saturated fat actually has more impact than dietary cholesterol on blood cholesterol levels, you should still limit your daily intake of dietary cholesterol to 200 milligrams—the amount in one small egg. There's no limit to the amount of egg whites you can eat, though, as long as they fit on the 25 percent of your plate devoted to protein.

LEGUMES

VERY LOW GI ≤ 30	
• Soybeans	18
• Edamame	20
• Chickpeas (garbanzo beans)	20
• Lentils	25
• Black beans	30

LOW GI ≤ 50	
Lima beans	32
Kidney beans	35
Chickpeas	35
White beans	35
Black-eyed peas	42

Legumes

Legumes—a group that includes beans, peas, and lentils—are one of my favorite functional foods and probably my top pick for an all-around health food. They're a good protein source and almost always low glycemic, making them a wonderful alternative for vegetarians or for anyone looking to meet their protein needs while lowering their intake of meats and saturated fat.

What else is great about legumes? They're full of riboflavin, niacin, folate, calcium, potassium, iron, and phosphorus. They're high in soluble fiber, which naturally lowers cholesterol. They're less expensive than meat and dairy products, and can be made into a wide variety of creative, flavorful dishes. In fact, when it comes to legumes, there's just no downside!

A cup of legumes gives you 110 to 150 calories of the best fuel you can buy. Choose from any of the varieties in the chart for the protein portion of your meal—all are low glycemic and do an excellent job of turning off your insulin pump.

A Word about Soy

One particularly amazing legume stands out—soy. Soybeans have twice as much protein as other legumes and provide nearly as many essential amino acids as animal protein—without all the saturated fat. They're a good source of calcium as well, making them a great alternative to dairy products. In addition, soy is full of naturally occurring isoflavones—phytonutrients that protect against cardiovascular disease and osteoporosis.*

*Lycan, T. W., Davis, L. M., Andersen, W. S, Cheskin, L. J., "The Health Effects of Soy: Benefits and Risks for Women," forthcoming.

A Habit of Health:

Legumes! Make daily consumption of legumes—beans, peas, or lentils—a part of your healthy eating strategy.

In fact, I think so highly of soy that it's my top choice for the protein component of our portion-controlled meal replacements (PCMRs) at Medifast®—and PCMRs are a great way to make using this healthy legume as your protein component a breeze!

Dairy Products and Cheese

Dairy products are the one protein source that can be quite high glycemic. Despite what the dairy industry would have you believe, dairy products can contribute to poor health—that is, if not selected properly. Whole milk dairy products are not only high glycemic but also high in saturated animal fat, a double unhealthy wallop that pumps up insulin while creating ready stores of fat.

True, dairy products are an excellent source of calcium—which has been shown to aid weight loss—but so are many of the fruits, vegetables, and whole grains you'll be eating. And calcium supplements offer the same advantage, without the fat and carbohydrates.

In fact, dairy products should be used sparingly and confined to low-fat, low-sugar servings during Phase I until you reach your optimal weight. Once you've reached your healthy weight, you may opt to include two to three servings of dairy a day—as long as you steer clear of whole-fat products and focus on skim (nonfat) or low fat. Good choices include nonfat yogurt such as Yoplait (6 ounces), nonfat milk (one cup), and cheese (1 ounce), especially low-fat cheeses such as ricotta or cottage cheese. Remember, though, that a 1-ounce serving of cheese is a very small amount—about the size of two AA batteries.

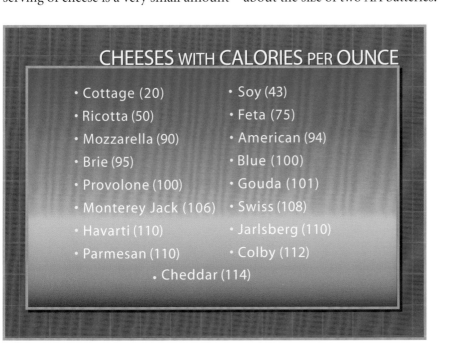

CHEESES WITH CALORIES PER OUNCE

- Cottage (20)
- Soy (43)
- Ricotta (50)
- Feta (75)
- Mozzarella (90)
- American (94)
- Brie (95)
- Blue (100)
- Provolone (100)
- Gouda (101)
- Monterey Jack (106)
- Swiss (108)
- Havarti (110)
- Jarlsberg (110)
- Parmesan (110)
- Colby (112)
- Cheddar (114)

Dr. A Says . . .

Learning to eat healthy for life is about much more than numbers on the scale. Don't forget to measure your other successes, like creating a new healthy recipe, walking farther than you thought you could, or enjoying an evening out while making good food choices.

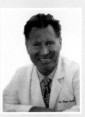

A 1-ounce serving of cheese is about the size of two AA batteries.

Seeds and Nuts: Your High-Octane Fuel Source

These health-giving, low-glycemic, protein-rich foods are also just chock full of healthy fats. But nuts and seeds are also extremely energy dense, meaning that they pack a lot of calories into a small amount. Those calories can add up in a hurry—in fact, a serving size is no more than a handful.

NUTS AND SEEDS WITH VERY LOW GI < 30	
• Peanuts	15
• Brazil nuts	15
• Pumpkin seeds	15
• Sunflower seeds	15
• Pecans	15
• Almonds	15
• Hazelnuts	15
• Walnuts	15

Nuts and seeds are about 15 to 30 percent proteins, with the remainder primarily made up of mono- and polyunsaturated fats—the healthy fats. They're also rich in thiamine, riboflavin, vitamin E, calcium, phosphorus, potassium, and iron. And as an added bonus, they're full of an amino acid that contributes to your body's ability to relax blood vessels, decrease blood pressure, and inhibit clot formation. The steady, powerful fuel they provide makes nuts and seeds great snacks for fueling breaks, with enough protein to give you a pleasant, long-lasting feeling of fullness. Just limit yourself to a small handful to avoid excess calories.

Recent research indicates that the walnut may be even more important than olive oil in creating the health-boosting effects of the popular "Mediterranean diet."

Starches

(25% of Your Plate)

Functional: Whole grain starches are a great slow-burning fuel, rich in fiber and loaded with B vitamins, calcium, potassium, and phosphorus. In their natural, low-glycemic state, they're critical for optimal health.

Dysfunctional: When refined and processed, starches are an energy-dense, high-glycemic poison that turns on your insulin pump and puts you in fat-storage mode.

It may seem dramatic, but it's true: your starch selections set the stage for success or failure.

Starches come in a vast array of options. Sadly, most of the options developed and promoted by the fast-food and processed-food industries are bad for you. Healthy starches, on the other hand, are a nutrient-rich source of slow-burning fuel and long-lasting energy.

When looking at starches, it's essential to consider their position on the glycemic index. Most processed and prepackaged starches score high on the index, meaning that they deliver large amounts of carbohydrates and must be avoided. Instead, shop for healthy, low-glycemic starches using my color-coded system—your reliable guide in this vast and sometimes confusing food group.

Healthy starch choices: Bread, pasta, noodles, and breakfast cereals made from grains such as rice, oats, wheat, barley, and rye. Potatoes, though a vegetable, count as a starch under my plan due to their high-glycemic, high-carbohydrate content.

Proportion of your meal: 25% of your nine-inch plate.

Portion size: About the size of a tennis ball.

Starch Choices

There's a wide variety of starches out there, many of which fall into the unhealthy, high-glycemic category. Just stay in the green and you'll be fine! (Note that I've included potatoes, actually a vegetable, in the starch section; because of their high-glycemic, high-carbohydrate content, they function more as a starch in most meals.)

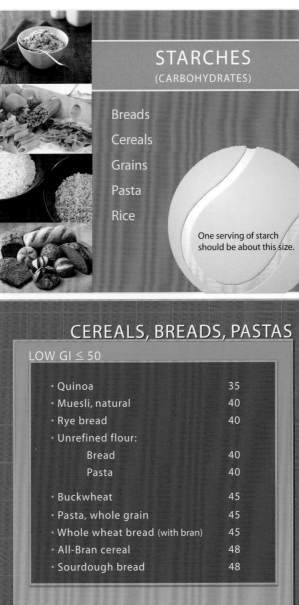

STARCHES
(CARBOHYDRATES)

Breads

Cereals

Grains

Pasta

Rice

One serving of starch should be about this size.

A healthy portion of starch is about the size of a tennis ball.

CEREALS, BREADS, PASTAS

LOW GI ≤ 50	
• Quinoa	35
• Muesli, natural	40
• Rye bread	40
• Unrefined flour:	
Bread	40
Pasta	40
• Buckwheat	45
• Pasta, whole grain	45
• Whole wheat bread (with bran)	45
• All-Bran cereal	48
• Sourdough bread	48

HIGH GI > 50	
• Oatmeal, from steel-cut oats	58
• Semolina (cream of wheat)	60
• Hamburger roll	61
• Couscous	65
• Cereals, refined	70
• Corn flakes	70
• White bread, enriched	71
• Bagel, white	72
• Dinner roll, white	73
• Kaiser roll, white	73
• Crackers	80

Your starch choices can set you up for success or failure—low-glycemic, whole grain starches are critical for optimal health, while refined and processed high-glycemic starches put you in fat-storage mode.

COMMERCIAL BREAKFAST PRODUCTS

- Kelloggs®

All-Bran	34
Frosted Flakes	55
Special K™	56
Nutri-Grain	66
Fruit Loops	69
Honey Smacks	71
Raisin Bran	73
Bran Flakes	74
Coco Pops	77
Corn Flakes	77
Corn Pops	80
Rice Krispies	82
Crispix®	87

- Shreaded Wheat   75
- Wonder Bread®   80
- Oatmeal, instant   82

PASTAS, POTATOES, RICE

LOW GI ≤ 50

Wild rice	35
Yams	37
Spaghetti, whole wheat	40
Spaghetti, durum	40
Basmati rice	50
Sweet potatoes	46
Brown rice	50

HIGH GI > 50

White pasta, cooked thoroughly	55
Potatoes, with skin, baked or boiled	65
Potatoes, peeled and boiled	70
Potatoes, mashed	80
Potatoes, instant mashed	88
French fries	95
Risotto	70
Rice cakes	85
Rice, precooked	90

Unhealthy Starches: A Habit of Disease

What about those choices so many of us make—the starches that poison your body? Unhealthy starches like the ones in the illustration below are convenient, inexpensive, readily available, and tempting, thanks to the food industry's heavy use of advertising. They fulfill a momentary need for comfort and satisfy cravings and hunger—for a short time, anyway. But they also rev up your insulin pump, turn on your fat-storage system, stimulate inflammation, and can lead to the myriad health problems that make up metabolic syndrome—the path to disease. In the end, they leave you with nothing but fatigue, excess weight, more cravings, and poor health. What's more, consuming unhealthy starches like these during Phase I of your weight loss will bring your fat-burning machinery to an abrupt halt for at least several days.

Once you've reached a healthy weight, your body should be able to tolerate some of these foods on occasion—but I recommend that you eliminate them permanently. You'll soon find that the meals I teach you to prepare using healthy starches will be just as convenient, taste much better, and bring you to a state of energy, vibrancy, and health.

Eating unhealthy starches like soda, french fries, candy, and doughnuts brings your fat-burning machinery to a halt.

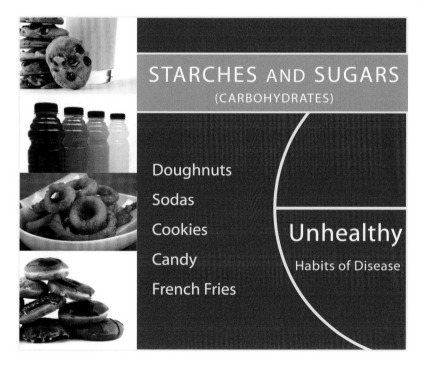

STARCHES AND SUGARS
(CARBOHYDRATES)

Doughnuts

Sodas

Cookies

Candy

French Fries

Unhealthy
Habits of Disease

Unhealthy Starch Choices.

Fats

Eating the right type of fats in the right amount can have a dramatic impact on your health and is an important component of our healthy eating strategy. The typical Western diet includes about 34 percent of its calories from fat, the vast majority from saturated, animal-based fat. According to the USDA, fat should make up between 25 and 35 percent of your daily caloric intake, with no more than 7 percent coming from saturated fat. (The Habits of Health will

Fat as a Percentage of Calories in Daily Diets. People in the U.S. get many more of their calories from fat than people in Japan or Africa, where diabetes, heart disease, and obesity are much less prevalent.

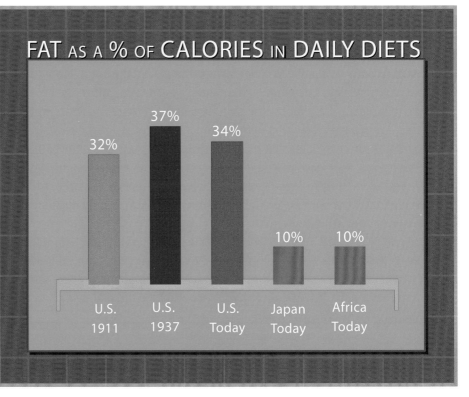

FAT AS A % OF CALORIES IN DAILY DIETS

- U.S. 1911 — 32%
- U.S. 1937 — 37%
- U.S. Today — 34%
- Japan Today — 10%
- Africa Today — 10%

Why does fat so easily lead to weight gain and disease?

- A gram of fat contains nine calories—more than double the calories in a gram of protein or carbohydrate.
- When combined with too many high-glycemic, processed carbohydrates, our bodies store fat calories at an accelerated rate.
- Calorie for calorie, fat is much less effective than protein or complex carbohydrates at satisfying your appetite and giving you a sense of fullness.

reduce your ingestion of fat below 25 percent.) It's no wonder that Western societies, which eat too much of the wrong fat, lead the world in heart disease, diabetes, obesity, and several types of cancer.

Take a look at the chart above, and notice how fat intake in the U.S. compares to that of other countries that have a lower incidence of these diseases.

Unhealthy Fats

The type of fat you consume has far-reaching effects on your health. In general, the fats to avoid are *saturated, hydrogenated,* and *partially hydrogenated* fats.

Saturated fats derive from animals and occur in high levels in foods such as hot dogs, hamburgers, bacon, and fatty meats.

Hydrogenated fats, also known as *trans-fats*, are found in most processed foods, where they're used to extend shelf life. Directly linked to heart attack and stroke, they've also been found to oxidize the brain, accelerating the loss of memory and cognitive function. In fact, they represent such a health hazard that progress has been made to ban hydrogenated fats entirely.

Partially hydrogenated vegetable oils were first developed with the launch of the low-fat, low-cholesterol craze in the 1980s, when saturated fats were found to contribute to heart disease and stroke. Polyunsaturated fats were known to be healthier than saturated fats, but they spoiled more easily—so food scientists devised ways to increase their stability by heating them and altering their molecular shape. Thus were invented partially hydrogenated vegetable oils, derived from corn, soybean, and cottonseed oils. These so-called "trans-fats"—which were unsaturated and had no cholesterol—were thought to be a healthier choice than butter. In the end, however, they were determined to be even more dangerous, causing oxidative stress, radical formation, and an inflammatory state.

Butter or Margarine?

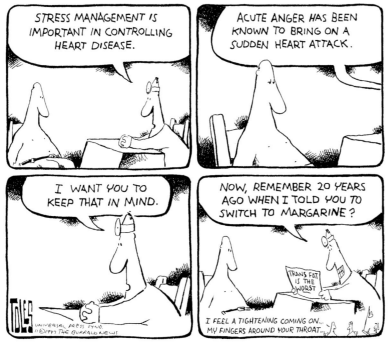

STRESS MANAGEMENT IS IMPORTANT IN CONTROLLING HEART DISEASE.

ACUTE ANGER HAS BEEN KNOWN TO BRING ON A SUDDEN HEART ATTACK.

I WANT YOU TO KEEP THAT IN MIND.

NOW, REMEMBER 20 YEARS AGO WHEN I TOLD YOU TO SWITCH TO MARGARINE?

TRANS FAT IS THE WORST

I FEEL A TIGHTENING COMING ON... MY FINGERS AROUND YOUR THROAT...

TOLES © 1997 *The Washington Post*. Reprinted with permission of UNIVERSAL PRESS SYNDICATE. All rights reserved.

Most types of margarine are full of unhealthy trans-fats. Butter, on the other hand, has no trans-fats—but it's loaded with cholesterol and saturated fat. So how does it all stack up?

Butter
- No trans-fats
- 7 grams of saturated fat per tablespoon (63 calories)
- 33 mg of cholesterol per tablespoon

Margarine
- No cholesterol
- Low in saturated fat
- High in trans-fats*

Remember that as a general rule—and a Habit of Health—you should limit yourself to no more than 10–15 grams of saturated fat and 200 milligrams of cholesterol per day (assuming your cholesterol level is in the healthy range).

*Semi-solid (tubs) and liquid margarines contain one-third as much trans-fats as solid (stick) margarine.

In the 1980s, the medical establishment believed that margarine was a healthier fat than butter. Today, we know that the trans-fats found in most margarine are just as unhealthy— or worse.

Are all margarines bad for you? No. Several types of semi-solid margarine are free of trans-fats, including brands such as Smart Balance and Benecol (though the latter cannot be used for cooking).

A Habit of Health:

Limiting your intake of saturated fat and cholesterol

- Limit your intake of saturated fat to 10–15 grams a day.
- Limit your intake of cholesterol to 200 milligrams a day (or lower if your cholesterol level is already too high.)

Top sources for healthy fat:

- Fatty cold-water fish, especially salmon
- Soybeans
- Olive oil
- Nuts, especially almonds
- Avocados, guacamole
- Flaxseed products

Healthy Fats

My plan makes it easy to stay within the USDA guidelines for fat intake by building in strategies for healthy fat consumption. You'll get about 20 to 25 percent of your daily calories from fat, mostly through mono- and polyunsaturated fats such as those found in olive, canola, and flaxseed oils. You'll also consume small amounts of fat through fish, skinless white poultry, and healthy lean and wild meats.

So what exactly are these healthy fats, and how do they serve as functional foods to support weight loss and put you on the path to optimal health? Healthy fats—what scientists call *essential fatty acids*—may also be known to you by the popular term *omega fats*. They're wonderful foods that have very specific and helpful roles in weight loss. Among other benefits, they turn off insulin, unload unhealthy triglycerides from your fat cells, increase your metabolism, and protect your muscle membranes and your brain against memory loss.

Note, however, that all fats and oils, while rich in health benefits, are a calorie-dense food—*with 120 calories in just one tablespoon.* Therefore, they should be used sparingly, particularly during Phase I, when it's important to maintain a lower energy intake.

Healthy Fats and Cholesterol

How exactly does eating "good fat" alter your cholesterol level and improve your health? A diet high in monounsaturated fat decreases your level of unhealthy triglycerides and LDL (the so-called "bad cholesterol") without decreasing HDL (the "good cholesterol").

Think of LDL as the trucks that deliver unhealthy fats and cholesterol to your blood vessels, and HDL as the trucks that cart them away. By increasing the amount of monounsaturated fat in your diet, you'll keep removing just as much of the bad stuff, while letting less of it in. And as you progress, I'll show you natural ways to continue bringing in those good HDL trucks and rid your body of even more unhealthy fats and cholesterol.

Cooking and Salad Oils

One benefit of oils high in monounsaturated fats is that when they're heated they develop fewer free radicals than polyunsaturated oils. That means they're great for cooking. Note, however, that olive oil—my favorite healthy oil for just about everything else—cannot be used for high-temperature cooking because its low smoking point will cause it to smoke, impair flavor, and become degraded. So if you're really cooking, peanut oil may be a better choice.

The Omega Fats: Omega-3, Omega-6, Omega-9

Think all omegas are alike? Think again. There are different types of omegas, some healthy and some not so healthy.

Omega-3 is the flagship of healthy fats. It can have a profound effect on your waistline, muscles, and brain, and can help you move quickly toward optimal health. As you can imagine, we'll want to make sure to provide you with the right amount. Fish is a great source of omega-3, which you'll learn more

COOKING AND SALAD OILS

	Omega Type	Monounsaturated	Polyunsaturated	Saturated
• Olive	O-9	75%	8%	17%
• Canola	O-6,9	55%	38%	7%
• Sesame	O-6,9	39%	43%	18%
Peanut	O-9	34%	45%	21%
Corn	O-6	20%	66%	14%
• Soy	O-6	19%	65%	16%
• Safflower	O-6	13%	79%	8%
• Sunflower	O-6	11%	80%	9%
• Coconut (unhealthy)	O-6	5%	2%	93%

The oils in the green shaded area are the healthiest.

Fats and oils are extremely calorie dense, and should be used sparingly.

about in the next chapter's discussion on buying healthy protein. Liquid flax-seed oil is another prime source. It can't be used as cooking oil, but it's great to use on salads or breads or added to soups.

Omega-6 is a healthy fat *if it's consumed in a 1:1 ratio with omega-3s.* Unfortunately, for the most part, our consumption of omega-6 far outweighs our intake of omega-3. Most vegetable oils, including soybean, corn, sunflower, and safflower oil, contain heavy concentration of omega-6. Increasing your use of olive and canola oil, and adding flaxseed oil to your diet, will help restore a healthy ratio and provide a better balance to support health.

Omega-9, another very healthy omega, is found in olives, avocados, and nuts. Olive oil, particularly extra virgin olive oil, is an ideal way to get enough omega-9. Use it for sautéing or to add a marvelous flavor to cooked foods and salads—just make sure you don't cook at very high temperatures, and, as with all oils, keep track of the amount so you don't consume too much!

Fiber

You've probably heard that fiber is an important part of a healthy diet. But the different types of fiber can be a little confusing. Here's a guide so you can be sure to include both types in your daily food choices. (There are about 3 grams of fiber per cup or piece of the foods listed below.)

Soluble fiber dissolves in water. Its benefits to your body include slowing the breakdown of complex carbohydrates and helping to reduce blood sugar. When you eat it in large enough quantity, it can help lower cholesterol as well.

Good sources of soluble fiber: Grains such as rye, barley, and oats; vegetables and fruits; legumes.

Insoluble fiber doesn't dissolve in water and is not absorbed or digested by the body. But it does reduce hunger (it's filling!), helps keep your gastrointestinal tract clean, and aids in regular bowel movements by pulling water into the colon.

Good sources of insoluble fiber: Brown rice; whole wheat breads and cereals; seeds; fruit and vegetable skins; legumes.

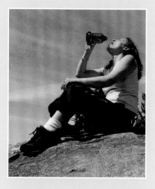

A Habit of Health:
Drinking plenty of water

Drink a glass of water as soon as you wake up, before every meal, and any time you feel the urge to put something in your mouth! (In addition to water's other wonderful benefits, it helps suppress appetite.)

Dr. A Says . . .

Liven up your water by adding a squirt of lemon or some fresh mint leaves. And try to start your day with a couple of glasses before you hit the coffee pot.

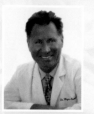

Water

What's water doing in a discussion of our major food groups? Water is a critical component of your body, making up between 55 and 60 percent of your weight. Your body can't store water—unlike fat—so you need to replenish it often. That's why drinking at least eight glasses a day is a core Habit of Health.

Water plays a key role in supporting health, particularly during weight loss, when it helps remove toxins and other unhealthy substances stored in your fat cells. Being well-hydrated helps all your organs and systems function properly. In fact, every function in your body takes place in water. It's the solvent that moves nutrients, hormones, antibodies, and oxygen through your bloodstream and lymphatic system, and removes waste. And of course it's essential to your kidneys' ability to filter and eliminate metabolic byproducts and toxins. If you don't drink enough, your body is forced to recycle dirty water, diminishing the efficiency of every metabolic function.

What you may not realize is that we actually lose nearly twelve cups of water every day: two cups through perspiration, six cups through urine, two to four through breathing—and nearly one cup through the soles of our feet! And in high altitudes or dry environments, you lose even more, so you can get dehydrated in a hurry.

During Phase I of your weight-loss plan, there are even more good reasons to make a conscious effort to drink your eight glasses a day. Here are a few:

- It's calorie free, but helps you feel full and satisfied.
- It keeps you from overeating. Studies have shown that when we feel hungry, 30 percent of the time our bodies are actually signaling for water.
- It facilitates the removal of toxins such as pesticides and preservatives from your cells.
- It prevents dehydration as your body eliminates excess salt and water from a diet of too much processed food.
- It minimizes or eliminates fatigue, lack of energy, headaches, and unclear thinking.
- It speeds up metabolism. A recent study showed that drinking two 8-ounce glasses of cold water increased metabolic rate by 30 percent for ninety minutes.
- It helps your liver convert fat to energy.
- It compensates for the loss of glycogen stores as you lose weight.

Water FAQs

What's the best source for my eight glasses a day? Plain water is the best beverage for quenching thirst—and it's cheap, calorie free, and contains no sugar, caffeine, or other additives. Tap water should be filtered first, though, to remove chlorine and other contaminants.

What about bottled water? Bottled water is fine, as are sparkling waters flavored with lemon or lime. Just make sure they haven't been enhanced with sugary substances and calories!

What about distilled water? Distillation takes out both impurities and minerals, including calcium, magnesium, and sodium, which may provide clinically important portions of your recommended dietary intake. I encourage you to check the mineral content of your drinking water, whether tap or bottled, and choose water most appropriate for your needs. If you do use distilled water, you should supplement your mineral intake through your diet in order to maintain proper health.

What about reverse osmosis? Reverse osmosis produces distilled water, so the above cautions apply. And because it removes all of the impurities, minerals, and toxins, its filter requires considerable maintenance and cost.

I'm just not thirsty. Do I still need to drink water? Don't use thirst to guide your water intake! Thirst is a late warning symptom of dehydration. Waiting until you're thirsty to drink means that your body must function at less than optimal efficiency for several hours.

How do I know if I'm not drinking enough? If you start feeling tired, have trouble thinking, develop a headache, or notice that your urine is darker than usual, these are late-stage signs that you need to drink more water! (Urine should be almost colorless unless you've just taken vitamins.)

Is it possible to drink too much water? No—not unless you have a specific medical condition that requires you to restrict your fluid intake, such as renal failure or severe congestive heart failure, or if you have performed intense physical activity in a hot environment, in which case you should consume an electrolyte-enriched drink.

Topping It Off with Herbs and Spices

Herbs and spices are a great way to enhance flavor without adding calories, fat, or other unhealthy substances. And many do much more than that—they actually help you lose weight while providing particular health benefits as well. Try these great choices:

- Toss foods with a simple mixture of sea salt, black pepper, olive oil, and vinegar.
- Add red pepper to an egg-white omelet to decrease hunger and increase metabolism.
- Add a pinch of turmeric, source of the substance curcumin, to add a hint of mustard flavor and reduce inflammation.
- Don't forget garlic, cilantro, parsley, and basil, which add so many flavors and have numerous health benefits.

That's it—my easy shopping system for long-term healthy eating and reaching an optimal weight. When combined with the PCMR system you learned about in chapter 7, you now have a comprehensive strategy for reaching and maintaining optimal health.

When you think of the hours we spend shopping for clothes, electronics, even pet supplies, it really makes sense to take the time to learn and use this simple system. Once you do, you can be sure that you're giving your body the best-quality fuel available, through foods that boost your ability to function and put you on the path to optimal health.

A Habit of Health:
Eliminating excess salt

Processed food is loaded with salt. Lowering your salt intake has important health benefits, including helping to lower your blood pressure. Here are some tips for eliminating excess salt from your diet.

- Follow the Habits of Health, including my Healthy Eating for Life system.

- Lower or eliminate your intake of processed foods.

- Don't add salt to your food.

- Fill your salt shaker with half salt, half pepper.

- Use salt-free seasonings.

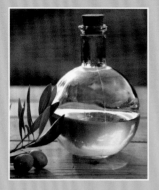

A Habit of Health:
Selecting and preparing
healthy foods

Chapter 10

Putting It All Together

Healthy Meal Plans for Optimal Health

You've learned about portion control, about the three major food groups, and about shopping for healthy foods with my color-coded shopping charts. Now it's time to put it all together to plan meals that are quick, convenient, affordable, portable, and most of all, healthy—and will help you reach your first goal:

A healthy weight!

Quick and Easy Tools for "Automatic Eating"

For most of us, eating processed, microwaved, or fast food is an easy alternative to preparing meals that seem too hard, too time consuming, and that leave us with a messy kitchen and a load of dishes. Cooking just doesn't seem worth it!

One of my goals is to make preparing healthy foods as easy as stopping into a fast food restaurant. First, let me introduce you to some of my own favorite tools that will make your new healthy eating strategy a breeze.

Portable cooker

These portable, self-contained countertop appliances make preparing portion-controlled meals a breeze! Portable cookers actually provide a miniature range that cooks your meals quickly (in about 3–10 minutes) without any dishes. Both the two-portion and four-portion models allow you to cook on a non-stick surface, eliminating the need for extra fat or oil, and the cooking process doesn't even require turning, so there's no hassle! And what's really great is that you can take this portable device to your workplace. I use my portable cookers all the time to make great-tasting meals.

Portable blender

This compact tool lets you mix up great-tasting fruit smoothies, healthy frozen shakes, and other tasty meals and snacks—without the mess.

Shaker cup or jar

This is a great way to quickly prepare portion-controlled meal replacements (PCMRs), which we introduced in chapter 7. PCMRs can be a useful part of your fueling strategy in the healthy eating plan as well.

Wok

The indispensable ancient Chinese tool for fast, healthy cooking.

Bamboo steamer

Make delicious steamed foods right inside your wok.

Zipper-style plastic bags

Pop extra meals and snacks into these to keep one jump ahead when you need to fuel.

Portable cooler

An insulated, lightweight cooler keeps prepared meals fresh and is easy to transport.

Why all this emphasis on quick and easy? Because humans react to hunger and stress, often in ways that don't promote health. We need to create an automatic eating system—my healthy version of fast food—to fuel your body before you cave in to cravings. Planning meals in advance and having them ready to go—and, perhaps most important, sticking to my every-three-hour healthy eating schedule—helps you stay in control. And what happens when you're in control?

- You'll reach a healthy weight over time.
- You'll develop permanent Habits of Health.
- You'll improve your health and possibly reduce your reliance on medications for certain weight-related health conditions.
- Your work performance will improve.
- Your quality of life will improve.
- You'll eliminate cravings.
- Your mental focus and energy will improve.
- You'll save money.

What are we waiting for?

Important: Before You Begin

Before you start your journey, I suggest you schedule a visit to see your primary care provider, usually your family doctor. No doubt your doctor will be excited that you've decided to lose weight and create health in your life. After all, it makes their job easier! In the appendix, you'll find a sheet of information to give your physician that explains this "health makeover" you're doing. It's also available for download at my Web site at www.habitsofhealth.net.

A special note for those with type 2 diabetes: Checking in with your doctor before you change your diet is particularly important if you have type 2 diabetes. As you switch to my low-calorie, low-glycemic diet, your blood sugar will lower immediately, and your level of medication will need to be reduced accordingly. The great news is that this is a signal of your body's initial step toward health. Your disease progression is being arrested! But do remember to watch your blood sugar closely in the beginning to make sure your medications are properly adjusted.

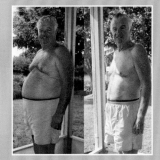

"Learning the Habits of Health changed my life forever!"

RON GOELZ
Over three years at optimal health

I lost 75 pounds on Medifast® and thanks to my weight loss, my doctor was able to reduce medications for blood pressure, cholesterol, and triglycerides. The Take Shape for Life™ support system in particular is invaluable, and is one of the key reasons for my success.

I've incorporated Dr. A's Habits of Health into my life and know I will remain optimally healthy for the rest of my life! ■

Results vary. Typical weight loss is 2-5 lbs per week for the first 2 weeks and 1-2 lbs per week thereafter.

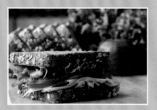

Dr. A Says . . .

Reduce your exposure
to pesticides by washing
and scrubbing fresh
produce, discarding
the outer layers of leafy
greens, and trimming
fat and skin from meat
and poultry.

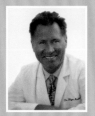

Your Customized Daily Meal Plan

So what does a day on your new meal plan look like? Remember the basic principles of reaching an optimal weight:

• Eat breakfast.
• Eat a small amount of food every three hours.
• Eat a healthy meal at dinner time.

To create your daily menu, you're going to design a healthy breakfast and dinner using your nine-inch plate, supplemented by four fueling breaks. Each of your two meals provides about 300 to 400 calories through:

• A combination of vegetables and fruits* (50% of your plate = small paperback novel of about 100 pages)
• A healthy, low-glycemic starch (25% of your plate = tennis ball)
• A healthy protein (25% of your plate = deck of cards)

* Remember to use fruits sparingly during the weight-loss phase and choose only those with a glycemic index below 30 (from the dark green section of the charts).

Your fueling breaks provide about 100 calories each. If you wish, you may add a second fueling break item at lunchtime (for a total of two 100-calorie items), or opt for a light lunch (a regular nine-inch-plate meal without the starch component). The PCMRs function as the perfect fueling, and you'll find a list with plenty of ideas and options for foods you can use for fueling breaks later in the chapter.

This eating strategy gives you a steady, balanced stream of energy throughout your waking hours, for a total of 1,200 calories per day. Let's go through a sample day's menu to see exactly what we're looking at.

7:00 a.m. Breakfast (300–400 calories)

Vegetable/fruit	strawberries/peaches	(small paperback)
Starch	¾ cup rolled oats	(tennis ball)
Protein	½ cup low-fat milk	(deck of cards)

10:00 a.m. Fueling break (100 calories)
  Handful of almonds (12) or PCMR

1:00 p.m.

  Option 1: Fueling break (100 calories) plus another fueling serving if needed

  1 cup vegetable soup and 4 Wheat Thins crackers

Option 2: Light lunch (200 calories)

Vegetable/fruit	½ tomato and 1 cup lettuce with oil and vinegar	(small paperback)
No starch		
Protein	5 ounces cooked turkey breast	(deck of cards)

4:00 p.m. Fueling break (100 calories)
    Yoplait nonfat french vanilla yogurt or PCMR

7:00 p.m. Dinner (400 calories)

Vegetable/fruit	fresh asparagus	(small paperback)
Starch	whole grain pasta	(tennis ball)
Protein	grilled salmon	(deck of cards)

10:00 p.m. Fueling break (100 calories)
    Frozen nonfat yogurt (3 ounces) or PCMR

What to Expect on Day One and Onward

So what can you expect after your first day on the meal plan? For one thing, you probably won't have any hunger pangs or cravings—and your energy level should be consistent, balanced, and high.

Your first experience is just a starting point. Over the next few weeks, it's going to get better and better. Your internal clock is being changed, along with your body's expectations. You're feeding your body healthy food (it likes that!) and giving it regular nourishment through small meals throughout the day—just what your ancient, 10,000-year-old programming wants. By feeding it smaller meals, you're giving your body the ability to process food without being overwhelmed and having to work too hard. And as a bonus, you'll rediscover your flavor palate as you move farther and farther from processed food with its excess sugar and salt!

Planning Your Fueling Breaks

Your fueling breaks are an extremely important part of your day and a critical component of my healthy eating plan. To make sure you always have healthy fuel on hand, it's a good idea to prepare these small meals ahead of time and bring them with you to work or wherever your day takes you. You can use the prepackaged PCMRs or you can prepare and transport whole foods. That's where the zipper-style plastic bags and portable cooler come in. Just fix up your day's worth of fueling breaks, pop them into the plastic bags, and take them with you in the cooler, together with an ice pack or two.

The following fueling break ideas are healthy, easy to prepare, and perfect for transporting. Each contains around 100 calories, making them ideal for the fat-burning state you want to encourage if you're working on reaching or maintaining your optimal weight. Remember, you can add one extra fueling break item at lunchtime if you wish, or opt to have a light lunch instead by preparing a regular nine-inch-plate meal without the starch component.

If you haven't reached your optimal weight yet, be sure to check the glycemic index of any snack before you choose it. It's important to eat only lower-glycemic snacks during weight loss—that is, foods that fall in the green zone (preferably dark green), with a glycemic index of less than 30.

Sample Fueling Breaks

- PCMR. These make excellent fueling breaks and assure that you're getting a 100-calorie, low-glycemic, nutrient-dense healthy food source.
- Cheese and tomato. One portion (size of two AA batteries) of natural cheese such as cheddar or Monterey Jack with one sliced tomato.
- Endive and tuna salad. One endive leaf with one tablespoon tuna salad, prepared with hummus in place of mayonnaise. Mediterranean Delights makes delicious, organic, low-fat hummus in flavors like tomato basil, and low-glycemic endive makes a handy container for the tuna salad.
- 3 oz mixed nuts (a small handful)
- 10 almonds and celery stick
- 29 pistachios
- 12 cashews
- 20 peanuts
- 2 tbsp sesame seeds
- 4 Brazil nuts. Great for getting your selenium!
- ½ sliced apple with 3 walnuts
- ½ apple with 2 tsp natural peanut butter. Make sure it's all-natural peanut butter: just peanuts and salt.
- ½ cup fresh strawberries with 2 tbsp light whipped topping
- 1 cup fresh cherries
- 1 medium apple
- ½ cup blueberries (high glycemic) or strawberries (lower glycemic) with a dollop of yogurt
- 1 orange
- 1 pear
- ½ peach with 2 tbsp yogurt
- 2 cups raspberries
- 30 raisins
- Fresh veggie mix. 1 cup broccoli, red pepper, cauliflower with 1 tbsp low-fat ranch dressing.
- 6 pieces basil, sliced tomato, and hummus. My wife Lori's creation: put a dab of hummus and tomato on top of a basil leaf—delightful!
- Herbal lentils and one tomato
- Celery sticks with 1 tbsp natural peanut butter
- 1 cup fresh spinach salad with olives
- ¼ cup egg salad with lettuce or endive
- Half small avocado
- Cauliflower (size of paperback)
- 1 cup tomato and cucumber soup
- ¼ cup guacamole. Combine avocado, tomato, lime juice, and hot pepper to taste.
- Basil, tomato, and hummus (1 tomato)
- Grilled portobello mushroom sprinkled with cheese
- 5 cherry tomatoes with one portion cheddar cheese (size of two AA batteries)

- ½ cup endive and cottage cheese spread. In a food processor or blender, mix cottage cheese, red pepper, fresh parsley, chives, and chopped jalapeno. Spread on endive.
- Eggplant pizza slice. Sprinkle a slice of eggplant with oregano and roast. Melt cheese on top.
- 1 cup vegetarian chili
- ½ cup edamame (soybeans)
- Half red bell pepper dipped in 3 tbsp hummus
- ½ cup cucumber slices
- 1 large dill pickle
- 1 carrabolla (starfruit)
- 2 cups baby carrots
- 3 celery sticks with 1 tsp natural peanut butter
- ¼ cup hummus and avocado dip with 3 celery stalks
- 1 cup mashed lentils and tomatoes
- Vegetables and dip. Choose either ½ cup cucumber slices, 6 celery sticks, 6 slices red pepper, or ½ cup raw broccoli florets and dip into 2 oz fat-free, sugar-free ranch dressing.
- 1 cup bean and chickpea salad. Toss diced celery, green pepper, cooked red beans, cooked chickpeas, and fresh parsley together with low-calorie balsamic vinaigrette.
- ⅓ cup low-fat cottage cheese with 4 olives
- Yogurt with ¼ cup berries. Yoplait Light plain yogurt is a great choice.
- ½ cup cottage cheese and ½ medium tomato
- 1 Yoplait Light Smoothie
- ½ cup low-fat cottage cheese with 5 strawberries
- 1 serving of string cheese
- 3 oz frozen nonfat yogurt
- 1 square 70% or higher dark chocolate with 5 almonds
- 1 whole deviled egg. Cut a hard-boiled egg in half, mix the yolk with hummus, and fill the egg.
- 1 cup of soup (cream of tomato, cream of chicken, chicken noodle, or vegetable)
- 1 slice Wasa crispbread with 1 oz smoked salmon
- 1 slice whole grain bread (such as Fiber for Life) with 2 oz fat-free turkey breast
- ½ cup couscous with celery sticks
- 4 slices Melba toast
- 1 slice Wasa crispbread and ½ sliced tomato

Once you've reached a healthy weight, you can add these to the list as well:

- 1 cup fresh mango
- 1 cup cantaloupe
- 1 medium banana
- 28 grapes

This list should help you get started on ideas for your own small meals. Remember, each one should be low glycemic and no higher than 100 calories.

> If you're short on time or just don't feel like preparing these 100-calorie meals, remember that PCMRs are an easy and great option for fueling breaks!

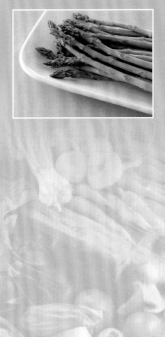

Planning Your Meals

When it comes to healthy eating, planning ahead is the key to success. The sample menus below—two weeks worth of healthy breakfasts, dinners, and fueling breaks—should give you a good start. Feel free to mix and match meals, or substitute fueling break ideas from the list above. Or make it easier on yourself by sticking to the sample menus for the first two weeks and, if you've enjoyed them, start the cycle again at week three.

Using these sample menus is a great way to learn how to prepare healthy meals—an important Habit of Health. And to top it off, you'll find recipes for all the evening meals in the appendix. Together, the meals I've planned for you are easy to prepare, give you lots of great flavors, and support your ability to stay at your optimal weight.

Note: Selecting a healthy, medically formulated PCMR can provide an excellent, nutritious, 100-calorie exchange for as many of the four fueling ideas as you desire. For more information on ordering your PCMRs, see the resource list on page 370.

Sample Meals

Recipes for all evening meal entrees can be found in the appendix.

WEEK ONE MENU

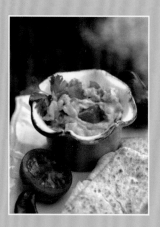

Day One

Breakfast

> Scrambled egg or omelet with ¼ cup mushrooms, ½ cup spinach, and 1 tablespoon parmesan cheese (optional)
>
> ½ grapefruit
>
> 1 cup green tea

Mid-morning Fueling

> 1 serving sugar-free Jello with ¼ cup cottage cheese

Lunch Fueling

> ½ whole wheat English muffin, toasted, with 1 teaspoon all-natural peanut butter

Mid-afternoon Fueling

> Veggies dipped into ½ cup low-fat ranch dressing

Dinner

> Mixed green salad with red peppers and cucumber
>
> Balsamic vinegar and olive oil
>
> Broiled cod (scrod) with lemon pepper
>
> 3 ounces whole wheat angel hair pasta tossed with chicken broth or bouillon, lightly sprinkled with parmesan cheese

Evening Fueling

> 1 medium hard-boiled egg

Day Two

Breakfast

> Sugar-free natural muesli
>
> ½ cup skim milk
>
> 1 cup raspberries

Mid-morning Fueling

    10 almonds

Lunch Fueling

    1 ounce fresh mozzarella

    1 sliced tomato on a bed of lettuce and basil, drizzled with olive oil and
        vinegar

Mid-afternoon Fueling

    Low-glycemic, 100-calorie protein bar

    1 cup coffee, black

Dinner

    Grilled herbed chicken breast

    Grilled zucchini and yellow squash mix

    1 slice sourdough bread

Evening Fueling

    3–4 ounces fat-free natural yogurt

Day Three

Breakfast

    1 slice rye toast with nonfat cream cheese

    1 orange

    1 cup green tea

Mid-morning Fueling

    ½ sliced apple with 2 teaspoons all-natural peanut butter

Lunch Fueling

    Fresh spinach with red peppers and minced garlic or onion and 1 table-
        spoon parmesan cheese, sprinkled with balsamic vinegar

Mid-afternoon Fueling

    10 almonds

Dinner

    Roasted pork tenderloin

    1 cup cooked cauliflower, mashed with 1 tablespoon parmesan cheese and
        garlic (optional)

    3 ounces cooked whole grain pasta with ½ fresh tomato and herbs, drizzled
        lightly with olive oil and tossed

Evening Fueling

    8 medium strawberries dipped in light Cool Whip

Day Four

Breakfast

    Poached egg

    ½ whole wheat English muffin

    Baked half tomato sprinkled with parmesan

Mid-morning Fueling

    1 cup raspberries

Dr. A Says . . .

Don't skip breakfast!
It's one of the keys
to successful weight
maintenance. In fact,
according to studies, 80
percent of people who've
maintained a 35-pound
or greater weight loss
make breakfast a part of
their day . . . every day.

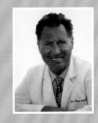

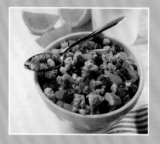

Lunch Fueling

> 1 slice whole grain bread
>
> Sugar-free fruit spread

Mid-afternoon Fueling

> ½ cup cherry tomatoes with balsamic vinegar and hummus

Dinner

> Montreal grilled beef
>
> Steamed asparagus
>
> 1 cup sautéed mushrooms with 1 teaspoon olive oil

Evening Fueling

> ½ cup fat-free herbed cottage cheese

Day Five

Breakfast

> ¾ cup rolled oats with ½ cup diced apples and raspberries and 1 teaspoon
>   sliced almonds
>
> ½ cup skim milk

Mid-morning Fueling

> 2 tablespoons sunflower seeds

Lunch Fueling

> 1 ounce gouda cheese
>
> 1 romaine leaf seasoned with ½ teaspoon olive oil and fresh black pepper

Mid-afternoon Fueling

> 1 cup bell pepper strips and cucumber

Dinner

> Herbed poached salmon
>
> Fresh steamed spinach
>
> 1 slice toasted rye bread lightly drizzled with olive oil

Evening Fueling

> 1 cup low-glycemic mixed fruit

Day Six

Breakfast

> 1 slice whole grain toast
>
> ½ cup low-fat cottage cheese with ½ cup blackberries

Mid-morning Fueling

> ½ grapefruit

Lunch Fueling

> Mixed green salad with herbed olive oil and red wine vinegar

Mid-afternoon Fueling

> 1 cup tomato soup with celery stalk

Dinner

> Sautéed chicken with lemon and capers
>
> Steamed broccoli

Evening Fueling

> Fat-free Yoplait vanilla yogurt

Day Seven

Breakfast

Omelet with chives, spinach, and Colby cheese

1 fresh sliced peach

Mid-morning Fueling

Cherries

Lunch Fueling

Alfalfa sprouts, olives, and tomato slices

Mid-afternoon Fueling

Carrot and cucumber sticks

Dinner

Grilled Chinese five-spice beef

Bok choy (Chinese cabbage)

Evening Fueling

Brazil nuts

WEEK TWO MENU

Day Eight

Breakfast

Baked eggs with chopped broccoli

1 slice whole wheat bread

Mid-morning Fueling

Nectarine

Lunch Fueling

Yoplait Light Smoothie

Mid-afternoon Fueling

½ cup edamame (soybeans)

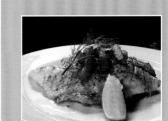

Dinner

Mixed green salad with red peppers, cucumber, balsamic vinegar, and olive oil

Marinated turkey cutlet

⅓ cup whole wheat pasta lightly drizzled with olive oil and sprinkled with parmesan cheese

Evening Fueling

½ cup fat-free cottage cheese

Day Nine

Breakfast

1 biscuit shredded wheat

½ cup skim milk

½ cup strawberries and ½ cup raspberries

Mid-morning Fueling

½ cup walnuts

Lunch Fueling

1 ounce fresh mozzarella

Slice of tomato

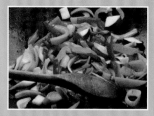

Mid-afternoon Fueling

Large dill pickle wrapped in a thin slice of turkey

Dinner

Sirloin and vegetable kabobs

Small green salad

Evening Fueling

1 medium pear

Day Ten

Breakfast

1 slice rye toast

1 teaspoon nonfat herbed cream cheese

2 ounces smoked salmon

Orange slices

Mid-morning Fueling

4 ounces low-fat yogurt

Lunch Fueling

Fresh spinach with red peppers and minced garlic or onion

Mid-afternoon Fueling

½ cup almonds

Dinner

Grilled sea bass with tomato salsa

Endive seasoned with fresh herbs and malt vinegar

Evening Fueling

1 ounce cheddar cheese

Day Eleven

Breakfast

1 hard-boiled egg

1 ounce lean ham

1 slice whole wheat rye bread

½ grapefruit

Mid-morning Fueling

1 cup strawberries

Lunch Fueling

2 cups tossed salad (lettuce, tomato, cucumber, 2 tablespoons low-cal salad
     dressing)

Mid-afternoon Fueling

½ apple with 2 teaspoons peanut butter

Dinner

Sautéed chicken with basil and lemon

Asparagus

3 ounces whole wheat linguini

Evening Fueling

½ cup fat-free herbed cottage cheese

Day Twelve

Breakfast

Cinnamon rolled oats oatmeal

½ cup skim milk

1 apricot

Mid-morning Fueling

1 hard-boiled egg and three strawberries

Lunch Fueling

1 ounce gouda cheese

1 romaine leaf seasoned with ½ teaspoon olive oil and fresh black pepper

Mid-afternoon Fueling

Red pepper strips dipped in 3 tablespoons hummus

Dinner

Seared sea scallops

Mixed field greens drizzled with balsamic vinegar

1 slice sourdough bread with a drizzle of olive oil

Evening Fueling

Mixed berries

Day Thirteen

Breakfast

1 slice whole grain wheat bread

1 cooked egg

Sautéed fresh spinach

1 cup green tea

Mid-morning Fueling

½ grapefruit

Lunch

Mixed green salad with herbed olive oil and red wine vinegar

Mid-afternoon Fueling

Sugar-free Jello with ½ cup raspberries

Dinner

Sautéed ginger beef

Steamed broccoli

3 ounces whole wheat spaghetti

Evening Fueling

Fat-free Yoplait vanilla yogurt

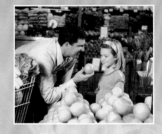

Day Fourteen

Breakfast

Omelet with chopped tarragon and cheddar cheese

½ grapefruit

Mid-morning Fueling

20 cherries

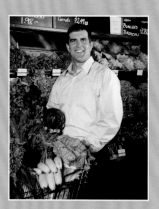

**Not Losing Fast
Enough? Low on
Energy?**
If your weight loss is
slower than you expect
or your energy level is
low, eliminate the starch
component and double
up on vegetables
until you notice
improvement. Avoiding
fruit for a couple of
days until your weight
loss picks up is often
helpful.

Lunch Fueling
 Alfalfa sprouts, olives, and tomato slice
Mid-afternoon Fueling
 Carrot and cucumber sticks
Dinner
 Balsamic glazed chicken with rosemary
 Herbed grilled portabella mushroom
 One slice whole wheat rye bread, toasted
Evening Fueling
 4 Brazil nuts

You now have two weeks of meal plans, as well as the recipes you need to prepare your evening meal. You can repeat the two-week cycle or mix it up with meals you like. And you'll find more selections available for download from the Web site at www.habitsofhealth.net.

Don't be afraid to experiment and become adventurous. You can make all kinds of healthy entrees, as long as you:

• Keep in the proper proportions of 50 percent vegetable/fruit, 25 percent starch, and 25 percent protein

• Use my shopping menus

• Stay in the green zones

• Choose from the food charts that contain "very low" and "low" glycemic selections

Remember, you can mix and match you fueling breaks too, as long as you stay within the guidelines.

• •

So there you have it—a very simple method to help you reach and maintain your optimal weight while learning crucial dietary habits, including:

• Eating every three hours
• Eating breakfast
• Making healthy food choices
• Eating low-glycemic foods
• Planning your meals

Once you have a handle on these habits, you'll have the framework for success—not only for weight loss but for a lifetime of maintaining your healthy weight and optimal health.

Checklists for Change

Before you begin your weight-loss plan, make sure you've taken these important first steps:

✓ You've created a microenvironment of health.

✓ You've gone shopping and stocked your pantry and refrigerator with groceries selected using the color-coded shopping system.

✓ You've taken the health assessment and if possible are using the workbook, *Living a Longer, Healthier Life: The Companion Guide to Dr. A's Habits of Health,* to plot your health path.

✓ You've created a structural tension chart for your first goal of reaching a healthy weight. (For more information, see chapter 4.)

✓ You've bought a journal and are regularly recording your daily eating habits and activity level. (See *Living a Longer, Healthier Life: The Companion Guide to Dr. A's Habits of Health* for more information on using a journal as a tool for tracking choices that support optimal weight and health.)

Once you're on the move, here are some tips:

✓ Get through your first few days of new healthy eating successfully.

✓ If you need some extra motivation, review chapters 3 and 4 on motivation for change, fundamental choice, and the discipline of daily choices.

✓ By day four you should feel great, with lots of energy as your body starts to respond to healthy fueling. After a week, if you're ready and feel good enough, start slowly increasing your daily activity.

✓ Drink at least eight 8-ounce glasses of water every day.

✓ Eat slowly.

✓ Use your support system. If you have a coach, call her or him. (See chapter 18 for more information on building a support system.)

✓ Make sure you're writing in your journal. This is a great way to monitor your progress and help you focus.

"Live at your optimum!"

RANDY GRAY

Over one year at optimal health

I started working with Dr. A at 217 pounds, with arthritis in my shoulder and soreness and swelling in my knees. Today, I've lost 40 pounds and four sizes in my waist—and I can play basketball or run for miles with no soreness. In fact, I'm the same weight now as when I played basketball as a freshman in college! Now I coach others to do just what I did, by guiding them every step of the way through this safe, effective, and easy-to-follow comprehensive system to optimal health. And you can do it, too. Learn the habits of lifelong health! ■

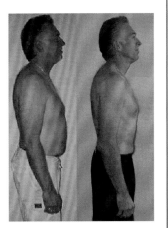

Results vary. Typical weight loss is 2-5 lbs per week for the first 2 weeks and 1-2 lbs per week thereafter.

If you're using the healthy eating system to knock off those couple extra pounds and have reached your healthy weight (with a body mass index below 25) you're ready to transition to your permanent schedule.

In Phase I, we've laid the foundation for a more efficient energy management system by teaching you how to control the types of foods you choose, your portions, and the timing of your meals.

You're now eating healthy, you're at a healthy weight, and you're ready to take the next step of your journey. As you transition to Phase II, we'll boost both your energy intake and your energy expenditure. The thread that connects each phase is the relationship between energy in and energy out. Let's take another look at the energy diagram. Notice that the colored boxes in Phase II highlight our three key focal areas: a healthy body mass index, or BMI (white), increased activity and exercise (green), and increased caloric intake (red).

Energy Management in Phase I: Moving into Transition. Before you transition to Phase II, you'll have decreased your daily energy intake (red line) as well as your body mass index, or BMI (white line). Once you've reached your healthy weight and BMI and have begun to develop the fundamental Habits of Health, you're ready to begin transitioning to Phase II.

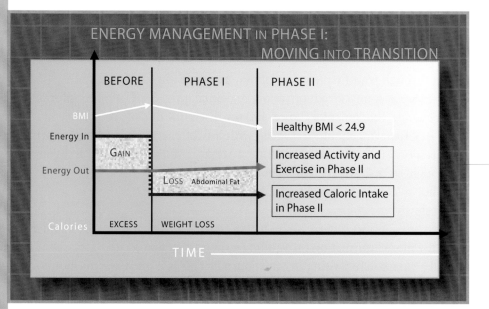

ENERGY MANAGEMENT IN PHASE I: MOVING INTO TRANSITION

	BEFORE	PHASE I	PHASE II

BMI
Energy In
GAIN
Energy Out
LOSS Abdominal Fat
Calories
EXCESS WEIGHT LOSS
TIME

Healthy BMI < 24.9

Increased Activity and Exercise in Phase II

Increased Caloric Intake in Phase II

In the next chapter we'll review the science of weight loss and maintenance, and teach you more great ways to control your energy intake and your insulin pump. There's a lot of great material there, but if you're at a healthy weight and eager to increase your calories, feel free to move right ahead to chapter 12.

Chapter 11

The Science of Healthy Eating and Weight Loss

Three Core Principles

My comprehensive healthy eating system aligns the cutting-edge of medical science behind three core principles essential for reaching and maintaining a healthy weight:

- Fuel control—Mastering calories and insulin
- Hunger control—Satiety: the science of fullness
- Waist control—Removing excess visceral adiposity (fat)

Let's look at each of these core principles, one by one.

Core Principle 1
Fuel Control—Mastering Calories and Insulin

The healthy eating system you're learning now is built around Habits of Health that give you the ability to control the quantity and quality of your energy intake. Most people aren't able to master this most fundamental principle even after a lifetime of struggle. You see, they're relying on their internal programming to select their food choices. But as we've discussed, that programming—which was optimal for a different time, when we needed to grab onto and hoard every calorie we consumed—is no longer helping us. Today, unlike 10,000 years ago, we have no system for disposing of all that excess energy. So if we consume more than we need to run our body, the extra calories get stored away—as fat. That fat around your middle is a symptom of an imbalance between your energy intake and energy output, with your intake set higher than it should be.

Here are the methods built into our system.

1. Portion Control

We have two important tools at our disposal to help us cut down the total amount of food we eat. The first, medically formulated portion-controlled meal replacements such as Medifast's®, are backed by a wealth of scientific research that documents their effectiveness. For many people, particularly those with busy lifestyles who need instant access to healthy, nutritious fuel, this high-quality "fast food" has become a permanent tool for weight maintenance, not just weight loss.

Nutrients we need
in relatively large
quantities are called
macronutrients,
while those we need
in relatively small
quantities are called
micronutrients.

The second, my nine-inch-plate system, is a simple visual technique that keeps you mindful of portion size for all three categories in our user-friendly system: protein, starch (carbohydrates), and fruits and vegetables.

2. Three-Hour Fuelings

Eating every three hours fits right into our nature as hunters and gatherers. Paired with low-glycemic eating, it turns off our insulin pump, keeps us at an even energy level, and helps us avoid wide swings in glucose (blood sugar) and other key nutrients. It also decreases the body's workload, and I believe will be shown to reduce dangerous oxygen radicals that lead to inflammation and disease. And, of course, it reduces the chances that you'll overeat due to cravings!

3. Fueling Percentages

Your body runs on three different types of fuels, or macronutrients—carbohydrate, fat, and protein. (A fourth type of fuel, alcohol, contains a significant number of calories but has no nutritive value.) Using these fuels in just the right proportions is a critical part of weight loss and optimal health. Let's look at each group, one by one.

Macronutrients as Fuel: Calorie Content in the Four Types of Macronutrients. Macronutrients—carbohydrates, fats, proteins, and alcohol—are the body's main fuel sources. The number of calories per gram differs, with fat containing the most calories, alcohol the second most, and carbohydrates and protein the least.

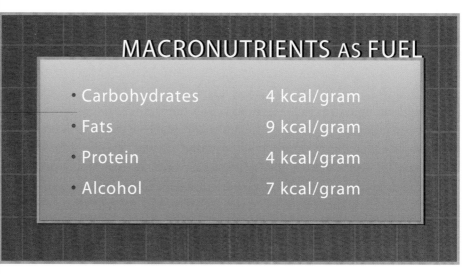

MACRONUTRIENTS AS FUEL

• Carbohydrates	4 kcal/gram
• Fats	9 kcal/gram
• Protein	4 kcal/gram
• Alcohol	7 kcal/gram

Carbohydrates: 50% of your daily calories

One of the primary drivers of my healthy eating system is the relationship between the carbohydrates you eat and your body's production of insulin, the key hormone in energy management.

When you eat carbohydrates, your blood sugar, or glucose, level rises, causing your pancreas to secrete insulin. This flood of insulin unlocks the gates that allow your body's tissues (especially muscle, your greatest energy consumer) to use glucose as an energy source. As a result, your blood sugar returns to normal. In a healthy individual, glucose level peaks about thirty minutes after a meal. Insulin levels rise accordingly, just behind the rising glucose level. It's a fine-tuned cycle that keeps blood sugar precisely controlled, as you can see in the chart on the next page.

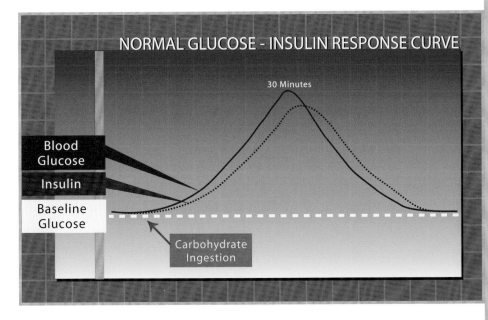

NORMAL GLUCOSE - INSULIN RESPONSE CURVE

30 Minutes

Blood Glucose

Insulin

Baseline Glucose

Carbohydrate Ingestion

Normal Glucose-Insulin Response Curve. In a healthy individual, blood sugar (glucose) levels rise and peak about thirty minutes after a meal. Insulin is secreted in response, at a precisely controlled level that lags just behind that of blood sugar.

When our insulin levels are too high for too long—a result of eating unhealthy, high-glycemic foods—we move quickly from a state of health to non-sickness and disease.

One of insulin's key roles is to determine whether the body takes more of its energy from carbohydrate or from fat. When insulin levels are low, as they are just after you get up in the morning, your body burns mainly fat. Having a healthy low-glycemic breakfast can keep you in this fat-burning state, as can a little early morning activity. When you follow this pattern, your body uses those healthy breakfast carbohydrates right away for energy, instead of storing them away as fat. Conversely, when insulin levels are high—for example, after you eat a high-carbohydrate meal—your body burns mainly carbohydrates and stores fat.

In fact, of the major food groups, carbohydrates (starches and sugars) are by far the greatest stimulators of insulin. That's why it's so important to eat low-glycemic carbohydrates, which don't raise blood sugar as much as high-glycemic carbohydrates do, and therefore put less demand on the pancreas to produce insulin.

Prolonged high levels of insulin can lead to diabetes in susceptible individuals. When that happens, the pancreas can no longer produce the right amount of insulin to control blood sugar (type 2 diabetes), and may eventually be unable to make insulin at all (type 1 diabetes).

Unfortunately, as we go about consuming our supersized meals in bliss, the damage begins without notice. Deep inside, high insulin levels are creating a state of inflammation, decreasing the flexibility of our blood vessels and causing premature aging of our cells. There are warnings to be had—poor sleep, low energy, headaches, thirst, cravings, hunger. But for many of us, these signs seem like nothing more than one more reason to stop at the fast food drive-thru or local drugstore to grab a soda and some painkillers. In fact, over 8 million Americans right now have diabetes *and don't even know it!*

The good news is that once you get your fueling mixture correct through my healthy eating program, you're going to feel unbelievably better. It will be like switching to high-performance fuel! And what's more, it has the power to prevent diabetes—or even stop it in its tracks.

Right now, over 8
million Americans have
diabetes and don't even
know it!

The Power of Low-Glycemic Eating

Remember, food can be used in one of two ways—as an energy source or stored away in fat cells. When you eat a high-glycemic meal, those cells respond by turning on the insulin and stimulating an enzyme that ramps up your fat-storage system. Low-glycemic eating, on the other hand, shuts down your fat factory. Let's see how that's going to work in Phase I.

Right now, you're probably eating too many calories, mostly from unhealthy carbohydrates like soda, bread, cookies, pizza, corn flakes, instant rice—any of a number of cheap, plentiful (and tasty!) high-glycemic foods. To find out just what happens to our bodies when we eat foods like these day in and day out, let's first take a look at the *glycemic index*—a great tool that makes it easy for you to choose carbohydrates that support health.

The glycemic index (GI), created in 1981 by Dr. David J. A. Jenkins, provides a standard for determining which foods raise blood sugar the highest, stimulating insulin production and weight gain. Using pure glucose, or sugar, as a reference point, Dr. Jenkins fed a variety of foods to his subjects and studied what happened to their glucose and insulin levels. Take a look at the chart below to see the results from eating pure glucose, which has a GI score of 100 on the 0–100 scale.

Note: The glycemic index of food is the percent area under the curve compared to glucose.

Glucose Reference
Curve: Glycemic Index.
When you eat pure glucose
(sugar) your blood glucose
(blood sugar) level rises
steeply and then falls.
Glucose has a score of
100 on the glycemic index,
a standard measure of
glycemic content in foods.
The glycemic index uses
a scale of 0–100.

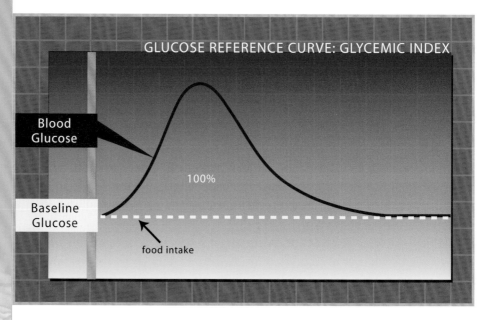

Now let's see what happens when you eat a low-glycemic food like lentils. (FYI, these small green legumes make a great-tasting soup.)

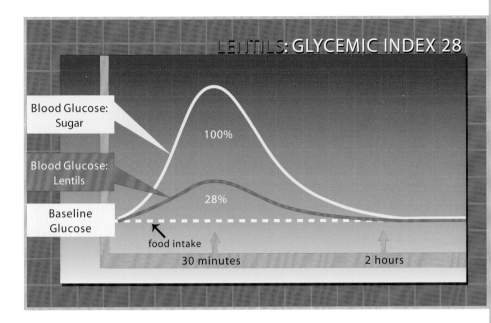

Lentils: Glycemic Index 28. Compare the rise in your blood glucose level when you eat lentils (green line) as opposed to pure sugar (yellow line). The curve is much less steep when you eat lentils, which have lower glycemic content.

As you can see, lentils raise blood sugar only 28 percent as much as glucose does, creating far less demand on the pancreas to secrete insulin.

Your body can handle high-glycemic food some of the time. But when you eat such foods daily, you create a chronic state of hyperinsulinism, the first step on the downward path to non-sickness and diabetes. Not to mention that this constant high level of glucose and insulin turns on fat storage and converts all that extra energy to... yep, fat. And what do you think happens after blood sugar level peaks? It drops, of course, to *below* normal. The result is hunger pangs and cravings that soon enough have us running for the next vending machine.

Here's a closer look at what happens when we eat high-glycemic versus low-glycemic foods.

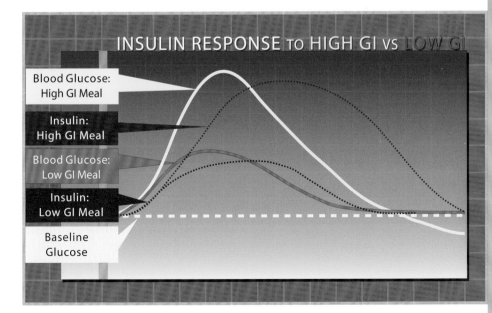

Insulin Response to High-Glycemic vs. Low-Glycemic Foods. When you eat low-glycemic foods (green line), your blood sugar and insulin levels don't rise as dramatically as they do when you eat high-glycemic foods (yellow line). As a result, you don't get a rebound effect that can cause your blood sugar to dip below normal between meals and lead to cravings and hunger pangs.

Now look what happens when we eat high-glycemic foods all day.

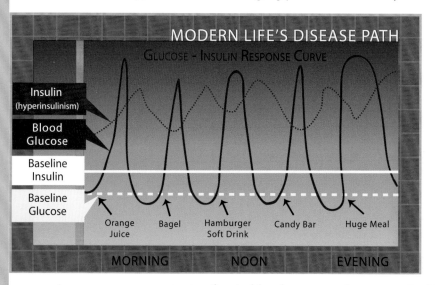

As you can see, constant spikes in blood sugar are interspersed with dips between meals that bring about cravings for yet more quick carbohydrates, and the insulin level remains elevated continuously. Today, over 45 million people in the U.S. alone suffer from hyperinsulinism as a result of Habits of Disease like these.

In Phase I, we're going to turn off your insulin pump right off the bat by limiting your intake to low-glycemic carbohydrates—foods that are 30 and under on the glycemic index (your dark green charts). Then we'll add nutrient-dense but lower-calorie fuel sources to help you feel full and gain control over your intake. It all adds up to a fat-busting, inflammation-soothing combo that would make Mother Nature herself proud!

Now let's turn to our second major food group—fat.

Fat: Less than 25% of your daily calories (less than 7% from saturated fat)

How big a role does fat ingestion have on blood sugar and insulin response? Let's take a look.

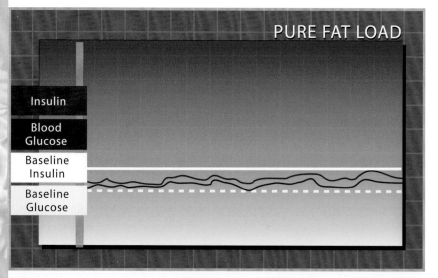

Pretty negligible, as you can see. Fat's role in weight gain and weight loss is related to its energy density rather than its effect on glucose and insulin. In fact, with nine calories per gram, *it provides over twice the energy per gram as carbohydrates!*

That caloric density helps explain why it's so easy to overdo our calorie intake by eating too much fat, and why doing so leads quickly to obesity—not to mention that fat tastes good and is easy for our bodies to store in virtually unlimited amounts. To help you keep fat in control, my healthy eating system encourages you to eat only healthy fats and to carefully monitor your overall fat consumption.

Protein: 20–25% of your daily calories

While protein provides energy, it's also our body's building block for cellular structure, immune function, and myriad health-giving processes.

Under my eating plan, in which every meal includes a highly digestible protein source, you benefit from a consistent supply of this important nutrient. This keeps your body from using muscle as a fuel source—a common problem on many other weight-loss plans. And regular protein means that your body has adequate building material for the repair and growth of critical support structures.

On top of which, studies have shown protein to be highly effective in spurring weight loss and maintenance—first, by helping you feel full, and second, by requiring more energy to digest than carbohydrates and fats do. You'll find out more about protein as a weight-loss tool in the next section, when we discuss *satiety* (the science of fullness).

The Role of Alcohol

Alcohol's not really a nutrient since it doesn't provide nutrition per se, but it does play a role in managing—or not managing—your weight. Not only is alcohol high in calories, it lowers inhibitions, making you more likely to overeat or to eat unhealthy foods. In fact, it can halt the fat-burning state in its tracks and diminish your ability to control your energy intake, and it should be avoided entirely during Phase I. If you do drink, you can resume doing so in Phase II—though you may want to change your drink of choice to red wine once you learn in Phase III and IV about the healthy, longevity-producing properties of some of its ingredients!

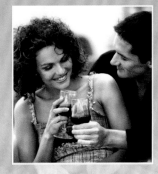

• •

Now that you've gained a better understanding of how your body uses the energy you feed it, let's take a look at some important techniques that can help you use that energy more effectively and fight hunger as you burn fat.

Satiety: (sə-tī′ĭ-tē) The
state of being full

Leptogenic: Likely
to cause someone to
become thin

Core Principle 2
Hunger Control—Satiety: The Science of Fullness

The emerging science of appetite control has given us a number of important ideas that can make your new *leptogenic* world—the world of thinness—that much stronger. Most of these principles are already built into your healthy eating strategies, so they should be pretty easy to grasp.

We'll focus on five principal areas that can help you fight hunger:

• Volumetrics
• Energy density
• Sensory-specific satiety
• Protein enhancement
• Fiber

Volume: The Key to Satiety

Research shows that we eat about the same volume or weight of food every day. So it makes sense, if you want to feel full quicker, to eat foods that are *low density* (that is, contain a lot of water) and *high volume* (meaning there's a large amount of food per calorie). Vegetables and fruits are good examples. In addition to being high in water content, they contain lots of nutrients, so they create a sense of fullness. That's why making foods from this group a large part of your meal—as you do when you use my healthy eating system—is so effective for weight loss and maintenance. With its color-coded listings and high percentage of vegetables and fruits, my system is designed to help you increase your intake of filling, low-density foods in the proper proportion.

Controlling Your Intake through Energy Density (ED)

Knowing the energy density (ED) of foods can help you choose ones that promote weight loss and maintenance—a particularly useful tool when you're choosing foods that aren't part of the glycemic index, such as meats. In fact, the ED number is already an important part of food labels on products in Europe and Canada.

But since we don't yet have this information on our food packaging, we need to calculate ED ourselves. To do so, divide the number of calories in one serving by the weight of that serving in grams. For example, if one serving of peanut butter contains 190 calories and weighs 32 grams, divide 190 by 32 for an ED of 5.9.

Once you have the ED, you can use this simple guide to determine which foods are good choices:

• **Best:** ED less than 1. Includes vegetables and fruits. Eat mostly foods from this group, which makes up 50 percent of our plate system.
• **Good:** ED between 1 and 2. Includes whole wheat pasta and skinless meats. These are also good choices.
• **Limit:** ED above 2. Choose these foods sparingly, but if you really want some, go ahead and enjoy them as a special treat.

When you use our healthy eating system, you'll automatically choose the right proportion of foods that help you feel full and minimize energy density. But for additional guidance, here's a diagram that categorizes some common foods based on their ED—another great tool to help you make healthy choices.

Foods with the lowest ED (the dark green section) are the best choice if you want to curb your appetite without adding a lot of calories. Foods with the highest ED (the dark red section) should be limited to those times when you really need to satisfy a craving. They're best eaten for taste—never when you're hungry.

FOOD GROUPINGS BY ENERGY DENSITY (ED) LEVEL

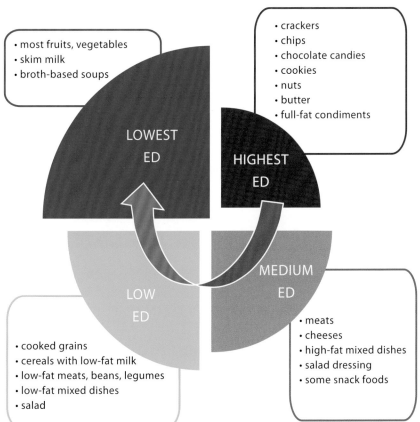

- most fruits, vegetables
- skim milk
- broth-based soups

LOWEST ED

- crackers
- chips
- chocolate candies
- cookies
- nuts
- butter
- full-fat condiments

HIGHEST ED

LOW ED

- cooked grains
- cereals with low-fat milk
- low-fat meats, beans, legumes
- low-fat mixed dishes
- salad

MEDIUM ED

- meats
- cheeses
- high-fat mixed dishes
- salad dressing
- some snack foods

Flavor Enhancement: The Food Industry's Dirty Little Secret

Did you know that flavor can either stimulate or suppress the brain's appetite control? While science is just beginning to understand how it all works, the food industry has been using this trick for decades, overloading our senses with processed foods filled with salt, sweet, and sour flavors to encourage us to overeat.

One classic way the food industry overstimulates our appetite centers is by masking ingredients. It may surprise you to find out that some cereals actually

Food Groupings by Energy Density (ED) Level. To feel satisfied while keeping calories in check, choose mostly foods from the *lowest*-ED section (dark green), followed by those from the *low*-ED section (light green). Eat foods from the *highest*-ED section (dark red) sparingly, and never when you're hungry.

A Habit of Health:
Avoiding foods with too
many ingredients

When you're shopping,
be sure to check the food
labels and avoid any
grocery items with lots
of ingredients. Studies
show that if a product
contains fewer than three
ingredients, you're less
apt to overeat.

• • • • • • • • • • • • • •

**Macronutrients Ranked
by Level of Satiety.** Which
types of foods make us
feel fullest? Protein is the
most filling, followed by
complex carbohydrates,
then fat. Alcohol is at the
bottom, making it a poor
choice when you're trying
to maintain your weight.

contain more salt than potato chips! As a result, we keep eating in order to satisfy our salt appetite center, even once our sugar senses are full.

Flavors can work the other way as well. Experts at Yale's Prevention Research Center found that people tend to feel fuller and stop eating sooner when a meal contains fewer flavors. So limiting the varieties of flavors that you eat may actually help you lose weight! The best way to do that? Limit your intake of processed foods and beat the food industry at its own game! Instead, let your color-coded shopping charts be your guide to buying healthy whole foods with flavors that are naturally satisfying and true.

Battle Hunger with Protein

Don't skimp on protein! Studies have shown that protein makes us feel fuller than other macronutrients such as carbohydrates and fats. A recent Washington School of Medicine study showed that participants on a controlled higher-protein diet (up to 30 percent of their daily intake from protein) felt less hungry than those on a lower-protein diet (as little as 15 percent protein). And when given as much to eat as they wanted, the higher-protein group lost considerably more weight than the lower-protein group.

Another benefit of protein is that your body uses more energy to break it down, and that means you're burning more calories just to digest it. So the total number of calories you need to maintain your weight might be a little higher if you eat the right amount of protein.

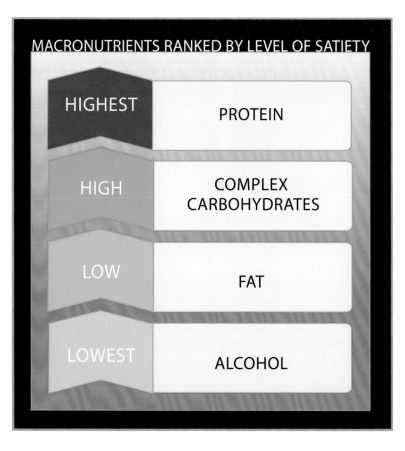

MACRONUTRIENTS RANKED BY LEVEL OF SATIETY

HIGHEST	PROTEIN
HIGH	COMPLEX CARBOHYDRATES
LOW	FAT
LOWEST	ALCOHOL

That's one reason we've been careful to include the proper proportion of healthy low-fat proteins in our healthy eating strategy (25 percent of your plate), as well as ample portions of low-density complex carbohydrates (50 percent of your plate). That way you know you're choosing the most satisfying and filling foods available.

Remember, though, that some high-protein foods can be extremely energy dense because of their fat content. Grabbing a handful of nuts may stave off hunger, but it comes at the price of high calories. Just be sure to keep your intake moderate.

Fill Up with Fiber!

Not only does fiber provide critical health benefits, it also fills you up so you're less tempted to overeat. As we discussed in chapter 9, both soluble and insoluble fiber are important. Let's go over the differences.

Soluble fiber slows the breakdown of complex carbohydrates, helping reduce blood sugar. In the right quantity, it can even help lower blood cholesterol. Soluble fiber is found in rye, barley, oats, vegetables, legumes, and fruits.

Insoluble fiber can't be absorbed or digested by the body, but it still provides a number of benefits, including reducing hunger and cleaning your digestive tract by pulling water into the colon, which stimulates regular bowel movements. Insoluble fiber is found in brown rice, whole wheat breads, cereals, seeds, vegetables, fruit skin, and legumes.

Are You Sure You're Hungry?

Stress, socializing, watching TV, eating out with friends—all of these can contribute to mindless eating.

Our three-hour fueling strategy should fulfill your body's energy needs most of the time. So if you find yourself wanting to eat outside of your planned meals and fueling breaks, you may well be responding to something other than hunger.

If so, remember the tools that keep you on your path. Eat slowly, paying attention to all the sensory input you're experiencing through your food. You'll feel full and satisfied sooner. In time, eating mindfully in this way will become second nature. Becoming more aware of your eating habits and experiences will help you stay focused and encourage you to make the best secondary choices to support your primary goals.

Could You Be Thirsty?

Sometimes when we think we're hungry, it's really a sign that our body's craving water. Here's a tip: Next time you feel hungry, grab a big glass of water and drink the whole thing. Wait fifteen minutes or so and ask yourself if you're still hungry. About 30 percent of the time, what we think is hunger is something else entirely.

Before Increasing Your Dietary Protein
Upping your intake of protein can put a larger load on your kidneys. If you have healthy kidneys and drink plenty of water, you can handle a moderate increase in daily protein intake. People with existing renal disease or severe diabetes, on the other hand, should check with their doctor before significantly increasing the amount of protein in their diet. To find out your protein cut-off point, divide your weight in pounds by two. The result is a good estimate of your upper limit of protein per day in grams.

A Habit of Health: Asking yourself if you're really hungry before you eat

A Habit of Health: Being aware of cravings

The vast majority of our taste satisfaction—95 percent—comes from the first three bites. So when you have a hankering for something sweet, salty, creamy, extremely energy dense, or full of high-glycemic carbs—you know, one of those Habits of Disease—don't just push that feeling away. Grab a tablespoon and take a bite. Just one. Wait a couple of minutes and ask yourself, Am I satisfied? Repeat up to three times over the next several minutes, while remaining in a mindful state. Ask yourself if continuing this behavior supports your primary goals.

You now have a comprehensive understanding of your healthy eating strategy and know how to use tools such as portion-controlled meal replacements (PCMRs), a nine-inch plate, the three major food components, and the color-coded system to stay on top of your energy intake and hunger for life.

A recent study showed that simply by decreasing portion size and energy density by 25 percent, people were able to maintain their healthy weight.* And now, so can you. Combine your new understanding of portion control and energy density with your knowledge of healthy protein, starch, and vegetables and fruits, and you have the Habits of Health to support a lifetime of healthy eating!

Core Principle 3
Waist Control—Removing Excess Visceral Adiposity

You now know a bit more about how the extra energy you take in leads to fat. But how exactly do you go about unloading this dangerous villain?

Many people think the answer is exercise. Well, that's true if you're close to your healthy weight and just want to maintain the status quo. But intense exercise simply isn't the best way to lose weight. And for someone who's overweight and out of shape, it's a downright terrible way! For starters, I've seen far too many overweight people strain their knees, develop tendonitis and lower-back pain, or worse from pounding the pavement in a desperate attempt to lose weight. Plus, it's not even effective! People join gyms in droves in January, but by April—when those very same gyms are a ghost town—they've resigned themselves yet again to being overweight.

In fact, holding off or at least cutting back on exercise for the first few weeks of Phase I is critical to reaching a fat-burning state and experiencing safe, effective weight loss. It's the difference between success and failure! Why? At this beginning stage, exercise can actually slow weight loss down by stimulating stress hormones. In addition, as your body uses up its glycogen stores and adjusts to a lower insulin level and salt intake during the first week, it will eliminate any excess water it was holding onto. The resulting decrease in blood pressure can make you fatigued, lightheaded, or dizzy if you exercise prematurely.

Besides, steering clear of exercise for now gives you time to learn and slowly begin applying important Habits of Health such as stretching, progressive movement, and eventually weight resistance training. It's all about sequencing you for success, and it's one of the elements that sets this program apart from many others. We use your early success to generate more success.

It just makes sense! Keeping you in a fat-burning state is the most efficient way I know to unload excess fat. Let's look at a couple of examples to help you understand just how this smart approach to weight loss works.

Our first example is a healthy male who weighs 167 pounds and has a BMI (body mass index) of 24. The chart on the next page shows you his energy-storage percentage for each major energy source.

*Rolls, B. J., et al., "Reductions in Portion Size and Energy Density of Foods," *American Journal of Clinical Nutrition* 83 (January 2006): 11–17.

Protein represents 18 percent of this man's energy stores, and is designed to be used for energy only in emergencies, such as starvation. Our program, unlike many diets, is designed to protect against a dangerously low protein level, which can lead to cyclical yo-yoing. *Glycogen,* your body's store of carbohydrates, is less than 1 percent in this man.

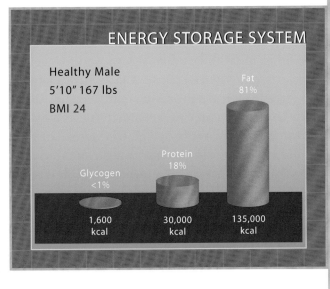

Fat, on the other hand, is plentiful and provides a rich reservoir of energy—over 135,000 calories in this example.

Now look at the chart below to compare this healthy individual to someone who through poor daily choices—perhaps as little as one soda a day!—has reached a BMI of 30 and is medically obese. At 209 pounds, he's accumulated 42 pounds of unhealthy fat, each of which contains the energy equivalent of 3,500 calories. His fat-storage facility has sequestered an excess 147,000 calories of energy!

This obese male has doubled his fat stores to a whopping 282,000 calories! He needs to offload all this extra energy before it precipitates a heart attack, stroke, or other health hazard!

Now, what if he were to try to do this through exercise alone, while maintaining his normal eating pattern? Let's see . . . running a marathon race consumes on average about 2,600 calories. Assuming for a moment that our obese friend here could even manage this level of activity (which I definitely wouldn't recom-

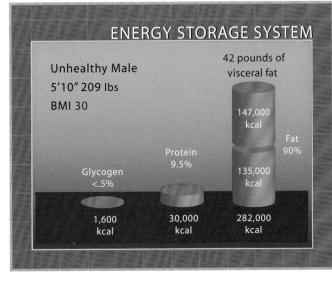

mend!), he'd have to run more than fifty-six marathons to burn off his excess weight. If he were to run one marathon a week, it would take him over a year to offload those calories—and that's using one of the most intense forms of exercise there is!

Energy Storage System: Healthy Male. This man has a healthy proportion and amount of fat, protein, and glycogen (carbohydrates) stored away.

Energy Storage System: Unhealthy Male. At 209 pounds, this obese individual has accumulated 42 extra pounds of dangerous visceral fat around his organs.

Let's contrast that scenario with our healthy eating strategy. We could help this same unhealthy man reach his healthy weight and offload those 147,000 calories of fat in less than sixteen weeks—safely, without significant loss of muscle, *and without exercise*. And we have a retrospective study performed by independent researchers from Johns Hopkins University to validate it!*

How? By inducing a natural fat-burning state while protecting, and even enhancing, the body's protein stores. First, you limit your energy intake through our portion-control system, lowering your total daily calories to below your current energy expenditure. This discrepancy causes your body to burn through its limited supply of stored carbohydrates (glycogen) in the first few days, while your low-glycemic, decreased-carbohydrate diet helps turn down your insulin pump. As a result, your body sends out signals that it needs energy. The ensuing hormonal changes convert your fat cells from storage centers to little fuel tanks full of triglycerides, a substance that the liver converts into useful energy through a process called *ketosis*—in other words, fat burning (not to be confused with *ketoacidosis,* an unrelated condition that occurs in diabetes). Once you enter this controlled fat-burning state, you can offload two to five pounds per week for the first two weeks and one to two pounds per week thereafter.

You can see why it just doesn't make sense to try to reach your healthy weight through exercise alone. A much easier, safer, and more effective method is to tap into this excess fat reserve and use it as an energy source. There will be plenty of time to add exercise once you're feeling better—and in fact, when the time's right I'll guide you through a progressive series of easy-to-learn steps to help you develop habits that support greater flexibility, cardiovascular health, and muscle strength.

Your New Weight-Loss and Health Path: Glucose-Insulin Response Curve. Once you begin to control your energy intake by eating frequent low-glycemic meals and snacks, your body's internal response will quickly level out, reducing the blood sugar spikes and dips that lead to cravings and the high insulin output that leads to dangerous inflammation and disease.

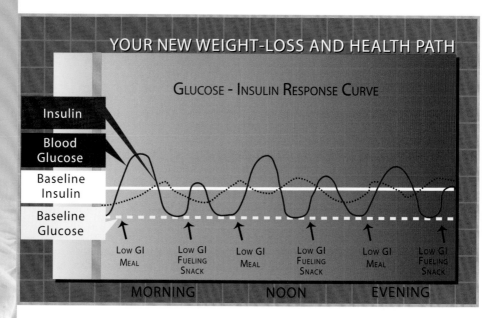

*Crowel, M. D., and Cheskin, L. J., Johns Hopkins University School of Medicine, "Multicenter Evaluation of Health Benefits and Weight Loss on the Medifast Weight Management Program."

In the meantime, our healthy eating system is designed to bring order to your day and restore function to your body. Just take a look at the illustration on page 144 to see the difference in your blood sugar and insulin level once you begin to unload excess calories, turn off your insulin pump, and turn on fat burning by mastering your energy intake!

Best of all, once you've reached your healthy weight, you can use this very same system (with expanded variety and calories) to maintain it. Soon, with the addition of my healthy movement program, you'll be burning enough extra calories to stay at your ideal weight indefinitely! It's all part of my balanced plan to move beyond weight loss to a state that supports you for life—in optimal health.

"You can't put a price on optimal health."

GREG REX

Over six years at optimal health

Even as a kid, I was teased for being chubby. To help control my weight, I got involved in high-endurance sports with the hope of being in shape to pursue my passion—surfing. But once I started working, I had less time for exercise, so I started dieting. Juice fasts, vegetarianism, food-combining, eating for my body type, high-protein, low-fat, you name it. Even when I did lose weight, I just gained back more.

At age 37, I weighed 233 with a BMI (body mass index) of 32. My life was totally out of balance. I was so heavy I couldn't even surf! So I hired a triathlon coach and trained five days a week for a year, but the scale didn't even move. After one year of all those disciplined workouts and trying to "eat less"—in other words, starving myself all day, exercising like crazy, and eating a huge meal at night—I lost just three pounds. I lost 53 pounds using the Medifast PCMRs and the help of my Take Shape for Life coach.

It's been six years now, and I'm still at my college weight and I am now living the Habits of Health. I sleep better now and have the energy of a 25-year-old. My body fat is between 14 and 16 percent,

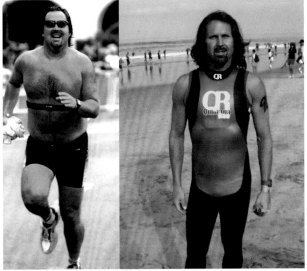

Results vary. Typical weight loss is 2-5 lbs per week for the first 2 weeks and 1-2 lbs per week thereafter.

down from 38. And best of all, I'm traveling the world surfing twenty-foot waves. You can't put a price on that! ∎

Dr. A Says . . .

Suffering from back pain? Maintaining a healthy weight is the number one way to strengthen and protect your back, according to the American Council on Exercise.

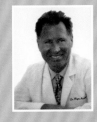

Share Your Success!
We love to hear from
folks who've made the
commitment to optimal
health and are turning
their life around. Share
your story at
www.habitsofhealth.net

Phase II
Learning the Habits of Health
The Foundation of Long-Term Success

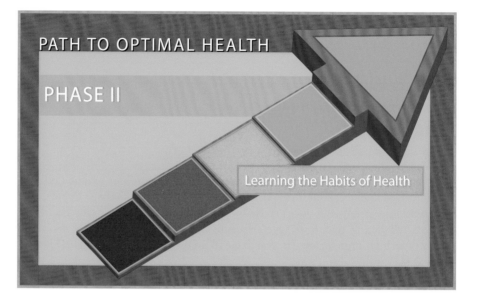

Congratulations on reaching your healthy weight! You've now positioned your body to operate efficiently, and I'll bet you're feeling better than you have in quite a while.

Why not celebrate your success by doing something you never thought you could do—like one client of mine who lost 150 pounds and went sky-diving on her sixtieth birthday to celebrate her new healthy body.

The Beginning of Your Journey

Most weight-loss systems (a.k.a. diets) end once you lose the weight—a recipe for yo-yoing and weight regain. But in our plan, reaching your healthy weight in Phase I is really just the beginning of your journey to optimal health.

Our focus during Phase II is to solidify this first important step. To do so, we're going to build on your early success by learning and reinforcing the Habits of Health that make it easier to maintain your new healthy weight as you take the next steps on your journey.

Before we start, let's review your energy management system as it looks now and find out how it's going to change during transition and throughout Phase II.

Your Phase II Energy Diagram

In Phase I, we helped you reach a healthy weight by reducing the total number of calories you eat and by teaching you to choose healthy, low-glycemic foods—a process that turned your body's fat-storage machine into a fat fire sale. Now we're going to shift our focus. By increasing both your caloric intake and your caloric expenditure, we're going to help you reach equilibrium—the state at which you're able to maintain your weight most efficiently.

Let's revisit our energy diagram.

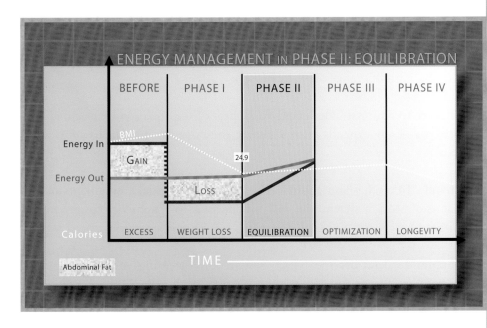

ENERGY MANAGEMENT IN PHASE II: EQUILIBRATION

| | BEFORE | PHASE I | PHASE II | PHASE III | PHASE IV |

Energy In — BMI — 24.9
Energy Out
GAIN
LOSS
Calories — EXCESS — WEIGHT LOSS — EQUILIBRATION — OPTIMIZATION — LONGEVITY
TIME
Abdominal Fat

Energy Management in Phase II: Equilibration. In Phase II, you'll reach a state of equilibrium—a balance between *energy in* (calories consumed, represented by the red line) and *energy out* (calories expended, represented by the green line). Your body mass index (BMI), represented by the dotted white line, will remain relatively stable at around 24.9. As you add healthy muscle, your BMI may rise slightly.

As you can see, in Phase II your *energy in* (red line) and *energy out* (green line) will meet at a natural set point—the point where you've achieved a proper balance between the calories you consume and the calories you expend. Reaching this set point puts you in complete command of your weight and is instrumental to both optimal health and longevity.

A Teachable Moment

Now that your palate has been cleansed of processed food, with its excess salt, fat, and high-fructose corn syrup, it's the perfect time to solidify the healthy eating habits learned in Phase I. As we expand your food intake, we want to make sure that these new habits have become automatic. If not, you'll be susceptible to *calorie creep*—an insidious increase in your daily intake. Unfortunately, our nutritionally polluted world makes it easy to slip. That's why it's all the more important to stay mindful and to lock in the Habits of Health through tools such as my healthy eating strategies and convenient medically formulated portion-controlled meal replacements.

Right now you're experiencing a creative, exciting, satisfying period of generative growth, on top of which you're about to add more variety to your meals.

Metabolism: The biochemical process by which your body converts food into energy. During metabolism, calories—from carbohydrates, fats and proteins—are combined with oxygen to release the energy your body needs in order to function.

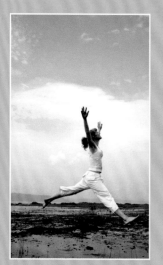

But this time of transition is also the period when most people who have lost weight fail.

The next seven chapters provide a protective blanket of new Habits of Health to help transform your lifestyle into one of permanent health. By the end of Phase II, you'll have learned the behaviors you need to support a lifetime of health!

Chapter 12 transitions you into my permanent healthy eating plan. You'll learn why most diets fail and how proper motivation (which you learned about in chapters 3 and 4) makes it easy to make the necessary adjustments to your energy management system and create a lifelong eating strategy. That includes dialing up your calories, increasing the amount of food you eat, and introducing a full range of healthy foods.

Chapter 13 addresses the "energy out" part of the equation by teaching you how your body expends energy, setting the stage for our Habits of Motion system.

Chapter 14 teaches you about NEAT and EAT, essential components of the Habits of Motion system that will provide an A-to-Z approach to movement for life.

Chapter 15 describes the NEAT System for increasing your daily activity without exercise or any demands on your daily schedule. This is a wonderful entry point for those who haven't been active, as well a great way to increase the energy expenditure of the seasoned exercise enthusiast.

Chapter 16 continues adding movement to your day through the EAT System, using a formalized walking program to begin increasing your muscular and skeletal strength.

Chapter 17 explores why sleep is critical to maintaining a healthy weight and helping the body recuperate, and provides tips for improving the quantity and quality of your sleep.

Chapter 18 discusses the importance of proper support, particularly in light of recent discoveries on the power of social networks to create health or disease.

By the end of Phase II, you'll have built a foundation of habits that will guide and support your health for the rest of your life. Let's start this phase by completing your permanent eating strategy to produce a lifetime of optimal health.

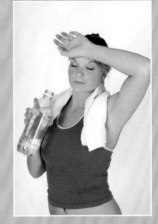

Chapter 12

Healthy Eating for Life

Your Transition to Permanent Health

Your discipline throughout Phase I has paid off. You've reached a healthy weight—the first important milestone on the path to creating optimal health. And that means you're ready to transition to Phase II. In Phase II, we'll start by expanding and developing the eating plan you used during Phase I to create a strategy you can use for life.

Phase II is also a time for learning how to make many daily choices that will assist you on your journey to optimal health. First, let's review the Habits of Health you've learned so far, which form the foundation for all your success to come.

Six of these beginning habits, which you're learning while you're losing weight, spell out the acronym BeSlim™—a tool I created at Medifast®/Take Shape for Life™ to help you understand the behaviors essential to maintaining a healthy weight.

"BeSlim"

- Breakfast
- Exercise
- Support
- Low-fat meals every three hours
- Individual plan
- Monitor

Now we're going to take these beginning steps and start developing them into your comprehensive long-term optimal health plan. Here's how.

> Breakfast. By now, you're in the habit of beginning each day with a healthy breakfast (which may be in the form of a portion-controlled meal replacement)—an important routine that's critical for long-term weight loss, according to the National Weight Control Registry.

> Exercise. As your weight has decreased, perhaps you've started adding more activity, using the stairs instead of the elevator, for example, or taking the dog for a walk. If you've been in Phase I for a while, you may have started learning my progressive movement systems for sustainable exercise, as outlined in chapters 13–16. Whatever your current level of physical ability, my plan is

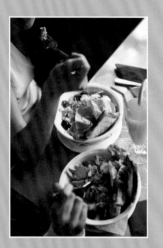

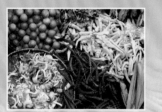

designed to give you an easy entry into the world of fitness. You've been hearing me talk about the relatively minor role exercise plays in weight loss. Well, that was true in the beginning of Phase I. But increasing your activity level becomes very important as you move from Phase I into Phase II and beyond. After the first three weeks of Phase I, your body is ready for increased motion. You're lighter, you have more confidence, you're physically healthier, you have the right motivation, and you're in better command of the beginning Habits of Health. My NEAT and EAT plans for physical movement are doable and fit your current level of health and fitness. Over time, these systems will put you on track for success!

> **Support.** I'm a big believer in seeking help on your journey to optimal health. While I can serve as your immediate mentor, having a live coach such as a health care professional or a trained health coach can add tremendous value. We'll discuss this further in chapter 18. Additionally, your family, friends, or weight-loss buddy or group can be helpful for encouragement and moral support.

> **Low-fat meals every three hours.** You're now in the habit of eating smaller meals every three hours—a very powerful Habit of Health. And low-fat, low-glycemic eating has been shown to be a key factor in long-term maintenance of weight loss. This is a great time to review the lessons of healthy eating. In fact, there will never be a better time. You're feeling better, you're tuned into the proper motivation and healthy choices, and you're learning how to choose and prepare foods that support your health.

As you learned in chapters 8–10, your permanent eating strategy includes meals that:

- Are low-glycemic
- Satisfy your hunger
- Control your caloric intake
- Contain low amounts of healthy fats
- Keep to a three-hour eating schedule

These basic behaviors form the key Habits of Health you'll need to keep in mind as you head into Phase II.

Now, as you begin your transition, we're going to expand the food choices available to you (while keeping within our healthy guidelines) and add calories to your meals until you reach equilibrium between your energy in and energy out. That's how we'll make our healthy eating system into a complete plan that teaches you how to eat for a lifetime of health.

> **Individual plan.** Now that you're past the initial weight-loss stage, you're ready to build a permanent plan that gives you control over your energy intake and long-term strategies for life.

> **Monitor.** You've gotten used to checking your weight weekly. Keeping an eye on your energy balance helps you make sure you're not loading fat. (See box, below, Monitor Your Weight and Measurements Regularly.)

Now that you've solidified your understanding of these key Habits of Health, let's look ahead to what's next—learning how to use these important new behaviors to maintain your weight loss and build optimal health for life!

The Two Keys to Maintaining Your Healthy Weight

There are two main reasons why most diets fail when used without other supports: a lack of understanding of energy balance, and a lack of understanding of proper motivation.

1. Energy Balance:
The First Key to Maintaining Your Healthy Weight

The fat cells in your body use energy. When you lose weight, you decrease your metabolic demands, and the amount of energy your fat cells use decreases significantly as well. As a result, you experience a lower level of daily energy expenditure. If you simply go back to your old, pre-diet eating habits (as dieters so often do), your energy needs will be out of balance, and your new, lighter body will be taking in more energy than it can use. And as a result, your weight can balloon. It's the classic yo-yo pattern, caused by an ever-widening gap between energy in and energy out.

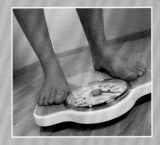

A Habit of Health:
Monitoring your weight
and measurements
regularly

Monitor Your Weight and Measurements Regularly

Regularly monitoring your weight and waist and hip measurements is an important surveillance tool and provides an accurate picture of your current reality. Remember, the scale and tape measure are your friends! Here are some tips:

- Set up a regular schedule for weighing and measuring. I believe that once a week is the most reliable schedule for tracking a trend, but daily is fine if you prefer.
- Weigh and measure yourself in as little clothing as possible.
- Weigh and measure yourself on the same scale and at the same time of day. Most people are at their lowest weight in the early morning.
- Use my favorite technique to check inches and weight: Monitor yourself regularly by trying on a favorite pair of jeans or pants whose proper fit you know well. If you have to get on the bed and hold your stomach in, you'll know you're putting on weight and need to adjust your calories accordingly!

Even worse are unbalanced diets that lower calories so severely that your body is forced to cannibalize its own muscle, or diets designed to fabricate weight loss by manipulating macronutrients such as fats and carbohydrates, producing an imbalance in the amount of energy you take in from each group. Diets like these are hard to sustain. The body isn't shy about letting you know it has a macronutrient deficit, and soon enough the cravings will begin. Even if you do manage to stay with one of these diets long enough to lose some weight, once the diet's over, it's off to the races to replenish that deficit. That's why a low-carbohydrate diet has no chance of long-term success. After all, nature knows best!

Medically formulated low-calorie meal replacements and my Healthy Eating for Life System deliver a proper balance of macronutrients in the form of healthy, great-tasting, low-glycemic foods that will keep you satisfied for a lifetime and protect your muscles from attack.

Optimal Daily Intake of Macronutrients for Long-Term Health. Your body needs a balance of **macronutrients**—carbohydrates, proteins, and fats—in order to run at its best. Some diets manipulate macronutrients, producing an imbalance of energy from each group. But these diets are hard to sustain.

Optimal Daily Intake of Macronutrients

Macronutrient	Energy per Gram	Percent of Total Daily Calorie Intake
Carbohydrates	4 kcal/gram	44–55%
Protein	4 kcal/gram	20–25%
Fat	9 kcal/gram	15–25%

2. Proper Motivation: The Second Key to Maintaining Your Healthy Weight

Many people go on a diet with the sole purpose of losing pounds—so when their weight-loss goal is reached, they think they're done. And they're glad, because their diet has been a period of great deprivation, and they can't wait to get back to their old way of life. But with our plan, reaching a healthy weight is just the first step on your path. Your underlying motivation is inspired by your fundamental choice—the choice of optimal health that you adopted during our preparation for this journey.

In *Living a Longer, Healthier Life: The Companion Guide to Dr. A's Habits of Health,* you'll find a number of exercises focusing on motivation and choice. This is a good time to take a look at those, if you haven't done so already, and make sure you have a firm grasp of the motivation behind your decision to lose weight and attain optimal health. These new habits are integral to your success as you review your current reality and prepare to move forward from where you are right now to where you want to be.

Your Current Reality

You're now at your healthy weight, equipped with habits that will serve you well for the rest of your life—a life that may indeed be longer and of higher quality as you align with your fundamental choice. Let's review these habits.

- You're eating smaller portions at regular intervals (every three hours).
- You're eating lower-glycemic carbohydrates, healthy proteins, and healthy fats and oils.
- You've learned how to plan meals in advance so you're no longer just reacting to hunger and your environment.

As a result, you've gone from an overweight fat-storing state to a healthy fat-burning state. Now it's time to move forward by solidifying your healthy eating strategies and continuing your journey toward optimal health.

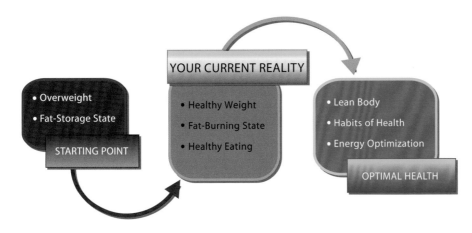

Your Current Reality.
As you enter Phase II, your current reality has shifted from your starting point. This transition brings you closer to optimal health.

Overview of Your Transition

The transition to your lifetime healthy eating strategy consists of two parts:

- Adding calories until you reach your set point (calories in = calories out)
- Introducing a full range of foods to support optimal health and maintain your healthy weight

Transition: A process or period marked by change. The passage from one state to another.

First, let's figure out your set point—the point at which the number of calories you take in is equal to the number of calories you use. The best way to do that is to figure out how many calories you burn in the course of a day. In other words, how many calories should you eat daily to maintain your healthy weight?

Determining Your Total Energy Expenditure (TEE)

Want to figure out how many calories you need to eat in Phase II to keep those jeans fitting just right? The most common method is to calculate your *total energy expenditure,* or TEE. Calculating your TEE as it is right now at your healthy weight will help us determine your optimal caloric intake during this phase. (We'll work on increasing that number in the next chapter as part of our overall Habits of Health strategy.)

Your TEE is determined by adding three figures:

- Your basal metabolic rate (BMR)
- Your physical activity level (PAL)
- The thermic effect of the food you eat (TEF)

Together, these show us how quickly your body is burning the fuel you're taking in, day in and day out.

Let's begin by looking separately at those three components.

Basal Metabolic Rate (BMR) is the energy you use for your basic bodily needs. Even when your body's at rest, it's using fuel to breathe, grow, circulate your blood, adjust your hormone levels, repair cells, and perform other functions. Typically, BMR is the largest portion of the TEE energy equation. Because the energy required by these basic functions remains fairly consistent, this number doesn't tend to change much.

Physical Activity Level (PAL) is the energy you use when you move—playing tennis, walking to the store, chasing after the dog. You have control of this number, and can change it quite a bit depending on the frequency, duration, and intensity of your activities.

Thermic Effect of Food (TEF) is the energy your body uses to process your food. Digesting, absorbing, transporting, and storing food all take energy—about 10 percent of the calories you use each day. For the most part, this number stays steady.

Take a look at the diagram below. You'll see that BMR is the largest energy user, accounting for 60–75 percent of your daily expenditure. PAL ranges from 25–30 percent, and TEF takes up 10–15 percent.

Total Energy Expenditure (TEE). To find out how much energy you use in a day—and therefore how many calories you should be eating—we're going to add up your basal metabolic rate, your physical activity level, and the thermic effect of the food you eat. Each of these three components accounts for a certain percentage of your total daily energy use.

TOTAL ENERGY EXPENDITURE (TEE)

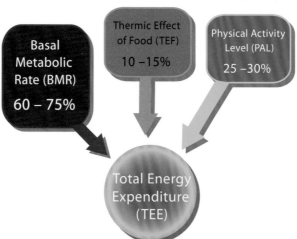

Basal Metabolic Rate (BMR) 60 – 75%

Thermic Effect of Food (TEF) 10 –15%

Physical Activity Level (PAL) 25 –30%

Total Energy Expenditure (TEE)

Calculating Your TEE

Now that you know what goes into your TEE, let's start figuring out your number. There are a couple of options available to help us, some more accurate than others. If you're not a math major or don't feel like getting out the calculator, you can start with a rough method to calculate your daily caloric needs. This initial number doesn't need to be exact, since it's only a starting point that you'll be adjusting as you monitor your weight throughout transition.

Option 1: The easy way to calculate TEE

To find out your TEE using the easy method, use the following formula:

Your current weight (in pounds) × 11 calories = TEE (daily caloric need)

This formula is based on a sedentary individual, so you'll need to adjust it as you step up your exercising, as follows:

Multiply your TEE by:
- 1.2 (for light exercise)
- 1.5 (for moderate exercise)
- 1.7 (for heavy exercise)

For example: 162 lbs × 11 kcal/lb = 1,782 kcal × 1.2 = 2,138 kcal/day (TEE)

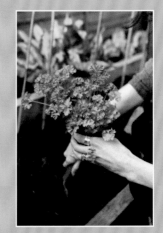

Remember to recalculate this number as you track your weight over the next several weeks.

Option 2: The harder but more accurate way to calculate TEE

To find out your TEE using the more accurate method, use the following formula:

$$TEE = BMR + PAL + TEF$$

First, let's break that formula down and find out how to calculate each part: BMR, PAL, and TEF.

1. Basal Metabolic Rate (BMR)

In the intensive care unit, I used various equations to calculate my patients' energy needs. This one, called the Mifflin-St. Jeor, takes into account differences in sex, height, weight, and age, for an accurate BMR:

Men:
10 × (weight in pounds × 0.455) + 6.25 × (height in inches × 2.54) − 5 × (age) + 5 = BMR

Women:
10 × (weight in pounds × 0.455) + 6.25 × (height in inches × 2.54) − 5 × (age) − 161 = BMR

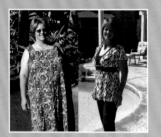

"I finally found out how to maintain weight loss forever."

KAREN KRUEGER

*Over two years
at optimal health*

My journey to optimal health began after a trip to Hawaii with my husband. What should have been a dream vacation made me feel like a beached whale! Something drastic needed to be done.

I learned about the system Dr. Andersen uses in Take Shape for Life to help people reach a healthy weight. I was impressed with the success stories I read online, and I thought, "What do I have to lose but fat?" I went from size 2X to size small and from 217 pounds to 126! I could never have imagined myself this size!

The program is so easy, the foods are convenient and portable, and they taste fabulous. And the best part of my journey? Through the Habits of Health I finally found out how to maintain weight loss forever and gain lifelong tools for optimal health! ■

Results vary. Typical weight loss is 2-5 lbs per week for the first 2 weeks and 1-2 lbs per week thereafter.

2. Physical Activity Level (PAL)

Your BMR is the amount of energy you expend if you're completely still. We need to modify your BMR to take into account the extra energy you expend as a result of your physical activity level (PAL). To do so, choose the *activity factor* from the Activity Factor Table below that most accurately describes your current activity level and multiply that number by your BMR. We'll call the result (your modified BMR) your EEpal, a number that represents your baseline BMR plus the extra calories you expend due to physical activity.

$$\text{EEpal} = \text{BMR} \times \text{Activity Factor (in other words, BMR + PAL)}$$

Activity Factor Table

1.2	sedentary
1.5	slightly active (light exercise or sports 1–3 days per week)
1.8	moderately active (job entails standing with some walking; moderate exercise or sports 3–5 days per week)
2.0	very active (job entails walking; strenuous exercise or sports 6–7 days per week)
2.2+	extremely active (physically strenuous job; very strenuous exercise or sports)

3. Thermic Effect of Food (TEF)

This final component calculates the amount of energy it takes for your body to process your food. While this number varies depending on the type of food you eat, it's generally about 10 percent of the total number of calories you consume. In other words:

$$\text{TEF} = \text{total calories consumed} \times 10\%$$

Now add that TEF to your EEpal (your modified BMR with PAL taken into account). In other words:

$$\text{TEE} = \text{EEpal [BMR} \times \text{AF]} + \text{TEF}$$

Adding together the three components you've just calculated will give you an accurate measure of the total number of calories you use in a day. And that's the same number of calories you'll need to eat in order to stay at your healthy weight.

Let's try out our formula using the following example:

- 46-year-old female
- 5 foot, 9 inches (69 inches)
- Sedentary
- Body mass index of 24
- 162 pounds (down from 206 pounds)

Here's our TEE formula: TEE = BMR + PAL + TEF

(or, for the purposes of our calculations, TEE = EEpal [BMR × AF] + TEF)

Now we'll plug in her numbers, starting with BMR.

1. BMR = 10 × (weight in pounds × 0.455) + 6.25 × (height in inches × 2.54) − 5 × (age) − 161

> = 10 × (164 × 0.455) + 6.25 (69 × 2.54) − 5 × (46) -161
> = 746 + 1,095 − 230 − 161
> = 1,450 calories per day

2. PAL (BMR modified for activity)

> EEpal = BMR × Activity Factor

This formula will tell us how much extra she burns on top of her BMR as a result of her level of activity.

> = 1,450 calories × 1.2 [sedentary]
> = 1,740 calories per day

3. TEF = EEpal (1,740 kcal) × 0.1 (that is, 10%)

> = 174 calories per day

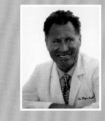

Now, if we take 1,740 calories (the modified increase in BMR as a result of activity, or EEpal) and add the thermic effect of food (TEF), which is 10% of that modified number, we get a total energy requirement of 1,914 calories per day.

> EEpal [1,740] + TEF [174] = 1,914
> TEE = 1,914 kcals/day

Let's say that she's currently eating 1,200 calories a day. The number of calories she can add and safely maintain her healthy weight is the difference between her TEE (the total calories she needs to maintain her weight) and her current level of calories:

> 1,914 calories per day − 1,200 calories per day = 714 calories per day

So the woman in this example would add approximately 714 calories to her daily intake.

Now that you know how to calculate your TEE, let's find out the best way to add foods and increase your daily calorie consumption to match it.

Your Transition Eating Plan

> *If you used the portion-controlled meal replacement (PCMR) system exclusively during Phase I,* you'll need to introduce new food groups as well as additional calories into your eating system. Read the next section, Transitioning from the PCMR System, to learn how to do this effectively.

> *If you're using the healthy eating system along with the medically formulated meal replacements,* you're already employing many of the principles of your permanent eating strategy. You can skip the next section, Transitioning from the PCMR System, and go right to the following section, Transitioning to Your Permanent Eating System.

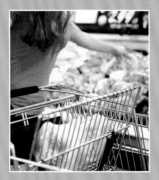

Transitioning from the PCMR System

If you've reached your healthy weight using portion-controlled meal replacements, you need to add the full range of food groups back into your diet as well as adding calories. You're already used to preparing a healthy lean and green meal along with your PCMRs, so this transition should be pretty easy for you.

We're going to introduce these new foods in a logical order that allows your digestive tract to become accustomed to them. Your starting point is five portion-controlled meal replacements and one lean and green meal, for a total of 800 to 1,000 calories a day. For the first four weeks of your transition, you'll increase your daily caloric intake incrementally each week by adding one of the four food groups that you avoided during Phase I.

Below is the schedule we use at Medifast to transition from weight loss into maintenance:

- Week 1: additional vegetables
- Week 2: fruits
- Week 3: dairy
- Week 4: whole grains

By the end of week four you will have added each of these four food groups and will be consuming approximately 1,350–1,500 calories.

The amount of time you'll spend transitioning to your calculated TEE is based on the total amount of weight you lost. Here's the schedule we'll use:

- If you lost less than 50 pounds, allow eight weeks to transition.
- If you lost 50–100 pounds, allow twelve weeks to transition.
- If you lost more than 100 pounds, allow sixteen weeks to transition.

For the purposes of this example, let's assume you've lost less than 50 pounds, meaning you'll need eight weeks to transition. Here's how the first four weeks should look:

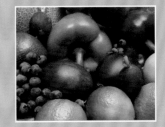

Week 1   Add vegetables (900–1,050 total calories per day)
- Add any vegetable from the green section of the charts.
- You're now eating five PCMRs, one lean and green meal, and one additional cup of vegetables.

Week 2   Add fruit (900–1,050 total calories per day)
- Drop one meal replacement.
- Add any fruit from the green section of the charts. (Fresh or frozen fruit is preferred, but canned may be used as long as it's not packed in syrup.)
- You're now eating four PCMRs, one lean and green meal, one additional cup of vegetables, and one medium-sized piece of fruit or ½ cup berries or chopped fruit.

Week 3   Add dairy (1,000–1,150 total calories per day)
- Dairy includes low-fat and sugar-free yogurt, milk, or lactaid product.
- You're now eating four PCMRs, one lean and green meal, one additional cup of vegetables, one medium-sized piece of fruit or ½ cup berries or chopped fruit, and ½ cup low-fat or fat-free dairy.

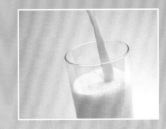

Week 4   Add whole grains (1,350–1,500 total calories per day)
- Drop one meal replacement.
- Whole grain choices include one slice of whole grain bread, ½ whole grain English muffin, ¾ cup high-fiber cereal, ½ cup whole wheat pasta, or ½ cup brown rice.
- You're now eating three PCMRs, one lean and green meal, one additional cup of vegetables, one medium-sized piece of fruit or ½ cup berries or chopped fruit, ½ cup low-fat or fat-free dairy, and one portion of whole grain starch.
- If you're exercising, add four ounces of lean meat, poultry, fish, or other protein.

Sample Daily Menu at Four Weeks

Breakfast: ½ cup high-fiber breakfast cereal (over 5 grams of fiber per serving) with ½ cup skim milk and 1 cup fresh strawberries

Mid-morning: Chai latte PCMR

Lunch: 4 ounces deli turkey; 2 cups salad greens with ½ cup total diced cucumber, tomato, and green pepper (plus 1–2 tablespoons reduced-calorie salad dressing if desired)

Mid-afternoon: Chicken noodle soup PCMR

Dinner: 4 ounces poached salmon with 1 cup green beans

Evening: Banana pudding PCMR with 1 teaspoon fat-free whipped topping

After the first four weeks, you will have introduced all four of the food groups you avoided during Phase I and will be eating approximately 1,500 calories. Over the following weeks, you'll continue to add calories until you reach your TEE, either by adding foods to one of your fuelings as outlined in the transition guide that came with your low-calorie, medically formulated meal replacements or to one of your meals using my color-coded portion-control system. For the woman in our example above, whose target TEE was 1,900 calories, that would mean adding 400 calories over the next four weeks. An easy way to do this is to add 100 calories each week until you've reached the permanent healthy eating schedule outlined in the next section.

If you'd like to understand this schedule a little better, go ahead and read the next section (which is tailored for those who are transitioning from the healthy eating system). If you prefer, you can skip that section and move directly to the following section, Planning Meals during Transition and Beyond. Either way, now is a good time to review chapters 8–10 as you adjust your diet and prepare to adopt healthy eating habits for a lifetime!

Transitioning to Your Permanent Eating System

In Phase I, if you used the healthy eating system to help improve your health, you learned how to eat every three hours, for a total of 1,200 to 1,300 calories per day. Using your nine-inch plate, you learned the right proportion of foods from the three major food components, and my color-coded, low-glycemic system helped you choose healthy carbohydrates, fats, and lean proteins, and showed you how to select your vegetables and fruits from the darkest green charts for the lowest-glycemic carbohydrates. This put you in a fat-burning state that helped you reach your healthy weight.

Now that you're transitioning to your lifelong eating plan, you no longer need to unload excess fat. Our new priority is to increase your daily calories until we reach a state of equilibrium between energy in and energy out. As part of that plan, we're going to add in some slightly higher-glycemic carbohydrates from the light green section of your color-coded charts. Eventually, you'll be able to choose from any of the carbohydrates on the green charts.

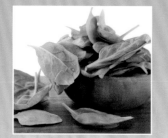

We're going to add calories back into your diet gradually in order to allow your body to adjust to this additional fuel. Let's take a look at your Phase I eating schedule, which taught you the basics of healthy eating.

	DR. A'S HEALTHY EATING SCHEDULE FROM PHASE I				
Breakfast	Mid-morning Fueling	Lunch Fueling	Mid-afternoon Fueling	Dinner	Evening Fueling
300 – 400 calories	100 calories	100 – 200 calories	100 calories	400 calories	100 calories

Transitioning into your permanent plan is simply a matter of adding about 100 calories to your daily intake for each week of transition, until you reach your Total Energy Expenditure (TEE). (If you lost more than fifty pounds, you'll want to go a bit slower, adding an additional 100 daily calories every two weeks of transition.)

Here's how your transition might look if your TEE is 1,900 calories per day.

Week 1 — add 100 calories to lunch
Week 2 — add another 100 calories to lunch
Week 3 — add another 100 calories to lunch, bringing it to a full 400-calorie three-component meal (using a nine-inch plate)
Week 4 — add 100 calories to the mid-morning fueling
Week 5 — add 100 calories to the mid-afternoon fueling
Week 6 — add 100 calories to breakfast
Week 7 — add 100 calories to dinner
Week 8 — monitor weight and adjust as necessary

(Note that I haven't added calories to the evening fueling. It's important to minimize the body's workload at night.)

Remember, PCMRs are an excellent way to add these incremental calories during transition, as well as after you reach your optimal daily caloric intake.

Here's an example of what the permanent eating strategy might look like for someone whose TEE is 1,900 calories.

	PERMANENT HEALTHY EATING SCHEDULE MODIFIED BY YOUR CURRENT TEE				
Breakfast	Mid-morning Fueling	Lunch Fueling	Mid-afternoon Fueling	Dinner	Evening Fueling
500 calories	200 calories	400 calories	200 calories	500 calories	100 calories

Dr. A's Healthy Eating Schedule from Phase I. This is how your daily intake looked in Phase I. Now you're going to add calories gradually until you reach your Total Energy Expenditure (TEE), the point where your intake and output meet.

Don't forget that PCMRs are a great way to add calories into your diet during transition and beyond.

Permanent Healthy Eating Schedule Modified by Your Current TEE. This is how your daily intake might look by the end of transition to Phase II if your TEE is 1,900 calories.

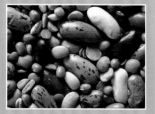

Your own permanent eating strategy may look different, depending on how many calories you need to take in each day for weight maintenance, based on your TEE. Remember, the total number of calories in all your meals and fuelings should equal the TEE you've calculated for yourself. You may need to adjust this number either up or down after the first couple of weeks to maintain your healthy weight and a BMI of under 25.

> Note: During the first week or so, you may gain a couple of pounds as you readjust your salt, water, and food intake. Don't be alarmed! If this trend continues for more than a few weeks, you'll need to stop adding additional calories or cut back on the number of calories in your dinner, lunch, or breakfast (in that order) until your movement plan gets underway and you start burning more calories.

Planning Meals during Transition and Beyond

Transition is a great time to add high-quality proteins, nutrient-dense starches, and a full range of fruits and vegetables to your diet. Just remember to continue your healthy eating strategies, including the following:

• Continue to use the PCMRs.

• Use a nine-inch plate for all your meals.

• Select healthy options from our three major food groups.

• Choose foods using the color-coded, low-glycemic shopping system. Stay with foods in the dark green sections (GI < 30) until you reach your new daily caloric allowance (your TEE), then add foods from the light green sections (GI = 30–50). Use foods in the red sections (GI > 50) only occasionally.

• Utilize the 100-calorie fueling choices from chapter 10 to add your additional daily calories.

• Utilize the menus from chapter 10 to create healthy meals, including the new 400-calorie lunch you'll be building over the first three weeks.

Here are some guidelines to follow as you add healthy foods into your diet from each of the three major food groups.

> *Don't Forget to Monitor Your Weight during Transition!*
> Your weight may fluctuate during transition as your body gets used to the additional carbohydrates, salt, and calories. Remember to monitor your weight vigilantly and adjust your calorie intake up or down if you fluctuate by more than a few pounds from your healthy weight. If you notice that you're gaining weight, cut back on calories a bit by recalculating your TEE and adjusting your intake accordingly.

Adding Calories from the Vegetable and Fruit Group

It's hard to go wrong in this category. All fruits and vegetables are healthy, low in calories, packed with vitamins and minerals, and provide fiber to help fill you up. On top of that, diets rich in fruits and vegetables may reduce the risk of some types of cancer and other chronic diseases.

By the end of transition, you'll have added a portion of fruit or vegetable to each of your six daily fuelings. You should be having at least two servings of fruit and four servings of vegetables per day.

Shopping tips:

- Choose fresh fruits and vegetables when possible, as outlined in chapter 9.
- If choosing frozen or canned fruits and vegetables, be sure they contain no added fat, sugar, or sauce.
- Include lots of salad greens in your diet.
- Add higher-glycemic choices such as corn, peas, and other fruits and vegetables *with caution*.
- When adding corn, keep the glycemic index lowest by buying corn on the cob with the husk intact.
- Sweet potatoes have a moderate GI of 46 (light green chart) when steamed, boiled, or baked.
- Yams have a GI of 37 and are high in fiber and nutrient dense.
- The lowest-glycemic fruits—citrus (orange, grapefruit, mandarins)—are great choices, as are stone fruits (apricots, plums, peaches, nectarines).
- Pineapple, watermelon, and cantaloupe can be eaten in moderate amounts.
- Berries are very low glycemic and a great choice as you add calories to breakfast, fuelings, and lunch.

As you begin adding your 100 calories per day following the transition schedule, make your selections primarily from the dark green color charts. This will keep your insulin pump turned off and give you some time to increase your energy expenditure as you begin my movement program in the next few chapters. Once you have reached your TEE and your weight is stable, you can start adding selections from the lighter green charts, and even a higher-glycemic choice on occasion.

How many calories?

- 1 cup cooked vegetables contains approximately 50–70 calories.
- 1 medium piece of fresh fruit contains approximately 80 calories.
- 1 cup of cubed fresh fruit contains approximately 80 calories.

Adding Calories from the Starch Group

Your starch selections have the biggest effect on your glycemic intake and require special vigilance as you complete your permanent eating plan.

As a rule, the more acidic a fruit, the lower its glycemic index because it slows down gastric emptying

Low-glycemic starches are a great steady source of nutrient-dense calories. You should have four to five servings a day, particularly if you're active. One serving equals one slice of bread or ½ cup of cooked rice, pasta, or noodles.

Healthy breads: Whole grains are high in fiber, nutrient dense, and contain vitamins and minerals. Good choices include:

- Pumpernickel
- Sourdough
- Stone ground or whole wheat
- Chapatis or other Indian breads made with chickpea flour

Cereals: Almost all commercial breakfast cereals are processed, which means that the grains have lost their structure and are no longer intact, making them high glycemic and poor choices. Good choices include:

- Rolled oats made into oatmeal (the gold standard of breakfast cereals!)
- Barley, bulger, and wheat bran
- Homemade muesli (fruits, nuts, seeds, rolled oats)

Pasta: Pasta is made from semolina grain. As long as you cook it al dente and serve it with a healthy protein, it's fine to have a cup of pasta. Choose a low-glycemic variety such as spinach rotini.

Rice: Rice is generally very high glycemic and should be avoided except in small quantities on limited occasions. Brown rice, which has a GI over 50, and long grain and basmati, with a GI around 58, are better choices than many other types of rice, which can have a GI approaching 100! Because sushi is served with seaweed, vinegar, and protein, its GI drops below 50.

How many calories?

- One slice of low-glycemic bread or ½ cup pasta or cereal contain approximately 80 calories.

Adding Calories from the Protein Group

As with starches, your protein selections should not come from processed or fatty foods, which not only add health-robbing saturated fats but also really pack on the calories.

Remember the tips for choosing healthy proteins that you learned in the healthy shopping guide in chapter 9.

- Eat red meat no more than twice a week, and make sure it's lean.
- Eat fish at least twice a week, and make sure it's fresh.
- Choose skinless, white-meat poultry.
- Choose low-fat or nonfat dairy.
- Don't forget nuts, seeds, and legumes.

*A Habit of Disease: Polluting Your Body
with Empty Calories from Processed Foods*

Sugar and fat: the non-nutritive agents

Today's average male eats almost 3,000 calories a day, and the average female around 2,000 calories a day. Amazingly, 40 percent of those calories come from refined, processed sugars and fats—primarily saturated animal fat. But when we fill up on calorie-laden fried foods and desserts, we leave ourselves very little room for the healthy, nutrient-rich foods our bodies need.

Where are our daily calories coming from? Let's look at a breakdown:

A Habit of Disease:
Polluting your body
with empty calories
from processed foods

A "WAIST"-LAND OF EMPTY CALORIES

	Males	Females
Daily Calorie Intake	3,000	2,000
Fat Calories	1,200 – 1,500	800 – 1,000
Sugar Calories	600	400
Total Fat and Sugar Calories	1,800 – 2,100	1,200 – 1,400
Remaining Calories	900 – 1,200	600 – 800

This means that the average male gets only 1,200 calories and the average female only 800 calories per day from foods that contain nutrients!

This dramatic nutrient deficit is a major reason that many of us have a constant desire to eat, despite our ample caloric intake. And that means more cravings, more overeating, and excess weight. It's yet another Habit of Disease taking us down the slippery path to non-sickness and sickness at a breakneck pace.

A Habit of Health: Choosing nutrient-rich foods

My healthy eating strategy ensures that you get nearly 100 percent of your calories from high-quality, nutrient-packed low-calorie PCMRs and whole foods. Eating this way helps you feel pleasantly satisfied—protecting you from the onslaught of nutritional pollution and supporting your goal of optimal health.

A Habit of Health:
Choosing nutrient-
rich foods

Legumes, including chickpeas, beans, soybeans, and lentils, are a wonderful alternative protein source—low glycemic, loaded with fiber and phytonutrients, and nutrient dense with vitamins and minerals. I recommend eating them at least twice a week or more as your main protein source.

How many calories?

- ½ cup legumes contain approximately 100–200 calories and is very low glycemic.
- A 4-ounce portion of lean meat contains about 250 calories.
- A 6-ounce portion of skinless white-meat chicken contains about 300 calories.

Choosing Right When You're Dining Out

Going out to eat has become a way of life. I certainly look forward to dining out with family and friends. After all, everyone needs an occasional pampered evening that's hassle free, with nothing to prepare or wash. You can make this indulgence a healthy one as long as you control your nutritional intake by following a few important guidelines.

Watch for Pitfalls

Look at dining out from the restaurant's point of view. Restaurants are in the business of making money and keeping their customers happy (so they can make more money). They want you to come back and bring all your friends. And fat, salt, and sugar sell.

A Habit of Health:
Avoiding fast foods

A Habit of Health: Avoiding Fast Foods

When I talk about dining out, I'm not talking about fast food restaurants. Fast foods make it nearly impossible to maintain a healthy weight. In fact, they're the masters of calorie creep, as anyone who's seen the movie "SuperSize Me" knows.

The bland, grey-looking stuff served in fast food restaurants—made palatable with the help of some synthetics from a fragrance company, no doubt—gives immediate gratification, loaded as it is with salt, high-fructose corn syrup, and animal fats, but it lacks much nutritional value. On top of which, that red and yellow color scheme is designed to attract you like a hummingbird to a feeder by stimulating your hunger and creating a stress response that can have a negative effect on your immune system.

So if you never enter another red and yellow establishment again, you'll have added another Habit of Health! If you find yourself having no other choice, then make the best of the situation and get a salad with grilled chicken and a low-calorie dressing.

More important, they have a secret weapon. What's the first thing that happens when you enter a restaurant? They ask you if you want a cocktail. And why not? After a busy day, a cocktail or glass of wine is the perfect way to relax. But after just one drink, the inhibitory neurons in our brain start to shut off. We begin to lose our ability to remember those primary and secondary choices we made so carefully. And with that, we lose our reason to avoid that 2,400-calorie Bloomin' Onion. Not to mention that the alcohol itself, with seven calories per gram, has almost double the calories of sugar and absolutely no nutritive value. Drink sparkling water with a slice of lime or a splash of cranberry juice instead of a cocktail while you wait for your meal. If you must drink alcohol, your healthiest choice is a small glass (five ounces) of red wine. But here's the key: *order your food first!*

If you know where you'll be eating out, call in advance and ask the restaurant to either fax or e-mail their menu to you, or look for their menu on the Internet. Decide in advance what you'll choose and stick to it. And try to choose restaurants that offer healthy dishes. In other words, stay away from the pizzerias and "all-you-can-eat" buffets!

If the timing of your dinner reservation means that you'll be exceeding your three-hour time period without eating, have a PCMR or a low-calorie snack before you go out. This will keep your appetite in check while you wait for your table and your food.

Once you're seated, ask for any bread or chips to be removed from the table or placed out of reach. Save your calories for more nutritious foods. And remember to keep that salad healthy by bringing your own low-calorie bottled salad dressing or a homemade dressing of balsamic vinegar, lemon, and a drizzle of olive oil. Restaurant dressings are full of fat, calories, and sugar.

Choose Healthy Cooking Methods

Scampi style, au gratin, broiled—what does it all mean in terms of calories? Here are some quick tips to help you sort the good from the bad.

Bear in mind that this is just a rough guide. There's no guarantee that items prepared in the preferred methods are really low in fat, since fats are often added in the cooking process (for example, grilled items may be brushed with oil, poached items may cooked in buttery liquid, baked items often contain oil or cheese, and marinara sauces often start with a base of oil). And if the cut of meat, fish, or poultry you choose is high in fat to begin with, it will likely still be high in fat after cooking, even using healthy cooking methods.

Stay away from cream sauces and soups, butter, oil, au gratin, breaded, Alfredo sauce, gravy, and anything battered or fried. Blackened entrees are usually dipped in butter or oil, covered with spices, and then pan fried.

Don't be afraid to take charge of your meal. Choose only lean cuts of red meat such as loin and flank. If you're having chicken, remember that white meat contains less fat. Ask for your meat, fish, or poultry to be prepared with minimal oil and butter or prepared "light." Have the chef trim all excess fat before cooking and be sure to remove the skin from poultry before you eat.

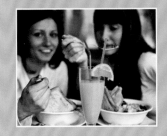

Try this tip! Check out menu selections on the restaurant's Web site before you go to avoid a potentially unhealthy environment or to preselect a healthy choice.

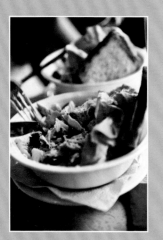

Request that vegetables be steamed with no added sugar or butter. Optimal cooking methods are baked, broiled, grilled, poached, or steamed. And of course, fresh is best!

Keep Portions in Check

Restaurant servings have gotten out of control. An occasional treat is fine, but if you eat out often, you need to develop an overall strategy for portion control. Here are a few tips.

- Visualize the divisions on the nine-inch plate.
- Order two appetizers instead of an entrée, such as soup and a dinner salad, or shrimp cocktail.
- Split a meal with your dining companion.
- Don't rely on the chef or waiter to serve you the proper amount of food. Surveys show that people generally eat everything that's put in front of them—whether they wanted it or not.
- Ask for a leftovers container right when you place your order. When your meal comes, eyeball your proper portion right away and put the rest into the box to take home.

PCMRs: The Healthy Fast Food—for Weight Loss and for Life

Medically formulated portion-controlled meal replacements (PCMRs) such as Medifast's are a convenient choice for your three-hour fuelings—especially if you don't have a lot of time to prepare food. These convenient low-fat, low-glycemic foods are loaded with vitamins and minerals, offer a careful balance of protein and carbohydrates, and provide you with a specific dose of calories so you don't have to worry about calorie creep. And because PCMRs are completely portable, they help ensure you're getting a proper fueling when it's not otherwise feasible. That's why I've used them myself for over six years now. They really help me to get in my five to six daily fuelings even if I'm in the midst of a busy lifestyle, traveling away from home, or just out and about and hungry. For more information on ordering your PCMRs, see the resource list on page 370.

Beginning Your Lifetime of Healthy Eating

You should now have a firm grip on the eating strategy that will support you for life. You understand the full range of healthy foods that will help you maintain your weight and set the foundation for optimal health. You've calculated your daily energy requirements and are starting to increase you caloric intake based on those calculations, adding calories gradually according to the amount of weight you lost.

As you learned in Phase I, you're eating every three hours, using my low-glycemic, portion-control system to keep a handle on your daily fuelings. You know how to use the system even when dining out, and you're savvier about avoiding the pitfalls of the restaurant environment.

It's not always easy to have a low-fat, low-glycemic, low-calorie meal on hand when you need it. That's why portion-controlled meal replacements (PCMRs) have been a lifesaver for many of my patients and others I've coached. As a high-quality, portable fast food, a medically backed low-calorie PCMR is just about unbeatable. It's a great tool as you continue your journey.

A recent study showed that simply by decreasing portion size and energy density by 25 percent, people were able to maintain their healthy weight.* And now, so can you. Combine your new understanding of portion control and energy density with your knowledge of healthy protein, starch, and vegetables and fruits, and you have the Habits of Health to support a lifetime of healthy eating.

Your transition to a sustainable and satisfying eating strategy is now complete. Let's turn our focus to the *energy out* portion of the equation and get your body moving.

"A dream come true."

EMILY PREATOR
Over eighteen months at optimal health

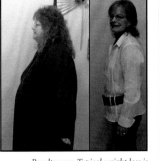

Results vary. Typical weight loss is 2-5 lbs per week for the first 2 weeks and 1-2 lbs per week thereafter.

Fifty-five years ago, this tiny baby girl had no clue her life would be filled with depression and unhappiness, living in a body larger than every other kid.

At age 42, morbidly obese with high blood pressure, I suffered a stroke. A few years later, I tipped the scales at 302 pounds. I tried diet after diet, always looking for the "magic pill." But any pounds I did manage to lose came off so slowly that I lost my motivation to continue.

Then I took a trip I'll never forget. I needed a seat belt extender for the airplane, and I couldn't even walk a few blocks without lots of rest breaks. I felt more hopeless than ever, and resigned myself to dying as the fat-bodied person I knew so well. Little did I know that the very next month would be the start of a dream come true.

My husband was determined to lose 25 pounds, and I thought it would help him if I tried the recommendations Dr. Andersen made to create optimal health too. "They probably won't work for me," I insisted... Well, Jerry lost his weight in ten weeks. And me? In eighteen months, I've lost 132 pounds and 131 inches following Dr. A's suggestions and Take Shape for Life! My stepson's in-laws didn't recognize me at his wedding—and was it ever wonderful fitting into the airplane seats and taking a walking tour of Philadelphia with ease!

I've begun to dream, and to live life. I've set and accomplished goals like going horseback riding and downhill skiing—physical activities I never could have considered before. I now use the Habits of Health, which Dr. A says are necessary to stay healthy. I work out regularly and enjoy being out in the world. And I've only just begun! I'm busy buying new clothes—having gone from a size 3XL to a 6 petit! I've never felt so alive and thrilled to wake up every morning! ■

Visit
www.habitsofhealth.net
for more information on
healthy eating for life.

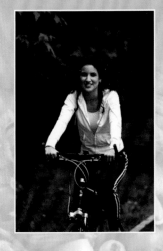

*Rolls, B. J., et al., "Reductions in Portion Size and Energy Density of Foods," *American Journal of Clinical Nutrition* 83 (January 2006): 11–17.

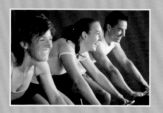

Chapter 13

Active Living : Inside and Out

In chapters 13 through 16, we'll focus on transitioning your body into a state of increased energy expenditure. In other words, we're going to get you moving and burning more calories both inside and out:

- *Inside* by building up the mitochondria (the energy users) in your cells and utilizing the natural thermic (energy burning) effect of food
- *Outside* by increasing your daily movement

Increasing your activity level—with exercise as the ultimate, though not immediate, goal—is essential to disease prevention and optimal health. But exactly what that looks like is different for everyone. As you've no doubt gathered by now, I firmly believe that the best way to integrate movement into your life is gradually, through a plan that's tailored to your current state of health, activity level, and weight.

Up to this point, we've targeted the energy-in side of the energy balance equation, because that's the most efficient way to reach a healthy weight. But to make your healthy weight last, and to continue your journey to optimal health, we also need to focus on upping your energy expenditure and physical activity level.

Unlike our ancestors, who had to continually search for food and hold onto every calorie they could, we've become so efficient at obtaining food and storing it away in our bodies that it's hard for us to unload enough energy to

---

Obesity and Rigorous Exercise: A Dangerous Combination

Not only is exercise alone ineffective for weight loss, it can be downright dangerous for those who are seriously overweight. In fact, asking someone who's out of shape and carrying an extra fifty pounds or so to go jogging, lift weights, or do circuit training is a recipe for disaster, leading all too often to back, neck, and knee injuries that can set them up for long-term failure—not to mention that the added stress on an already overworked cardiovascular system can have serious, even deadly, consequences.

Our approach, by contrast, features a movement plan that can be customized to all levels of health, weight, and fitness—beginning with activities that help you maintain your healthy weight and progressing to ones that move you toward optimal health.

> ### The Three-Day-a-Week Workout:
> ### Inefficient for Weight Loss, Great for Health
>
> What's wrong with intense, muscle-burning workouts? As long as you're in shape and can do them, nothing. . . they're just not very efficient at creating weight loss. Think of it this way: there are 168 hours in the week. The average three-day-a-week workout uses just 2 percent of those hours. Our energy management program, on the other hand, will help you tap into all 168!
>
> A lot of weight-loss programs tout intense workouts as an essential part of fitness. Unfortunately, that sort of rigorous exercise leaves most overweight people discouraged and believing they just don't have what it takes to maintain a healthy weight.
>
> Intense exercise can be a valuable tool *if it's introduced properly and customized to meet each person's ability.* Otherwise, it's unlikely to succeed long term. In the next chapter, we'll create a functional plan to increase your exercise level at a pace that makes it easy to incorporate into your life and easy to sustain. That's the way to ensure that these health-giving activities become permanent Habits of Health.
>
> *Already exercising?* You've got a great head start! Now, by adding my motion plan to your regular routine, you can harness those 100+ hours you're not already using for exercise. You'll pick up some great ideas to improve your fitness level and see a dramatic boost in your energy expenditure!

Physical Activity? Exercise? What's the Difference? You may think of the terms *physical activity* and *exercise* as one and the same, but it's important to make a distinction. *Physical activity* happens anytime your body's in motion. As you'll see later in the chapter, that motion can be voluntary or involuntary. *Exercise*, on the other hand, is planned movement that's more vigorous and leads to improvements in overall fitness.

keep our weight stable. And for many of us, the thought of working out in a gym three days a week, as most plans recommend, is far from appealing.

Relax! I know that workout gear probably isn't your preferred uniform. And in fact, an intense three-day-a-week workout isn't a good starting point for most of us. It's certainly not the easiest, most efficient entry point, and unless you're an exercise enthusiast, you should actually delay formal workouts until we've moved you a little farther up the path toward optimal health.

The Habits of Motion

My approach to physical activity takes a much broader outlook than exercise-focused plans do. Rather, it's based on creating habits of active living. We begin by stabilizing your healthy weight (without a lot of weight lifting and aerobics), then proceed to gradually introduce the foundational principles of the Habits of Motion. Throughout, we ensure that you're using the most efficient means possible to maintain your healthy weight. Fortunately, the most efficient way is also the easiest and safest way for you to start your movement plan!

I'm a firm believer in the motto "you need to crawl before you can walk." My plan gives you time to build your foundation by assimilating some basic principles of physical activity. When you're ready, we'll move into some more advanced techniques at a pace that makes sense for you.

After age twenty, we begin losing muscle cells at an ever-increasing rate. They're replaced with fat cells, which burn far less energy.

Thermogenesis: The process by which the body generates heat, or energy, by increasing the metabolic rate above normal. Thermogenesis can be activated by a variety of mechanisms, including supplements, nutrition, exercise, and exposure to cold.

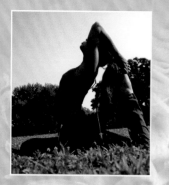

At the center of my plan is getting you to move your body like you did when you were a kid. Now that we're adults, life just seems to get in the way of getting out, playing, and having fun. Combine that with our terrible eating habits and sedentary jobs, and it's easy to see why we've just stopped moving. So we're going to start with baby steps, based on your current reality, and crawl our way back to energy equilibrium, fitness, and optimal health. We'll start by looking at all the many little movements that make up your day, and putting them to work for us.

As I teach you the Habits of Motion, I'll be focusing on two major objectives:

1. Stabilizing your weight by increasing your energy expenditure, primarily through physical activity
2. Optimizing your health through carefully paced exercises

We'll accomplish our first goal by teaching you how to become more active, through movements centered within the symphony of your daily job, chores, plans, and activities. But first, in order to help you understand how to harness your body's own energy, we're going to revisit an old friend: TEE.

Increasing Your Total Energy Expenditure (TEE) through Thermogenesis

Activity and *exercise* have different roles in our system. Introducing each of them correctly and in the right sequence is critical to making your new energy plan a permanent Habit of Health.

One big difference between exercise and physical activity is that exercise is generally done for a short period of time—usually just a few hours a week. Physical activity, on the other hand, can be integrated into your daily life in a much more organic and complete manner (see The Three-Day-a-Week Workout, page 171). Our main objective in increasing your activity is to put all your waking hours to work upping your energy expenditure. By tapping into the thousand different ways your body is active, we'll start increasing your total energy expenditure (TEE) even if your current activity level is minimal.

In the last chapter, we figured out how to find your energy equilibrium point by calculating your TEE. By learning how many calories you burn in a day, you established a starting point that tells you how many calories you need to ingest in order to maintain your healthy weight.

Now we're going to look at the three components that make up TEE and find out how to increase each one. After all, we're energetic creatures. Together, we're going to turn up your metabolic furnace and increase your ability to burn calories in a whole variety of simple ways you probably never even thought about. It's simple, it's scientific, and there's a name for it—*thermogenesis*.

Remember the TEE equation?

$$TEE = BMR + PAL + TEF$$

Let's break that down into parts and show you how to turn up the heat!

Basal Metabolic Rate (BMR)

As you may recall from chapter 12, Basal Metabolic Rate (BMR), which measures our body's basic functioning, accounts for the majority of the calories we expend—on average between 65 and 70 percent of TEE. It's calculated when the body is in a neutral, resting state—after a night of restful sleep, in a temperate environment, on an empty stomach—the point at which our organs are using the least amount of energy. Because many people think of this as a passive measurement, it's assumed that BMR is difficult to change. However, nothing could be further from the truth.

In fact, as the biggest component of our metabolic pie, BMR offers us a wonderful opportunity to tap into a thermogenic energy source that burns energy 168 hours a week. How? By ingeniously increasing the activity level and even the size of our organs to boost energy consumption. Let's look at two organs that are open to this process and have the biggest appetite for calories—our muscles and our brain.

Muscles in the Basal Metabolic State

When we think of consuming energy using our muscles, we're usually thinking of working out or performing some sort of physical activity. That's the type of energy use we'll discuss in the Physical Activity Level (PAL) section. This is an entirely different matter—here, we're talking about the energy your muscles use even when you're lying in bed in the morning, dreaming about sleeping in.

Unlike your bones, immune system, lungs, and other organs whose energy requirements are fairly fixed, the basal metabolic contribution from your muscles varies. And most of that variation—75 percent, in fact—is based on how much lean body mass you have.

How does it all work? It really comes down to tiny mitochondria, the little energy factories of our cells. Mitochondria work very hard taking the nutrients we consume and converting them into energy to power the machinery of our cells. In the case of our muscle cells, mitochondria are highly influenced by the work the particular muscles are performing.

Our bodies generally have the highest proportion of mitochondria when we're in late adolescence, after which point they start to diminish. Beginning at age twenty we lose about a pound of muscle each year. And what do those muscle cells get replaced with? You guessed it—fat cells.

Now here's the kicker: Each pound of muscle consumes around fifty to seventy calories a day. Fat, on the other hand, consumes much less energy—less than 10 percent of the energy that muscle uses. That means that as we lose muscle over the years, our energy expenditure decreases. And when energy expenditure decreases, fat accumulation increases.

That's why this loss of muscle mass and muscle strength—known as *sarcopenia of aging*—is linked to pre-obesity and obesity and contributes to a decrease in both BMR and PAL. Not to mention that having weak, flabby muscles plays a large part in our downward spiral to non-sickness and disease. But the good news is that this muscle deterioration is reversible.

A Habit of Health: Lowering room temperature to 68°

Being in a cooler environment is another way to increase your BMR and help you burn more calories. And as added benefits, you'll suffer from fewer respiratory issues and burn less fuel—so you'll be helping the planet while you help yourself!

We've all *heard of* exercise, and many of us *talk about* exercise, but the reality is that 60 percent of Americans don't take part in any kind of regular physical activity—and 25 percent get no activity to speak of at all!

NEAT (Non-Exercise Activity Thermogenesis) can have a huge effect on your daily TEE (and therefore on your daily calorie consumption). In fact, even minor changes in daily non-exercise physical activity can increase TEE by 20 percent.

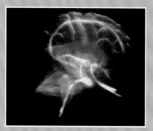

In Phase I, we emptied a whole bunch of those inefficient fat cells by decreasing your fat stores, especially around your organs. In Phase II, we're not only going to focus on increasing your lean muscle mass—we're actually going to work on increasing the size of the mitochondria in each cell, through specific techniques you'll learn in chapter 15. And in doing so, we'll tap into an energy expenditure system that's at work 24/7.

This behind-the-scenes increase in BMR sets the stage for long-term weight maintenance and permanent health. And as an added bonus, in addition to benefiting from increased energy expenditure during rest (BMR), your newly enhanced muscles will burn more energy when you're in motion too.

Your Brain and BMR

You may not think of the brain as a big calorie burner, but in fact our brains consume an incredible amount of energy (which explains why more than a few minutes without oxygen can have catastrophic consequences).

In fact, our brain accounts for about 25 percent of our BMR. What's more, the amount of energy consumption decreases with age as our brain atrophies, just like our muscles. That is, unless we do some active intervention.

Researchers are systematically unraveling the hidden secrets of the brain, including ways to keep our brain healthy and our memory intact. One of the most important discoveries they've come up with is that our brain cells and neurons have an amazing ability to develop in size and connectivity as we age. Activating new pathways and engaging in new activities are important ways to exercise your brain.

By learning the Habits of Health, you're already stimulating your brain by exchanging previous behaviors with new, healthy cognitive activities. And that's just the beginning. Even changing the way you do simple everyday activities—brushing your teeth with the opposite hand, for example, or driving home using a different route—stimulates the brain and actually increases your metabolic rate.

Another important way to stimulate brain waves and increase energy consumption is to tap into music and motion. In fact, combining music and rhythmic movement such as dancing or rowing can improve many aspects of our health, even decreasing systemic inflammation.

So you see that BMR is far from fixed. By focusing on the Habits of Health, you can actually increase the size, capacity, and metabolic function of your brain and muscles, even when you're resting. You'll learn how to give your body a workout in the next few chapters; then in chapter 25, I'll show you how to give your brain a workout too!

Muscles: The Secret Endocrine Organ

Did you know that having responsive, lean muscle is critical to maintaining healthy levels of insulin and glucose? And that unhealthy insulin and glucose levels are big contributors to a whole range of diseases? That's why reversing *sarcopenia*—loss of muscle mass and strength—is a big focus on our journey to optimal health.

Physical Activity Level (PAL)

Your Physical Activity Level (PAL), which accounts for 25 to 30 percent of TEE, is the part of the TEE equation that's easiest to change. That's why PAL has such a central role in helping you control your weight—both directly, through movement, and indirectly, by increasing the amount of calorie-burning muscle in your body.

PAL is made up of two parts: planned physical activity (what you probably think of as exercise) and the voluntary and unconscious movements you make as part of your everyday life. As we plan an activity program customized to your age, fitness level, and lifestyle, it's helpful to consider these two categories separately. One handy way to break it down is through the acronyms EAT and NEAT.

EAT and NEAT

EAT (Exercise Activity Thermogenesis) consists of the planned physical activities we perform in order to increase our energy expenditure and improve our overall fitness. It's what we do when we say we're "working out." These may range from the minimal task of going for a brisk walk to Herculean feats, like when Lance Armstrong expends 9,000 calories a day at the Tour de France. But despite all our talk of exercise today, for the vast majority of us, EAT is actually negligible. In fact, even exercise enthusiasts will find that EAT's contribution to daily calorie consumption pales by comparison to the power of NEAT.

NEAT (Non-Exercise Activity Thermogenesis) consists of the voluntary and unconscious movements we make as we go about our daily lives—by working, doing chores, or just through the silly little motions that happen. As I sit here writing, for example, I'm consuming extra calories just tapping my foot. It's easy, and it happened naturally as a result of getting into the beat of a great song on my iPod. NEAT is highly variable, ranging from about 15 percent of total daily TEE in very sedentary people to more than 50 percent in people who are highly active. Let's focus on two areas that contribute to your daily NEAT: work time and non-work time.

Our society's decreased activity level—and resulting decrease in NEAT—has been blamed to a great extent on a shift from manual labor to sedentary desk jobs. This has certainly been a major contributor. But look beyond the workplace to our cars, remote controls, snow blowers, elevators, and myriad other labor-saving devices we feel we must have. No wonder we're turning into something along the lines of those muscle-atrophied Star Trek creatures with huge heads and marshmallow bodies!

In the end, the compounding effects of those small daily choices have much more impact on weight maintenance than any exercise program. Formal exercise, including weight resistance training, circuit training, and aerobic exercise, is great for your health, and we'll introduce it to your life as you aim for the summit of optimal health—but in terms of weight maintenance, it's just icing on the cake.

Instead, in Phase II we'll focus on those everyday ways to increase daily energy expenditure—things that are available to each of us, all the time. But first

"Leisure-time sedentariness has resulted from the availability and volitional use of pervasive mechanization. When the energetic cost of non-work mechanization is estimated experimentally it approximates to 100–200 kcal/day: *a caloric deficit that potentially could account for the entire obesity epidemic.*"[*]

Dr. A's translation: Put down the remote, shovel your walk, open your cans with a manual opener, use the stairs, and take your dog for a walk, and you'll maintain your healthy weight. Take a friend and your dog for a walk and you'll help cure the epidemic!

*Levine, J. A., Levine Lab, Mayo Clinic, mayoresearch. mayo.edu/mayo/research/ levine_lab.

Eating lean protein
You've already learned that lean protein fills you up faster than other types of foods. But now there's even more reason to eat this super-food. Compared to other macronutrients, your body uses almost twice as much energy to break down and convert protein to fuel. In fact, a protein-based meal elicits a thermic effect of close to 30 percent of the total calories consumed—meaning that 600 calories of food burns up 180 calories just to eat!

Drinking ice water
Switching your daily dose of water (eight 8-ounce glasses) to ice water can burn an extra 74 calories a day. That may not seem like much, but it adds up to a whopping 7.7 pounds of fat per year! Not to mention that too little water can lead to sugar cravings, fatigue, irritability, and foggy thinking, and that dehydration significantly slows down fat burning. All the more reason to keep up this important habit of health!

let's spend a few moments finding out how to increase energy expenditure by selecting foods that actually boost your TEE from the *inside*.

Thermic Effect of Food (TEF)

Like BMR, this third component of TEE—the energy we use digesting and processing our food—is usually considered a fixed quantity that's not easy to change. But like BMR, it can be modified to boost your total energy consumption. The timing of your meals, the amount of food you eat, and the content of your food all have a big effect on energy expenditure. Let's start putting this forgotten component to work! Here are just a few ideas:

- **Eat every three hours.** While further documentation is needed, this great Habit of Health may actually contribute to an increase in TEF by causing your body to start up its metabolic machinery more often.
- **Choose lean protein.** Protein is a complex fuel that must be broken down into amino acids before it can be used. That takes energy—almost twice as much energy as your body uses to process carbohydrates and fats. (For more information, see sidebar, Habits of Health: Eating lean protein.)
- **Drink cold water.** Switch to ice water and up your TEF. Drinking just one 8-ounce glass of ice water burns 9.25 more calories than drinking a glass of room-temperature water. (For more information, see sidebar, Habits of Health: Drinking ice water.)
- **Seek out naturally thermogenic foods.** Several naturally occurring substances increase your energy expenditure, including caffeine, polyphenolic compounds (found in green tea), and capsaicin (found in red pepper, mustard, ginger, and cinnamon). Other substances with a thermic effect include selenium, chromium, alpha lipoic acid, L-carnitine, L-tyrosine, and calcium carbonate. We'll discuss these types of substances in greater detail later in the book, when you enter Phase III.

You now understand how these three components—BMR (your body's metabolic rate), PAL (your activity level), and TEF (the energy you use to burn food)—can be modulated to increase your total energy expenditure (TEE).

In the next three chapters, we'll outline a progressive plan to increase your daily energy expenditure, incorporating each of these important components. Our primary focus will be to incorporate the Habits of Motion into your life, slowly but steadily, to help you tap into a new life of motion.

Chapter 14

First Steps

Introduction to Dr. A's Habits of Motion System

The numbers speak for themselves:

- 60% of us get no regular physical activity.
- 25% of us get no activity at all.
- 50% of those who begin exercising quit within six months.
- One year after purchase, 90% of all exercise equipment is unused and relegated to a coat rack or cat perch.

What does it all mean? That until you've gotten your weight under control, increased your flexibility, developed a more active lifestyle, and organized your daily choices to support health, the honest truth is that launching yourself into a full-blown exercise program just isn't likely to be successful.

That's why, in this chapter and the next, we're going to focus on simple movements and activities that you can incorporate into your daily life right away, regardless of your current health, weight, or fitness level. They're easy, they'll help you maintain your weight, and they serve as the transition to a more healthy, active lifestyle. These Habits of Motion are the foundation of a total movement program that I'll be teaching you in these next few chapters—a program that you can use for life, starting right now.

The Problem with Exercise

When I was about five years old, my dad, following the belief system of the time, introduced me to swimming by throwing me into the deep end and proudly shouting, "Swim!" This wasn't uncommon back then; you may have even gone through a similar experience.

It's not unlike what happens when an out-of-shape, overweight individual starts an intense exercise program. Those millions of people who are convinced—mistakenly—that they must undergo vigorous exercise to lose weight suffer the same fate I did fifty years ago when I was thrown into deep water.

The aerobics revolution of the 1970s didn't help either. The idea of running a marathon to become "aerobically optimized" simply creates too high a barrier for most people. Thirty years later, we're still trying to overcome the notion that you have to exercise intensively in order to be healthy and fit. As you can tell from the bleak statistics above, the vast majority of us simply can't keep up.

Exercise: Planned movement that's vigorous enough to improve overall fitness

Can Lifestyle Changes Cure Obesity?

The answer from medical science is a resounding "yes!"—*if* we can overcome the barriers in our way. According to diet researcher Dr. Michael Dansinger of Tufts–New England Medical Center, "Most able-bodied persons who can find a way to overcome the monumental logistical and psychological barriers that prevent the full application of lifestyle change can reverse obesity within months."* It might sound simplistic, but the solution to the obesity crisis may actually depend on finding a way to implement lifestyle recommendations in just the right dose to foster meaningful and permanent change.

*Dansinger, M. L., and Schaefer, E. J., *Journal of the American Medical Association* 295: pp. 94–95.

And of course, many of us just don't like the gym experience and will find any excuse to avoid it—not enough time, too hard, boring. Many of these excuses are the result of our own, sometimes mistaken, perceptions, but just as many are logical and real. But in the end, if we can't overcome our psychological and logistical barriers to exercise, any success will be fleeting at best.

The Habits of Motion: The Key to Energy Expenditure

Our plan is about something very different. It's about simplicity. It's about weaving movement into the tapestry of your everyday life, about ramping up at your own pace, within your own comfort level, by finding little nooks and crannies in your routines that lend themselves to movement. And it's designed to be incorporated into your busy schedule without any additional time commitment. Whether you're 200 pounds overweight and currently inactive or a weight lifter with 8 percent body fat, the Habits of Motion can profoundly and permanently enhance your health and your life.

How? Just look around at today's environment. Our sedentary jobs keep us bent over a computer screen for hours at a time. Energy-saving devices such as elevators, escalators, and cars (you can barely find a sidewalk these days!) are robbing our bodies of flexibility, energy expenditure, and muscle. But by

Barriers to Exercise. There are plenty of reasons to avoid exercising—some based on our perception and some based on logistics. Unless we can overcome each of these barriers, we won't stay with it.

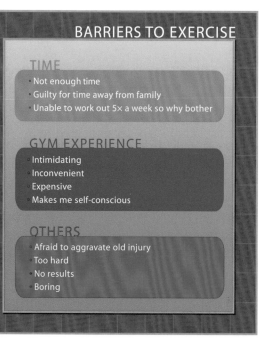

BARRIERS TO EXERCISE

TIME
• Not enough time
• Guilty for time away from family
• Unable to work out 5× a week so why bother

GYM EXPERIENCE
Intimidating
Inconvenient
Expensive
Makes me self-conscious

OTHERS
• Afraid to aggravate old injury
• Too hard
• No results
• Boring

tapping into your daily movements, even incrementally, you can create enough additional motion to offset the obesigenic effect of this automated world. Working within your existing daily routine, my plan taps into all your myriad natural movements, enhancing their quality and quantity to increase their contribution to energy expenditure.

Think of it as a basic course in movement. It's the way children go about their day. They don't go to the gym or lift weights or think about how many calories they're burning. They just play! That natural motion is just what we're going to restore. But don't worry—I won't make you get on the monkey bars!

Activity Thermogenesis (AT): Your Daily Energy Burn

You may recall from chapter 12 that Physical Activity Level (PAL)—the part of Total Energy Expenditure (TEE) that has to do with your body's motion—is the key *modifiable* area of energy expenditure. That's why we'll be focusing on PAL as we boost your calorie-burning mechanism and convert you from an energy-conserver to an energy-user.

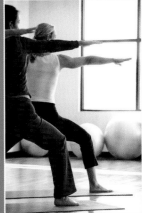

Another term that's used to describe this process is *activity thermogenesis (AT)*—the process by which the body generates heat, or energy, as it moves. AT is the energy used by our muscles to move and support our body. From the time you get up in the morning until you go to sleep at night, every movement you make requires energy. Our movement plan teaches you how to enhance your energy expenditure by adding movements that increase thermogenesis. Combined with your new healthy eating plan, this movement plan (in which, you may be pleased and surprised to learn, active exercise plays only a small role) provides a total system of healthy, balanced energy management for a lifetime of health.

Now let's revisit the two components of activity thermogenesis—EAT and NEAT.

EAT: Thermogenesis through Exercise

EAT (Exercise Activity Thermogenesis) consists of those activities performed expressly for the purpose of improving fitness—in other words, exercise. EAT activities—such as sports, workouts, and jogs—usually take place at a specific, planned time, and may range in intensity from a walk in the park to a grueling triathlon.

As you may recall, EAT takes up less than 2 percent of our weekly time, making it a less-than-effective way to burn energy. In addition, exercise stimulates several metabolic pathways, a process that may actually make you want to eat more. This state, known as *compensation,* is particularly prevalent among women when they start exercising.

What it comes down to is that the scheduled exercise that makes up EAT simply can't be counted on as a reliable way to maintain energy balance—at least not in the beginning, when successful weight loss leads to a corresponding drop in daily energy use (less mass means less calorie consumption, remember?).

Now, that's not to say that EAT doesn't play an important role in long-term health. In fact, exercise is a critical part of reaching optimal health, and

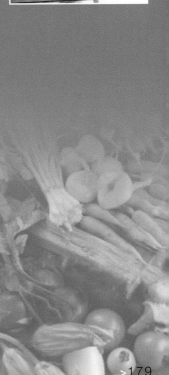

**Exercise: A Key
Player in Advanced
Energy Balance**
While exercise
comprises only a small
part of our daily activity
(if it's done at all), its
ability to build muscle
can help increase
your calorie-burning
potential. In chapter
16, we'll look at some
specific EAT activities
that build more and
bigger muscle cells to
fan your metabolic fire.

> *EAT: Your Graduate Degree in Optimal Health*
> The exercise that makes up EAT is critical for reaching optimal health. It builds muscle, increases energy expenditure, boosts your immune system, and is especially effective at lowering inflammation. It's sometimes said that if we could put exercise in pill form, it would be the world's most prescribed medicine. In my opinion, it's the best longevity medicine there is—if it's properly introduced in a schedule and dosage that makes sense.
>
> EAT is like your graduate degree in health. First, you need your prerequisites—and that's where the small, daily movements of NEAT come into play. Once you've incorporated NEAT into your life, we'll begin to block out some time for planned exercise. But even at that point, sessions of moderate length and intensity will do the trick. In fact, on most days, a thirty-minute walk is all you need to achieve the same benefits that the rigorous exercise enthusiasts of the past would have had you do!

in chapter 16, I'll teach you some simple, easy ways to make exercise a part of your busy life. The problem is that EAT only works if you do it—and few of us actually do.

Think of it this way: EAT is like going to graduate school for your advanced degree in health. First, you need the prerequisites—and that's where NEAT comes in. NEAT forms the basis of the first part of my movement system, setting the right foundation for a progressive movement plan that's easy to learn and apply and that prepares you for your climb to optimal health. After all, if you're going to continue moving forward, a mobile, flexible body and an active lifestyle make great starting points.

NEAT: Thermogenesis through Everyday Movement

NEAT (Non-Exercise Activity Thermogenesis) is made up of all of the movements your body makes outside of planned exercise. Compared to EAT, it's actually a much more efficient way to fight calorie creep and a more important contributor to energy expenditure. It's also much easier to do—in fact, you're already doing it.

Think of NEAT as your exercise training wheels, or as the movement version of the portion-controlled meal replacements—an easy way to begin offloading excess calories and get your energy in balance without making a big time commitment. I'll start by giving you a short undergraduate class on NEAT before introducing the Habits of Motion system.

Harnessing NEAT

What do sitting, standing, walking, talking, toe tapping, guitar playing, dancing, singing, shopping, gum chewing, and fidgeting have in common? They're all part of NEAT. As we search for solutions to the *real* energy crisis in our lives (offloading the excess energy we eat, that is), something as simple as changing our posture can have a dramatic effect on our energy balance.

Exercise for Long-Term Health

Once you've got the basics of NEAT (daily, non-exercise activities) under control, we'll slowly but surely integrate EAT (planned exercise) into your life—in ways that are easy, simple, and fun to do. Why? Because along with helping you maintain your healthy weight, regular moderate exercise can:

- Help prevent heart disease, strokes, diabetes, and other chronic disease
- Boost your overall mood
- Lower high blood pressure
- Reduce stress
- Strengthen muscles, bones, and joints
- Improve metabolism and increase your energy level
- Strengthen your immune system while decreasing CRP levels and inflammation
- Help prevent depression
- Increase bone density and help prevent osteoporosis

But NEAT can be hard to measure, especially since it's made up of so many diverse activities. Unlike the exercises of EAT, which are limited in duration and can be measured using metabolic equivalents (METs)—a technique I'll introduce in chapter 16—the many little movements that comprise NEAT are going on all the time. So how do we know if they're having any effect?

When Dr. James A. Levine and his innovative Mayo Clinic team (see sidebar, page 182, Can Standing for One Hour a Day Cure Obesity?) did their groundbreaking research on NEAT, they outfitted their test subjects with an array of equipment with names like *inclinometer* and *triaxial accelerometer* to continually measure body posture and movements, and had their subjects drink radioactive water to track NEAT's contribution to energy expenditure. This painstaking work gave us a good indication of just how much energy our daily low-level movements consume, in comparison to inactivity. Some of their results are shown in the chart below.

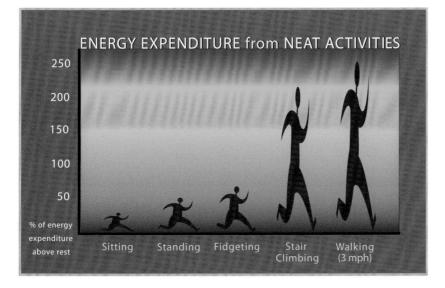

Energy Expenditure from NEAT Activities. When Dr. James A. Levine and his team of Mayo Clinic researchers measured the non-exercise (NEAT) activities of their subjects (see sidebar, page 182, Can Standing for One Hour a Day Cure Obesity?), they found out which ordinary activities generate the greatest energy expenditure.*

*Levine, J. A., "Nonexercise Activity Thermogenesis (NEAT): Environment and Biology," *American Journal of Physiology, Endocrinology and Metabolism* 286: E675–E685.

YOUR JOURNEY TO OPTIMAL HEALTH

Can Standing for One Hour a Day Cure Obesity?

A team of researchers at the Mayo Clinic, led by Dr. James A. Levine, spent ten days studying groups of mildly obese and lean volunteers—all self-proclaimed couch potatoes. They discovered that the obese group stayed seated for about 2.5 hours longer per day than the lean group—burning on average 350 fewer calories per day. The team's groundbreaking research showed that as humans overeat, the activation of NEAT burns enough excess energy to keep us lean. When NEAT fails to activate, on the other hand, the result is weight gain. And as we've learned from the work of James Hill,* a mere 100 to 200 calories per day of excess intake may well account for today's obesity epidemic.

*Hill, J. O., et al., "Obesity and the Environment," Science 299: 853–855.

Measuring NEAT in this way is all well and good, but not very practical for everyday life—unless you're prepared to get hooked up to a lot of wires and wear space-age underwear! Luckily, there's another, simpler way to measure NEAT, which I'll teach you in the next chapter when I introduce the NEAT System, part of my Habits of Motion system.

But first, let's look at the various kinds of NEAT we'll be tracking as we work on upping your daily energy expenditure.

Occupational NEAT and Leisure NEAT

Work makes up a big portion of our day and presents a very different set of obesigenic conditions and challenges. According to the National Sleep Foundation, the average person spends forty-six hours a week at work. Combine that with transportation to and from our workplace, and *fully one-third of our time* is spent on the job. Although what we do when we're working isn't always under our control, there are a number of potential openings for our motion plan even during working hours. That's particularly important today, with the advent of the computer and a resulting reduction in manual labor, which has cut movement out of our working lives dramatically. We'll discuss ways to "sneak" movement into your work day in chapter 15.

What about leisure time? That's an area where we do have control. But an increasing number of energy-saving devices have crept into every nook and cranny of our lives. Far from making our lives better, most of these so-called "advancements" are actually robbing us of our daily activity and our health. In fact, experiments have shown that the energetic costs of non-work automation are between 100 and 200 calories a day. That alone could account for the entire obesity epidemic!

Given what we now understand about the importance of normal, daily motions and weight control, it's all the more important to just say no to excess automation in your life. Don't let the machines steal your health!

The good news is that even an act as trivial as chewing gum can increase your energy expenditure 20 percent above your resting level—and that means 20 percent more calories burned. What a great ad for sugar-free gum that could be! A mindless motion like fidgeting can raise energy expenditure 20 to 40 percent. And strolling along while shopping at the mall, even at a slow pace of one mile per hour, doubles your energy expenditure. Pick up the pace to two or three miles per hour and you'll nearly triple it.

Movements like these are key components of my Habits of Motion system. Making it easy for you to measure, track, and increase the calories you burn is all part of my long-term plan to make motion—in all its forms—an integral part of your life.

> **Warning:** Consult your doctor before beginning this program. The instructions and advice presented here do not substitute for medical consultation. As with any exercise program, if at any point during your workout you begin to feel faint, dizzy, or have physical discomfort, stop immediately and consult a physician.

Dr. A's Habits of Motion System:
A Movement Plan for Life

Before introducing this active living system, I need to put on my physician's coat and take a moment to fill you in on your responsibility. Any time you change your level of activity, it's important to be evaluated by your primary care physician first. That's why I suggest you get a complete physical, taking into account any pre-existing health conditions like knee or joint problems, arthritis, or high blood pressure and discussing with your doctor how these conditions may be affected by an increase in movement. Heeding this warning is particularly important if you've just lost a lot of weight and are out of shape.

That's the first step. I also suggest you go slow at the beginning and pay attention to any signs of discomfort—though you can be assured that in the first part of my movement plan we'll only be adding mild activity in order to keep your heart rate in a safe range.

Got the green light from your physician? Great! Now let's go over the basics of my Habits of Motion system as we prepare to add movement to your life.

Tools for Success

Before you get moving, it's worth investing in a few simple devices to help you monitor your activity, track your progress, and stay safe.

Heart rate monitor. Heart rate monitors cost between $25 and $100, and are well worth the investment. Usually worn on the wrist, with a monitor around your torso, they provide an easy way to measure your heart rate automatically—though a watch with a second hand can be substituted. We'll be using a heart rate monitor to evaluate your physical response to increasing levels of movement, beginning by creating a target heart rate to guide us as we slowly condition this most important muscle in your body.

Stopwatch. Most heart rate monitors also function as stopwatches. We'll be using this to measure your NEAT activity and other movement routines.

Pedometer. A pedometer enables you to count your steps as you begin your movement program and monitor your progress as you move forward. As part of my movement plan, you'll strap a pedometer on from the moment you get up out of bed until you hit the pillow at night. That way, we can tally your total steps per day and use that figure to determine how many calories you're burning through NEAT. I suggest you buy the least expensive pedometer you can find that's accurate, reliable, and easy to use, though if you really want to go all out, you can buy a wrist GPS system that monitors your speed and distance and even tells you how to get home! (For more information on buying a pedometer, see the appendix or visit the Web site at www.habitsofhealth.net.)

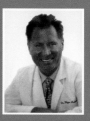

Staying Safe While You Move: Evaluating Your Heart Rate

Your heart is the most important muscle in your body. As you increase your physical activity, your heart will be working a bit harder, just like your other muscles. That's why monitoring your heart rate is so important.

If you have a heart rate monitor: Just strap it on and read the results!

If you're measuring your heart rate by hand: Sit down in a quiet space and measure your heart rate by counting your pulse for one minute (alternatively, count your pulse for ten seconds and multiply by six, though this measurement may be slightly less accurate). To take your pulse, place your index finger and third finger on your radial artery (located on the inside of the wrist below your thumb). ***Warning:*** *Do not use the carotid artery (side of the neck). Doing so can cause a stroke in individuals with occult plaque.*

Three Important Heart Rate Measures

Resting Heart Rate (RHR). The number of times your heart contracts per minute, measured when you're at rest.

Maximum Heart Rate (MHR). The highest number of times your heart can contract per minute during maximum physical exertion. MHR is most accurately determined with a cardiac stress test, but for our purposes we'll use the following formula:

$$MHR = 220 - your\ age$$

For example, the MHR of someone fifty years old is 170 beats per minute (220–50).

Target Heart Rate (THR). Between 50% and 85% of your maximum heart rate. As we increase your movement using NEAT, we'll check your THR to make sure we're not raising your heart rate too quickly. Once you're on pace and adding NEAT, we'll also use your target heart rate to maximize your cardiovascular fitness level.

On Your Mark, Get Set. . .

We're going to equip you with the knowledge and skills you need to add movement to your life in baby steps, through a logical schedule that slowly but surely builds Habits of Motion to last a lifetime. We'll start at the beginning, with a plan that's slow and easy, yet flexible enough to suit the needs of even a more advanced mover. It's a plan that's safe for all ages, that minimizes time commitment, that's effective, and most important is sustainable over time— and by that, I mean for the rest of your life. Until now, a plan like that just didn't exist!

In the next two chapters, I will unfold a system that will give you all the Habits of Motion you need to maintain a healthy weight and proceed up the path to optimal health. We'll begin in chapter 15 by putting NEAT movement into your daily life, and continue in chapter 16 by adding EAT—progressive, scheduled movements that fit your lifestyle. By the end, you'll have a complete system that will enable you to develop muscle and fitness at a pace and schedule you can stick with.

Let's take our first steps!

Chapter 15

· ·

Dr. A's Habits of Motion

Part 1: NEAT System

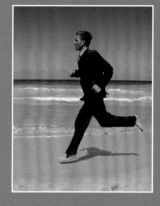

The NEAT System is designed for everyone. It's easy, it's effective, and you can do it. You already are—we're just going to make you NEATer!

NEAT is a bit like the story of the tortoise and the hare. By making small daily choices, you can win the race of weight maintenance and set the stage for exercise *at your own pace.* My NEAT System adds motion to every aspect of your day, but so gradually that it won't seem like much effort at all. That makes it particularly helpful for people who aren't used to exercising, for those with a BMI (body mass index) above 30, or those with medical conditions (cleared by a doctor first). It's a system you can do right now and continue doing into your 90s and 100s.

Just by making these little NEAT motions a part of your daily routine, you'll soon accomplish your primary goal of offloading a couple of hundred calories each day, and that's going to help your energy management system function flawlessly—indefinitely. Best of all, it's safe. There's no intense exertion involved (though we'll keep a close watch on your target heart rate just to be extra sure). It's important that you feel comfortable and protected as you start creating a more mobile, fit world for yourself. And now that you've lost some weight and are feeling better, you're ready to go!

Managing NEAT: The Six S's of Success

The NEAT System helps you take control of your body's energy balance by harnessing the movements you make in the course of your daily activities— the way you move your body, for example, or the way your perform everyday tasks at work and at home. To help you keep track of these motions, I've divided NEAT into six categories that represent the movements and postures that typically fill our days. Together, they serve as a training system to help you transform NEAT into an integral Habit of Health.

The six NEAT categories:

- *Stance*
- *Standing*
- *Strolling*
- *Stairs*
- *Samba*
- *Switch*

Exercise and Your Heart: The Benefits of Taking It Slow
It's a well-known medical fact that an unfit, sedentary lifestyle causes cardiovascular disease. Combine that with too much excess weight, and jumping too quickly into exercise can be a recipe for disaster. Although the risk is low, sudden death and heart attack are more likely to take place during exercise. That's why it's so important to ramp up slowly using the NEAT System, and to continue monitoring your heart rate. By the time you progress to the active exercising of EAT, your heart will be stronger than ever.

NEAT: It's in the Genes
Some people just have naturally high levels of NEAT. It's in their genes! They're more active by nature, and usually thinner as a result. But luckily, environment is more critical than biology when it comes to NEAT, and that's why the NEAT System arms you with the knowledge and techniques to augment your daily motion. When you consciously perform these small movements and activities daily, they soon become second nature, making the Habits of Motion part of your world.

These six categories cover the full range of muscle energy expenditure in your everyday life (outside of the scheduled exercises that make up EAT, that is). As part of my system, I'll teach you to track each one individually so you can be sure you're doing the most you can to increase your daily calorie burn. We want to make sure, especially in the beginning, that you're targeting behaviors from all six categories.

By making these small changes, you set the foundation for all the movement to come as you ascend the path to optimal health. Soon your NEAT behaviors will become automatic, and you'll never again struggle to burn calories.

Keeping Track: NEAT Activity Sheets

I know that keeping track of your daily activity can get tedious, but it is helpful—especially in the beginning as you evaluate your current level of motion and begin to make progress. I've made it a bit simpler for you by creating NEAT activity sheets tailored to the six NEAT categories. You'll find these in the appendix, as well as in the companion workbook and on the Web site at www.habitsofhealth.net.

It's important to use these tools right off the bat to record your starting point, and to continue using them as your activity increases. But don't worry—within a month of using the NEAT System, you'll internalize your new behaviors and will no longer have to think about them consciously or keep track of each movement. They'll just come naturally! That's when you know you've truly adopted these important Habits of Health.

Now let's find out exactly what we mean by *movement* as we explore the six NEAT categories—our S's of success!

Stance (Posture)

When the muscles that support your body's core axis—the chest, shoulders, back, legs, and abdominals—are aligned properly, they create balance throughout your body. Focusing on these foundational muscles helps you

---

Start Where You Stand: Silent NEAT

Want to burn sixty extra calories a day without lifting a finger? You can by paying attention to the first two S's.

The first two NEAT categories, *stance* and *standing*, may not seem much like movement at all. In fact, they're really just baseline body positions. But if you could put on a pair of electron X-ray glasses and observe your muscles at the microscopic level, you'd be amazed to see that your muscle cells are in continuous motion. At their most microscopic level, your muscles are made up of tiny units called *sarcomeres.* These tiny sarcomeres expend energy constantly as they slide back and forth, keeping your muscles at just the right tension to do their job. By focusing on your body position and effort, we can put more demand on these muscle fibers, and at the same time improve your overall health.

burn more calories and provides great training for your transition to the EAT exercises to come.

This focus is particularly important when you're sitting—a position we find ourselves in a lot in our automated world, especially at work. Computers, cubicles, meetings, commuting, and the mechanization of manual jobs all reduce our natural mobility, not to mention TVs, game boys, remotes, drive-thru fast food (a deadly double whammy!), cars, and shuttles. As you proceed through the six S's, you'll find some great ways to get up and move, starting by simply reminding yourself to get out of your seat whenever you can. But as this first NEAT category shows, even if you are stuck sitting you can still increase your energy expenditure and enhance your health.

In fact, sitting is one of the best times to work on your posture and core axis alignment. Start by using a proper chair that helps you sit up straight. Now flex your stomach muscles and take deep, slow breaths. (We'll discuss deep breathing more thoroughly in chapter 19.)

NEAT ideas:

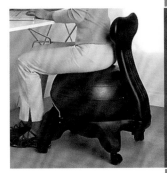

At work: Focus on sitting up straight in meetings. Get up and move around as much as possible, but when you must sit at your desk try using a balance ball chair, which forces you to use your core muscles for support.

At home: Focus on sitting up straight while watching TV or riding in the car (even better, get up and move any time you can!).

Measuring tools: Stopwatch and NEAT activity sheets.

Evaluation: Measure the minutes per day you spend focusing on core position (stomach in, shoulders back) while sitting, standing, or in motion. Count how many times you get up from a sitting position to move around.

Goal: Add two additional minutes of focus on core position per day.

Target: Thirty minutes of focus on core position per day. Additional target: use balance ball chair all day at work.

Energy expenditure: 1 kcal per minute of core position focus; 10 kcal per hour of balance ball; 1 kcal per instance of intentionally getting up from a sitting position when you would otherwise have continued to sit.

Potential: 60 kcal per day.

NEAT points*: 1 per minute of core position focus; 10 per hour of balance ball; 1 per instance of getting up from sitting.

* NEAT points represent energy expended *above* the amount you would expend resting. 1 NEAT point = 1 kcal.

By making small changes in each of the six NEAT categories, you're making *secondary choices* that support your *primary goal* to increase healthy movement.

Balance Ball Chair. Sitting on a balance ball chair forces you to use your core muscles for support, which burns more calories.

A Habit of Health: Increasing NEAT by flexing your stomach muscles while you sit up straight

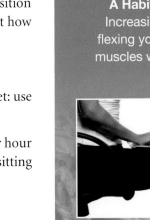

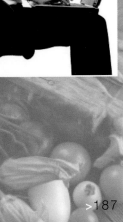

Can a "Walk and Work" Desk Cure Obesity? Researchers at the Mayo Clinic think so. In a recent study, Dr. James A. Levine replaced normal desks with workstations attached to a treadmill. By using the treadmills at a slow pace (around one mile per hour) for two to three hours per day, Levine's obese subjects burned 100 calories an hour. That's as much as 66 pounds in one year!

Standing

Merely moving from sitting to standing can substantially increase your energy consumption. When you stand, you begin to use weight-bearing NEAT—and one of the great advantages of weight-bearing NEAT is that the heavier you are, the more calories you expend. It's actually more effective the more you weigh! That's good news, because it means that if you're overweight, you can start off slow and still receive the benefits of increased movement. And although you'll begin to burn fewer calories per minute as you lose weight, you'll easily compensate for that decrease by being in better shape for more activity.

NEAT ideas:

At work: Get out of your chair as much as you can. Stand when talking on the phone, using a mobile phone with an earpiece or a portable headset, even if you have to buy it yourself (remember, you're investing in your health!). Get rid of comfy couches and get a "standing desk."

At home: All of the above, plus stand while you prepare meals, wash dishes at the sink, iron clothes, watch TV, and read the paper.

Measuring tools: Stopwatch and NEAT activity sheets.

Evaluation: Measure the minutes per day you spend standing.

Goal: Add ten additional minutes of standing per day.

Target: Two hours of standing per day.

Energy expenditure: 1 kcal per minute of standing.

Potential: 120 kcal per day.

NEAT points: 1 per minute of standing.

Strolling (Walking)

When I talk about walking in terms of NEAT, I'm referring to anything outside of a formal walking program. That includes going to the water cooler, delivering a memo to your boss, or shopping for that new dress at the mall. Remember, the point of NEAT is that it takes place *within your normal routines*, so it doesn't require a lot of extra time or effort.

As we get older, we typically take fewer steps per day. After age sixty, most people are down to around 4,500 steps. Our goal is to increase your daily step count to over 10,000, achieved mostly through NEAT and supplemented if necessary through my EAT System walking program, which I'll introduce in the next chapter. We want to keep you walking right into your eighties, nineties, and beyond!

NEAT ideas:

At work: Walk around the room when you're on the phone, walk to work or park your car farther away, talk to coworkers in person rather than by e-mail or phone, have walking meetings, choose the farthest restroom and water cooler, have your lunch (or fueling) in the park, try out a "walk and work" desk.

At home: Take the dog for a walk, meet people face to face rather than shouting from the other room, go to the mall and window shop, park your car as far as is safely possible from your destination, walk on the beach instead of sunbathing, pass on elevators, escalators, and drive-thrus. Get off the couch!

Measuring tools: Pedometer and NEAT activity sheets.

Evaluation: Measure your steps from the time you get out of bed in the morning until you lay down again at night.

Goal: Add 100 additional steps per week.

Target: At least 10,000 steps per day (a mile is about 2,000 steps).

Energy expenditure: As with other weight-bearing activities, the leaner and fitter you are, the fewer calories you expend per step. Your gender also comes into play, as does the pace at which you walk. Use the following chart to help you calculate how many calories you burn walking at a moderate pace (three miles per hour).

ENERGETIC STEP VALUE (ESV)		
(steps required to burn 1 kcal)		
Body Mass Index BMI	ESV (Female)	ESV (Male)
18 – 24.9 Healthy	36 steps per kcal	28 steps per kcal
25 – 29.9 Overweight	30 steps per kcal	24 steps per kcal
30 – 34.9 Class I Obesity	24 steps per kcal	20 steps per kcal
35 – 39.9 Class II Obesity	18 steps per kcal	16 steps per kcal
Over 40 Class III Obesity	12 steps per kcal	11 steps per kcal

To calculate the calories you burn from walking:

1. Take the number of steps you've *added* since beginning the program. (Let's say 2,000 more steps per day.)

2. Locate your correct BMI and gender from the chart above to find your Energetic Step Value (ESV). (Let's say a woman with a BMI of 38, for an ESV of 18 steps per kcal.)

3. Divide your steps per day by your ESV (2,000 ÷ 18 = 111) = 111 kcal or 111 NEAT points.

That's the number of calories you're burning each day just through the extra steps you take!

Potential: 100–300 kcal per day.

NEAT points: 1 per kcal burned.

Boost Your Motivation!
- Wear comfortable shoes, even to work—if your feet are comfortable, you'll walk more.
- Remind yourself to walk by putting up a poster of yourself or someone else having fun moving.

Energetic Step Value (ESV). Locate your BMI in the left-hand column of the chart to find out how many steps you must take to burn one calorie. This number is your Energetic Step Value (ESV), which you'll use to calculate the total number of NEAT points you earn from walking.

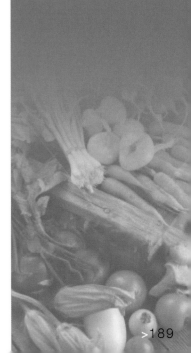

Boost Your Motivation!
Paint or decorate your
office stairwells to make
them more attractive
for walking.

Stairs

Stairs are a great way to accelerate NEAT. In fact, climbing just one flight of stairs is the equivalent of walking 100 steps. That means that climbing ten flights of stairs gives you the same benefit as a half mile of walking (and there are around 2,000 steps in a mile!).

When you climb stairs, you're actually lifting your total mass against gravity, making this one of the most effective NEAT activities available. Speed isn't critical here, so it's a great activity if you're overweight—and since it's a weight-bearing activity, you burn more calories the heavier you are.

Another great benefit of stairs is that they're readily available. Even when it's raining or cold outside, you can use stairwells where you work or in any multistory building. Just say no to elevators, and watch your NEAT increase!

One final note of caution: stair climbing is a moderately intense activity. If you're overweight or relatively inactive, see your physician first, start slowly, and pay attention to any signs that your body needs to take it easier. The good news is that if you add your NEAT activities in the order I've suggested, you should be fine by the time you begin stair climbing.

NEAT ideas:

At work: Take the stairs instead of the elevator or escalator (especially in bad weather, when you can't walk outside). Use the restroom or water cooler on a different floor. Take a stair break instead of a coffee break.

At home: Walk the stairs at the mall, ballpark, or department store.

Measuring tools: NEAT activity sheets.

Evaluation: Record the flights of stairs you climb (up and down) in a day. One flight of stairs is about fifteen individual stairs.

Goal: Add one additional flight of stairs per week.

Target: Ten flights of stairs per day.

Energy expenditure: Use the following formula to calculate how many calories you burn per flight of stairs *or* use the chart below to estimate (remember, each NEAT point equals one calorie).

NEAT Points per Flight of Stairs. Locate your BMI in the left-hand column to find out how many NEAT points you earn for each flight of stairs you climb.

NEAT POINTS PER FLIGHT OF STAIRS	
Body Mass Index BMI	NEAT Points per flight (up and down)
<25	3
25 – 30	4
30 – 35	5
35 – 40	6
>40	7

.022 kcal × number of pounds you weigh × number of flights

(For example, if you weigh 150 pounds and climb 10 flights of stairs per day: .022 × 150 lbs × 10 flights = 26 kcal.)

Potential: 25–50 kcal/day.

NEAT points: 1 per kcal burned, *or* estimate from the chart at left.

Samba (Dance)

Here, we're looking at movement generated by your body's natural rhythm. What do I mean by that? Put on a song you like and watch what happens. You might start tapping your pencil or your foot, or even singing at the top of your lungs!

There's a term for music's capacity to lift us up this way—*ergogenic*. An ergogenic aid is anything outside your body that boosts physical or mental performance, either by increasing your capacity to perform, removing psychological constraints to performance, or speeding your recovery after exertion. For the EAT System activities in the next chapter, we'll use music to distract you from any discomfort and enhance your performance. And as you'll see in chapter 19, music and rhythm can even help decrease inflammation.

For the purposes of NEAT, though, we'll be focusing on music's ability to enhance motion by amplifying brain arousal, a phenomenon that researchers have shown may actually increase the intensity of your activity—and that means you're burning more calories. In my book, whatever gets you moving is a great way to increase NEAT, especially when it's so much fun to do!

NEAT ideas:

At work: Turn on your iPod at lunch, go outside, and get in motion.

At home: Use music to augment everything you do on your own, from gardening to cleaning (avoid music in situations where it would prevent you from interacting with others, though, since talking also increases NEAT). Go dancing! Start with ballroom and work your way up to tap dancing, square dancing, and eventually more intense dances such as jitterbugging and hip hop.

Measuring tools: Stopwatch and NEAT activity sheets.

Evaluation: Measure the number of minutes you listen to music per day and the number of hours you dance per week.

Goal: Add ten additional minutes of music per day; work up to an hour or more of dance per week.

Target: Ninety minutes of music per day; one hour of dance per week.

Energy expenditure: 1 kcal per minute of up-tempo music. For dance, use the following formulas to approximate.

> *Slow to moderate dancing* (waltz, foxtrot, slow dancing, samba, tango, mambo, cha-cha): 3 kcal per minute.

> *Fast to intense dancing* (disco, folk, square, line dancing, Irish step dancing, polka, contra, country, ballet, modern, twist, jazz, tap, jitterbug, African): 5 kcal per minute.

Potential: 10 kcal per day for music; 20–30 kcal per day for dance (at an average of one hour of dancing per week).

NEAT points: 30–40 per day.

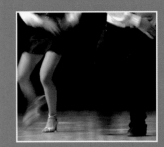

Dr. A Says . . .

Stay on track while you're staying with friends or family by asking them to join you on a walking tour or offering to cook a healthy meal.

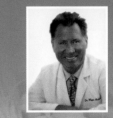

Switch

Switch means doing things by hand instead of by machine. That includes dishwashers, electric knifes, snow blowers, remotes, computers, and all the other automatic devices that steal from your energy-use account at an ever-growing pace. Your goal is to burn an extra thirty calories per day doing tasks by hand that you previously had machines do for you.

Warning: Do not extend "switch" to movements that can cause repetitive injury or exacerbate a current conditions such as tendonitis.

NEAT ideas:

At work: Take notes and sharpen pencils by hand.

At home: Put away the appliances and start doing kitchen and other indoor chores by hand. Take out the garbage, rake leaves, shovel snow, wash your car by hand, and mow your lawn with a hand mower (your neighbors will love the peace and quiet!).

Measuring tools: Stopwatch and NEAT activity sheets.

Evaluation: Record the amount of time you spend performing tasks using manual labor instead of a machine.

Some NEAT Pointers

- To maintain your healthy weight, aim to burn about 200 calories a day through NEAT activities.

- Be good to your heart! As you add new NEAT activities or increase your level of effort, keep checking your heart rate, especially if you feel lightheaded or weak. Make sure it's in the 50–60 percent range until you feel comfortable. Once you're on your way to becoming fit, this will no longer be required, except as part of your EAT System program.

- Don't be discouraged if you still have a lot of weight to lose—it can actually work to your advantage. The more you weigh, the more calories you burn with each movement, particularly when it comes to weight-bearing activities such as walking, stair climbing, and dancing. Pretty NEAT, huh?

- Get comfortable with NEAT before you move on to more vigorous exercise. The EAT System exercises you'll learn in the next chapter are ideal for maximizing fitness and creating optimal health, but it's important to take it slow. If you're worried about gaining your weight back, I can assure you that our NEAT System is the great equalizer to a sedentary life!

Goal: Add one or two substituted manual tasks per day.

Target: Ten substituted manual tasks per day.

Energy expenditure: 1 calorie per minor manual task (for example, opening a can using a manual opener); 3 calories per minute for manual chores (for example, raking).

Potential: 40 calories per day.

NEAT points: 1 per minor task; 3 per minute for chores.

Tracking NEAT: Your NEAT Activity Sheets

Now that you know how to evaluate, measure, set goals, and increase NEAT, it's time to put the NEAT System to work to help you keep your daily energy use and intake in perfect balance.

Before You Begin

Before you begin integrating all of these NEAT new activities into your life (once you've been cleared by your doctor, that is), you need to record your starting point. Knowing where you are right now will help you determine which of the six S's are going to give you the biggest boost when it comes to burning extra calories. Remember, we're only looking for 200 additional calories of energy expenditure per day. That's all! NEAT, like all the Habits of Health, doesn't require you to make extreme changes in your lifestyle.

To get a true baseline, you'll need to track your NEAT activity for seven days *before* implementing any changes. To do this, turn to the NEAT activity sheets located in the appendix. (They're also available in *Living a Longer, Healthier Life: The Companion Guide to Dr. A's Habits of Health* and on the Web site at www.habitsofhealth.net.)

As you'll see, there are three types of NEAT activity sheets:

• NEAT Scoring Sheet
• NEAT Activity Log (daily and weekly)
• NEAT Goal Setter

Just track your NEAT points for the day and week in the NEAT Scoring Sheet and Activity Logs (using your stopwatch and pedometer); you'll enter those figures into the Goal Setter.

Goal Setting for NEAT

Roughly speaking, your goals for this initial stage of your lifetime movement plan are as follows:

• 120 NEAT points per day for the first thirty days.
• 200 NEAT points per day for the second thirty days.

Depending on your current lifestyle and activity level, I suggest you focus on adding one additional activity per day for the first week, then one additional activity in each category starting the second week.

Dr. A Says . . .

Keeping track of your daily activity, how you feel before and after working out, and what keeps you motivated can help you learn what works and what doesn't—so if you should start to plateau, you'll be better able to get yourself out of it and keep moving forward!

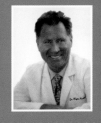

If you're sedentary, have a lot of weight to lose, or have a medical condition, proceed at a pace that's doable, doesn't overtax you, and is within your physician's guidelines. Remember, we're not in a hurry. Your healthy eating plan is improving your condition daily, and it's just fine for your movement plan to advance at a speed that works for you. If on the other hand you want to go faster and you're already in good shape, go ahead!

Moving Forward: From NEAT to EAT

By the end of the second month using my NEAT System, you'll be burning 200 more calories each day than you are right now, just by enhancing your normal, everyday activities. And that increase in energy expenditure means you'll be able to offset the natural decrease that occurs as you lose weight—the key to healthy weight maintenance! But just as important, you'll increase your flexibility, mobility, and total daily motion, to make your whole body stronger.

This initial series of activities is the first step in your movement program for optimal health. Now let's look at my scheduled exercise plan, beginning with walking, to help you prepare for your graduate degree in movement.

"My life is a whole new adventure!"

LISA CASTRO

Nearly five years at optimal health

Shortly before I began the journey to optimal health in 2003, I was diagnosed with connective tissue disease, worsened by stress. I was so fatigued and achy that I had to will myself out of bed every morning. I knew I needed to take better care of myself, but I just didn't have the time or the energy.

Within three months of starting the journey, I lost almost 25 percent of my body weight, going from a size 12 to a size 0 petite—and that's despite having low thyroid. In fact, the nurse said I have results that others would envy!

I use the Habits of Health all the time. I eat five to six small, low-fat, balanced meals each day,

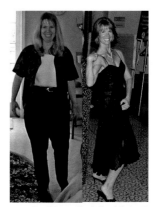

Results vary. Typical weight loss is 2-5 lbs per week for the first 2 weeks and 1-2 lbs per week thereafter.

and practice a regular exercise routine. The amazing benefits have been that I don't hurt any more, and I now have the energy to exercise regularly. It's amazing what good nutrition can do! I've gone from dreading the thought of getting out of bed, to feeling excited about the future and eager to seek new experiences. My husband and I are enjoying our lives so much now that we have the freedom to pursue our dreams and the regained health to achieve them! We call it our mid-life *improvement*—no crisis here! ∎

Chapter 16

Dr. A's Habits of Motion

Part 2: EAT System

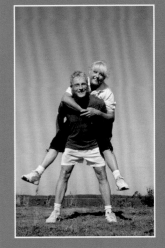

Exercise Activity Thermogenesis (EAT): Planned movement that's vigorous enough to improve overall fitness. Any activity performed deliberately to enhance the body's conditioning—ranging in intensity from a walk in the park to a triathlon.

The NEAT System showed you how to burn an additional 200 calories a day without making major changes in your activity level or daily routine. And you were able to put this user-friendly system to work right away to help maintain your weight, increase your flexibility and mobility, and build a healthier lifestyle.

But as you know, we have an even higher goal. We want to create optimal health. That's why you need the second part of my movement plan—the EAT System. EAT helps you optimize your health through specific, regularly scheduled exercises that boost your energy expenditure and significantly improve your all-around health, from your heart and immune system to your mental aptitude and sex life. As a result, you'll work better, feel better (EAT can decrease your need for medication and arrest the progress of disease), and even live longer. In fact, EAT is our most important predictor of longevity. It's the type of movement we didn't want to rush you into, but now that you're well on your way to a healthy weight and have increased your daily movement, it makes sense to add this powerful health-enhancing plan to your life.

Built to Last

My philosophy is that it's best to incorporate activities of *moderate intensity*, based on the premise that you're going to use them until you reach the end of a full, thriving life.

And although the EAT System will take a bit of time out of your day, it's specifically designed to minimize your daily commitment by giving you the most effective results in the least amount of time possible.

Best of all, it's part of a long-term strategy to reach and maintain optimal health for the rest of your life. It helps you rehabilitate, condition, enhance, and protect the very organs that help your body move—your musculoskeletal and cardiovascular systems. Optimizing these two systems through exercise ensures that you can enjoy great health into your eighties, nineties, and maybe beyond!

In fact, exercise becomes even more important as we age. By the time we reach our sixties, the average number of steps we take in a day declines by as much as 25 percent. One tragic result is an increased prevalence of hip fractures among the elderly due to falls. These fractures—which are much more common in people whose balance and strength are diminished from lack of physical activity—lead to death within a year among up to 40 percent of sufferers.

But it doesn't have to be this way. By optimizing your body systems and making use of the advances in life extension that you'll discover through the Habits of Health, you should be able to increase your shelf-life and support your health for at least 100 years.

That's why I don't recommend aggressive exercise programs. They're just not sustainable! Either they're too difficult to keep up or, worse, they cause injuries that put your future capability at risk. Instead, the EAT System, like all the Habits of Health, is designed to teach you small steps you can do right now and will want to continue doing for life. Think of it this way: if you want your car to offer you reliable transportation, you treat it with loving care by warming it up before you drive it and changing the oil regularly. It's really no different for your body!

Thirty Minutes a Day, a Lifetime of Health

That's all it takes! Thirty minutes a day of moderate activity for a lifetime of health and longevity. And that's because the NEAT System is already contributing the lion's share of your daily energy expenditure through your 10,000 steps a day and the other S's. The EAT System builds on this foundation by increasing your energy expenditure even more as you train and optimize your cardiovascular and musculoskeletal systems.

By adding EAT into the picture, you position yourself to achieve the Habits of Motion system's three core goals:

- Increasing energy expenditure to create a consistent balance between energy in and energy out.
- Optimizing cardiovascular health so that your heart, lungs, and blood vessels can deliver enough oxygen to keep your cells functioning properly, especially your brain cells.
- Building a strong, healthy support system of bones and muscles to help you stay active, keep fit, and maintain a healthy weight.

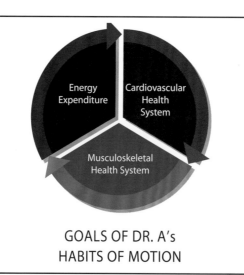

Goals of Dr. A's Habits of Motion. Our movement system has three goals: energy expenditure, cardiovascular health, and musculoskeletal health. These three components work together to support each other and help your entire body achieve optimal health.

GOALS OF DR. A's
HABITS OF MOTION

> *Weight Training: The Calorie-Burning Gift*
> *That Keeps On Giving*
>
> There's a lot more to muscle building than meets the eye. Not only does weight resistance training burn calories both during and after exercise, but the long-term results of weight training—more muscle—help you continue to burn extra calories 24/7. That's because muscle is the most important determinant of Basal Metabolic Rate (BMR), the rate at which your body processes food and burns it for energy. Adding a pound of muscle can increase your daily BMR—the amount of calories you burn in a day—by fifty to seventy calories.

Cardiovascular Health

I spent twenty years as a critical care physician helping patients with wounded cardiovascular systems do what healthy systems do naturally—deliver oxygenated blood to all the cells in the body.

Just twenty to thirty minutes of walking a day at a moderate pace is all you need to keep your heart, lungs, brain, and blood vessels healthy so they can support your entire body indefinitely. You can reach that goal by walking about one and a half miles at a pace of three to four miles an hour, or by doing other things you enjoy, such as riding a bike, swimming, skiing, or walking nine holes with a pull cart for your clubs. That's a far cry from Richard Simmons Sweatin' to the Oldies! (Though aerobics are fine too, if that's what gets you going!)

Musculoskeletal Health

As we discussed previously, sarcopenia—a degeneration of muscle mass and strength sometimes referred to as osteoporosis of the muscles—is a serious condition that affects people who don't use their muscles regularly for lifting and moving. It creates flabby, weak muscles that then lead to more inactivity, ultimately stressing all the organ systems. But by devoting just a little time each week, you can recondition your muscles and increase both their number and size. That's why the EAT System includes two thirty-minute weight resistance sessions each week to support healthy weight, physical appearance, and overall fitness.

> *Maximum Heart Rate (MHR)*
>
> The highest number of times your heart can contract per minute during maximum physical exertion. To determine your MHR, subtract your age from 220.
>
> *Target Heart Rate (THR)*
>
> Between 50% and 85% of your maximum heart rate.

Swim for Your Life! Swimming and other water exercises are great ways to meet your movement goals and are especially beneficial for the elderly, those who have arthritis, or anyone who's recovering from an injury. The buoyancy of water reduces your weight by about 80–90 percent, minimizing the amount of stress on your weight-bearing joints, bones, and muscles, while still giving you a workout in all three key areas of our movement system: cardio, strength training, and flexibility. Check out your local community recreation center or health clubs in your area to see if they offer swim classes and pool memberships.

**Walking:
A Wonder Drug?**
Studies have shown
that walking just thirty
minutes a day can have
a dramatic positive
effect on your health by:

• Lowering your risk for
depression

• Eliminating your need
for medications

• Reducing breast
cancer risk by 30%
and increasing
survival rates by 70%

• Lowering your
blood pressure and
preventing injury to
your cardiovascular
system by keeping
blood vessels open
and flexible

• Increasing survival
rates from heart
attack by 80%

Before You Begin: Staying Safe

Before you start your EAT program, make sure you know the ground rules for protecting your body from injury and staying safe.

• **Keep it slow.** Use slow, careful movements for weight training and other strengthening exercises. At the beginning, keep your heart rate at 50–65 percent of your maximum heart rate.

For example, if you're fifty years old:

$220 - 50 = 170$
$170 \times .50$ (in other words, 50%) = 85 bpm (beats per minute)
$170 \times .65$ (in other words, 65%) = 110 bpm (beats per minute)

So your target heart rate range is between 85 and 110 bpm (beats per minute) throughout your daily activity.

As you progress and begin to feel more comfortable, you can aim toward 65 or 75 percent, and eventually 85 percent once you're optimally fit.

• **Stretch it out.** Help prevent injury by stretching your major muscle groups, preferably directly after your daily EAT activity. Add some extra stretching for a few minutes each day to keep your muscles flexible, improve your balance, and increase your range of motion.

• **Cool it down.** After each session, allow your musculoskeletal and cardiovascular systems to return to their baseline state. I'll teach you some great stretching techniques to add to each workout.

Ready? Let's start your EAT System, beginning with our EAT Walking Program.

The EAT Walking Program

Since you're already walking as part of your NEAT System activities, adding this natural, low-impact, safe, and simple activity in a more scheduled version should be a breeze. All you need is proper clothing, comfortable shoes, and your pedometer, and you're on your way!

You may be wondering how the NEAT walking you're doing differs from the kind you'll be doing in EAT. Basically, while adding steps through NEAT helps you burn more calories, it's not intense enough to produce fitness. The EAT Walking Program, on the other hand, is designed with fitness in mind, so you get essential cardiovascular benefits. And because walking is convenient and easy to do, you're more likely to keep at it so it can become part of your long-term plan for sustainable health.

Here are a few general guidelines to make your first experiences with the EAT Walking Program pleasant and successful:

• **Where to walk.** Choose a route that's safe; avoid roads used by motor vehicles. Walking outside will enable you to get fresh air and sunshine, but if you prefer you can walk indoors on a track or treadmill. Upbeat music or television can help combat boredom.

- **What to wear.** Wear comfortable, loose-fitting clothing, preferably layered to respond to changing weather conditions. Avoid plastic or rubberized fabrics that trap moisture and heat. When walking in low light, wear bright clothes or clothing with reflective tape.

- **About shoes.** Invest in walking shoes that give you the proper support and traction to maintain good balance and posture. A well-fitting shoe should allow your feet to roll inward and outward slightly to absorb impact. It's a good idea to get professional advice from a store that specializes in exercise footwear to be sure the shoe matches your individual motion and keeps your musculoskeletal system in the proper position for pain-free walking. Remember, you'll be walking over 1,500 miles a year as part of the Habits of Health—for many years to come!

Stepping Out: Your First Day

> **Warning:** Do not begin the EAT program until you've lost weight and have become comfortable with the NEAT program. As with starting any new activity, consult your physician first.

The best way to build success is to start slow. Clear your pedometer and set a goal for your first walk. It doesn't have to be long, just five to ten minutes.

As you walk, pay attention to any discomfort you may be feeling—perhaps in the fit of your shoes, and especially any shortness of breath or chest discomfort. If you find yourself unable to carry on a conversation without catching your breath, slow down or stop until the feeling passes. Don't worry, you'll be able to pick up the pace soon. In the meantime, signs such as these will help us monitor and guide your progress. For some extra help finding your comfort zone, try a handy self-evaluation tool called the Rate of Perceived Exertion scale (see box, page 200).

Keep at a slow pace until your muscles feel warm and relaxed. If your heart rate is at the low end of your target zone (say, 65 percent) and you're not experiencing shortness of breath, you can begin to pick up the pace.

> *Just thirty minutes of moderate physical activity each day—say, walking one and a half miles at three to four miles per hour—supports cardiovascular health.*
>
> *(Based on guidelines from the American College of Sports Medicine, Centers for Disease Control and Prevention, American Heart Association, U.S. Surgeon General, and U.S. Dietary Guidelines 2005.)*

Important Rules for Stretching

- The best time to stretch is directly after your walk.
- Never stretch cold muscles.
- Problem areas may be stretched prior to your walk, but only after you've warmed up.
- Don't bounce when you stretch.
- Ease into a stretch slowly and hold gently. Stretch to the point where you feel a gentle pull, but never to the point of pain.
- Hold each stretch for 30 to 40 seconds. If you have problems with a particular area, stretch that area twice. (Hold for 30 to 40 seconds, release, then stretch again.)

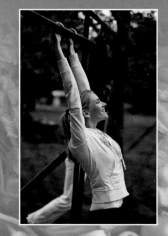

**EAT Walking Program
Key Points**

- Begin by walking twenty minutes a day, including five minutes for warm up and five minutes for cool down.
- Add five minutes each week, or as much as you're comfortable with.
- Work up to a brisk pace of around four miles per hour.
- Work up to around 20,000 steps per week by week ten (depending on your level of fitness and weight-loss goals).
- Your long-term goal is to walk for thirty minutes a day, five days a week.

Rate of Perceived Exertion (RPE)

Have you ever felt uncomfortable while exercising, or pushed beyond what seemed like an appropriate level? The Rate of Perceive Exertion (RPE) scale is a handy self-evaluation tool that helps you determine your comfort zone so you can keep your exercise sessions at a level that's more likely to prevent injury and promote long-term success.

To use RPE: Using a 0–10 scale, rate how much exertion you feel while exercising, with 0 being the equivalent of sitting quietly in a chair and 10 being akin to running up a steep hill. The recommended RPE range for most people is usually between 3 and 5. Remember, you're rating how hard you *feel* you're working, not how fast your pace actually is.

RATE OF PERCEIVED EXERTION

Borg Scale	RPE
0	nothing at all
0.5	very, very light
1	very light
2	light
3	moderate
4	somewhat hard
5 – 6	hard
7 – 8	very hard
9	very, very hard
10	maximum exertion

Adapted from Borg, G. V., "Psychological Basis of Perceived Exertion," *Medicine and Science Sports* 14 (1982): 377–81.

Here's a goal to set for your initial walking sessions. You can use either the amount of time or the number of steps to keep track.

Warm up	5 minutes at 1 mph	(about 160 steps)
At pace	10 minutes at 2 mph	(about 665 steps)
Cool down	5 minutes at 1 mph	(about 160 steps)

This twenty-minute session of around 1,000 steps (about a half mile) will consume approximately fifty calories if your BMI is 30.

Once you finish, spend about five minutes stretching. At right, you'll find two stretches for your hamstrings (the muscles in the back of the upper leg) and calves. As you practice these, make sure to follow my rules for stretching (see box, page 199).

Getting in Stride: Moving into Your Program

You've just completed the first step in what may well be the first successful long-term exercise program you've ever done. Now let's talk about progressing at a pace that builds a lifetime of health.

Your goal each week is to add five minutes of moderate walking (three to four miles per hour), until you're walking five days a week for thirty minutes each day. That's around 20,000 steps, or ten miles each week.

To keep track of your progress, use the EAT Walking Program Daily Tracking Sheet on page 202 and in the appendix (also located in the companion workbook and at www.habitsofhealth.net.) Just enter your daily minutes, steps, miles, and calories burned in the appropriate boxes.

To figure out how many calories you've burned, locate your Energetic Step Value (ESV) on the chart below and divide your total number of steps by your ESV. For example, according to the chart, the ESV for a woman with a BMI of 35 is 18. If she takes 20,000 steps in a week, she'll divide 20,000 by 18, for a total of 1,111 calories. That's 222 calories for each day of walking, on top of the extra 200 calories burned through NEAT!

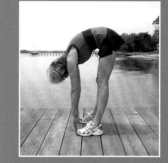

Hamstring and Lower Back Stretch. Slowly bend forward from your waist with your knees slightly bent. Reach for the floor and hold. Bend only as far as is comfortable.

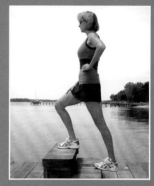

Calf Stretch. Stand on a stair or step with your right foot on the higher step and the front half of your left foot on the lower step. Slowly relax your left ankle, allowing the heel to drop below the step. Hold for 10 seconds. Repeat on the right foot.

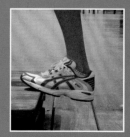

ENERGETIC STEP VALUE (ESV)

(steps required to burn 1 kcal)

Body Mass Index BMI	ESV (Female)	ESV (Male)
18 – 24.9 Healthy	36 steps per kcal	28 steps per kcal
25 – 29.9 Overweight	30 steps per kcal	24 steps per kcal
30 – 34.9 Class I Obesity	24 steps per kcal	20 steps per kcal
35 – 39.9 Class II Obesity	18 steps per kcal	16 steps per kcal
Over 40 Class III Obesity	12 steps per kcal	11 steps per kcal

Energetic Step Value (ESV). Locate your BMI in the left-hand column of the chart to find out how many steps you must take to burn one calorie. This number is your Energetic Step Value (ESV).

EAT WALKING PROGRAM DAILY TRACKING SHEET

Day	Warm-Up	Time	Cool-Down	Steps	Miles*	Calories
Day 1	5 minutes	10 minutes	5 minutes	1,000 steps	.5 mile	50 kcal
Day 2						
Day 3						
Day 4						
Day 5						

*1 mile = 2,000 steps

Once you've completed a week on the program, enter the week's data on the EAT Walking Program Weekly Tracking Sheet, below and in the appendix (also located in the companion workbook and on the Web site at www.habitsofhealth.net.)

This will help you get a big-picture view of your progress and keep you motivated.

EAT WALKING PROGRAM WEEKLY TRACKING SHEET

Week	Steps per Day		Steps per Week	Miles*	Comments
	Actual	Recommended			
1		1000 day	5000 week	3.5 mile	A little tired but energized by the end of the first week
2		1200 day			
3		1400 day			
4		1600 day			
5		1800 day			
6		2000 day			
7		2500 day			
8		3000 day			
9		3500 day			
10		4000 day			

*1 mile = 2,000 steps

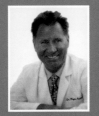

Picking Up the Pace: Advancing Your Program

The goal of the EAT Walking Program is to boost your cardiovascular and musculoskeletal health now and for years to come. It's a solid program that you can stay with for life just as it's outlined above. But you can also adapt the program to increase your level of fitness by adding hills, distance, and speed.

The best way to boost your workouts is by increasing their duration, rather than their intensity. My thirty-minute guideline is merely the baseline required to maintain fitness without cutting too much into your daily commitments. If you have time for more, that's great.

If you'd like to intensify your workout, burn more calories, and strengthen leg and buttock muscles, try walking up hills or raising the incline on your treadmill. It will help as you walk uphill to lean forward, shorten your steps, and pump your arms. Or to increase your cardiovascular fitness, try carrying lightweight dumbbells or wearing ankle weights or a weighted vest—but please don't attempt this until you're up to 20,000 steps per week and at a point where walking has become a Habit of Health.

As you step up your intensity, remember the basic principles of cardiovascular fitness:

- If you're unable to carry on a conversation, slow down.
- Keep your Rate of Perceived Exertion (RPE) below a six.

Once you've reached your EAT Walking Program goal of 20,000 steps per week (on top of the steps you're taking as part of the NEAT System) and have been walking five days every week for at least a month, you're ready to add the other essential component of the EAT System: resistance training.

The EAT Resistance Program

Does the thought of weight training conjure up images of sweaty, grunting muscle-heads in tank tops spending hours at the gym lifting huge amounts of weight? This type of boot-camp workout is not only unnecessary, it's downright unsafe. And it has no place in a sustainable health plan.

The EAT Resistance Program is something else entirely—two thirty-minute sessions a week specifically targeted to add strength to your musculoskeletal system (bones and muscles). The goal is to turn your underused, sarcopenic muscles into lean, efficient, healthy tissue that can support you for a lifetime.

Despite the negative effects of years spent in an environment of "labor-saving" devices, you can improve your muscle and bone strength in just a few months if you approach it correctly. The EAT Resistance Program, like all the Habits of Health, is easy to learn, doable, and sustainable. That makes it very different from programs that expect you to spend hours at the gym trying to

**Boosting Your
Walking Workout**

- Lean forward slightly from your hips to increase momentum, pace, and intensity.
- Tighten your abdominal muscles and buttocks to burn more calories.
- Flex your toes to engage your leg muscles and increase your speed.
- For a more energetic stride, swing your arms with your elbows bent ninety degrees, shoulders rounded and relaxed.
- Keep your focus about twenty feet in front of you to straighten your posture and help you walk tall.

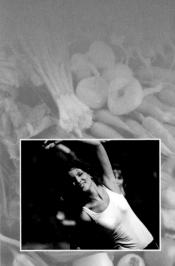

---

*Healthy Eating, NEAT, and EAT:
Working Together for Total Health*

Most exercise programs try to do too much. They promise weight loss, cardiovascular performance, and muscle enhancement—and deliver none very effectively. The Habits of Health, on the other hand, focus on a variety of small daily choices to create first healthy weight, then optimal health. We're not relying on exercise for weight loss—you're already doing that through the fat-burning healthy eating system. Energy expenditure is taken care of through the NEAT System, the EAT Walking Program covers cardiovascular health, and the EAT Resistance Program completes the picture by serving as a muscle and bone reconditioning program to help you retain your full range of movement for life!

You'll complete the EAT Resistance Program on the two days each week that you're not walking as part of the EAT Walking Program. Together, these two programs provide a complete cardiovascular and strength-training system in just thirty minutes a day.

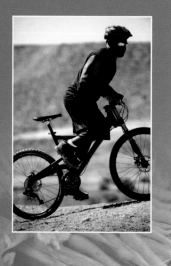

> ### *Avoiding "Lock Out": A Key to Effective Exercising*
> It's common to "lock out" your joints during an exercise, for example by straightening your elbows during a push-up or your knees during a squat. But this transfers the weight onto your bone structure and away from working muscles, and is not recommended. Avoiding "locking out" helps you increase tension and maintain a high level of intensity throughout your repetitions. In fact, the key to effective, long-term muscle development is moving the muscle slowly through the full range of motion and holding it at the point of maximum contraction just before lock out.

learn difficult exercises. And because the program only takes two days a week, it's a perfect complement to the five days you spend on the EAT Walking Program. Together, these two components provide you with a complete cardiovascular and strength-training system that takes only thirty minutes a day!

The Science of Healthy Muscles

Creating healthy muscles begins with the sarcomere, the microscopic muscle cell unit that creates all motion. As the functional unit of the muscle, a sarcomere works like a ratchet. When you contract your muscles, the filaments slide together, shortening the muscle. When you relax your muscle, the ratchet is released and the filaments move back to their original position, returning the muscle to its original length. By doing this over and over, you create little micro-tears that the body then repairs, making the muscles stronger and larger as a result.

This is traditionally accomplished by lifting weights repetitively until the muscle grows fatigued and tears occur. To facilitate this, some schools of thought have you lift more weight, and some have you do more repetitions. The time, degree of effort, and results of these techniques are all over the board.

My goal was to develop a safe, effective technique that anyone could use and sustain long term. That led me to my alma mater (home of my beloved Gators), the University of Florida. In the 1980s, researchers at the University of Florida School of Medicine discovered that moving a muscle group *slowly* through the full range of motion improves strength, bone density, and overall function. It's that slowness that's particularly important, as it eliminates gravity and momentum, causing the muscle to work more completely. As a result, the muscle is forced to develop more fibers and grow more quickly. Holding the muscle just as it's reached its point of maximum contraction reinforces the effect. And as an added benefit, slow and controlled movement minimizes the chance of injury, making it ideal for long-term practice.

Putting Science to Work

The EAT Resistance Program uses this science of slow contractions and relaxations, along with maximum hold time, to help you build muscle quickly and maintain it indefinitely. We'll focus on working your core muscles to improve your overall stance and posture, maximize energy consumption, and provide you with a platform to carry you into old age in top shape.

To create complete musculoskeletal health, we're going to work your core muscles and upper and lower extremities in rotation through slow, continuous repetitions that also work your cardiovascular system. That means you'll be getting cardiovascular benefits even on the days you're not walking! You'll then stretch each muscle group to maintain your full range of motion and flexibility.

This program is easy to learn and safe to do because it requires only moderate weights, when it uses weight at all. In fact, I've used these very techniques my whole life, both through everyday movements and through isometric exercises, and I can attest that they've enabled me to maintain my strength without ever setting foot in a gym. And if they work for me, they'll work for you too!

Before we begin, let's go over the core principles of the EAT Resistance Program:

- Muscle groups are moved slowly through the full range of motion in order to eliminate gravity and momentum and work muscles more completely. *Improves strength, bone density, and overall function.*
- Movements are held at the point of maximum contraction just before lock out to enable the muscles to grow fatigued and encourage them to recruit more muscle fibers. *Builds muscle.*
- Focus is on the core muscles. *Improves overall stance and posture and maximizes energy expenditure.*
- Movement is continuous. *Boosts cardiovascular health.*
- Muscles are stretched to the full range of motion after each muscle-group movement. *Promotes long-term flexibility.*

Equipping Yourself

Ready to go over the equipment and weights you'll be using? Take a look in the mirror. That's right! The most important piece of equipment is you!

By putting you at the center of your workout, I hope to eliminate any excuses you might have about driving to the gym, buying exercise equipment, or being short on space in your home. In fact, all I suggest you buy in the way of equipment is a mat, a balance ball, and, as your fitness increases, a pair of dumbbells.

Why don't I want you to use exercise machines? My program teaches you a complete system that you can use anytime, anywhere, for many, many years to come. And since my goal is to give you better balance, strengthen the muscles that stabilize your spine, and equip you to perform the movements you need for everyday life, it just makes sense to make *you* the principal piece of machinery!

Once you've made some initial progress, a few simple free weights—dumbbells, medicine balls, and vest and ankle weights, for example—will help you a lot more than machines and cables that isolate muscle groups and move your body in just one plane. After all, that's not how we move in real life. The movements you'll practice through the natural form of resistance training that I teach are much better preparation for unloading the groceries, taking out the trash, hoisting your kids, and walking the dog.

Music: Your Secret Weapon for Long-Term Motivation
You already know that music can boost your energy expenditure as part of NEAT. It's also a great motivator for workouts and can even help your muscles heal faster. In fact, it's been shown that people who listen to music during exercise have a better chance of staying with their program, thus enjoying such long-term benefits as enhanced quality of life and lower incidence of coronary heart disease—not to mention that music reduces pain and discomfort from stress and anxiety.[*]

*Maslar, P. M., "The Effect of Music on the Reduction of Pain: A Review of the Literature," *The Arts in Psychotherapy* 13: 215–219.

Choosing a Trainer
A certified personal trainer can help you get the most out of your exercise program by speeding up your learning curve, ensuring you're performing each exercise correctly, and adding a measure of accountability. After all, we all work a bit harder when someone's watching our progress! If you do choose to hire a trainer, just make sure they're a full-time professional who's certified by a reputable organization such as one of the following:

- American College of Sports Medicine (ACSM)
- National Academy of Sports Medicine (NASM)
- American Council of Exercise (ACE)
- The National Strength and Conditioning Association (NSCA)

If you do want to use weight-training machines, by all means give them a try—just make sure you stay safe by getting in great shape first. But if what you want is to increase your coordination and strengthen your core, stay with the basics.

What about Joining a Gym?

The EAT Resistance Program is designed to be completely doable from your home, with just you, this book, and the accompanying workbook as the principal equipment. In fact, you can do these exercises anywhere that provides you with thirty minutes of uninterrupted private time.

That being said, there can be advantages to going to a gym. You'll be surrounded by fellow exercisers whose motivation and knowledge can be helpful if you're new to working out, and many gyms provide professional trainers who can help you get started and ensure you're doing the movements correctly. In fact, hiring a trainer—either at a gym or in your home—is a good investment that I highly recommend if you haven't been exercising regularly or received training in the past. Then, once you're comfortable with exercising, you can begin working on your own.

A gym also gives you access to cardiovascular equipment that you can use to fulfill your EAT Walking Program requirements in bad weather or when you'd just like a break from your routine. I recommend doing thirty minutes on an elliptical cross-trainer, which gives a great workout to the cardiovascular system as well as the upper and lower body. Other equipment can be used to complement your EAT Resistance Program once you've reached a more advanced level.

All in all, there's much to gain from an EAT-friendly facility that gives you time to exercise away from distractions, hundreds of interruptions, and the family dog. That being said, I don't use a gym myself and manage to stay in shape in the comfort of my home. And so can you!

Your EAT Resistance Program Session: An Outline

Each EAT Resistance Program session works either your upper body or your lower body, along with your core muscles. Our major areas of focus are as follows:

Upper body
- core (upper)
- chest
- latissimus dorsi (back)
- shoulders
- arms

Lower body
- core (lower)
- thighs
- gluteals
- hamstrings
- calves

In the appendix, you'll find exercises for each of these muscle groups, as well as coordinating stretches. I recommend starting with the level one exercises and advancing only once you can do both rotations at a Rate of Perceived Exertion (RPE) of two or less (see box, page 200).

Your Weekly Routine

Once you get going with the EAT Resistance Program, you'll complete two thirty-minute sessions each week, consisting of:

1. A five-minute warm-up.
2. Five repetitions of five selected movements (a total of ten minutes), followed by a rotation of five different exercises that work the same muscle groups.
3. A five-minute stretch of the muscles you've worked.

Let's break that down to get a better picture of just what you'll be doing in each session.

Warm-Up: Five minutes

Prepare your body to work out through five minutes of slow to moderate movement that increases your cardiac output, carries blood to your muscles, lubricates your joints, and helps prevent injury.

- Walk in place while swinging your arms.
- Mentally walk through the resistance movements you'll be performing in your resistance rotation.
- If you're at a gym, use any type of cardio equipment (treadmill, exercise bicycle, Stairmaster) at a moderate pace.

Resistance Rotation: Two rotations of ten minutes each

Challenge your muscles to grow healthier through short, intense workouts that stimulate all your muscle fibers. Strengthen your bones and build lean, efficient muscle—not bulk—through slow, focused movements that utilize the full range of motion.

- Choose a set of five exercises (one rotation).
- Begin each exercise with a slow consistent contraction (eight seconds), hold in place just before lock out (four seconds), then relax the muscle as you slowly return to your starting position (eight seconds)—for a total of twenty seconds per exercise.
- Immediately begin another repetition, for a total of five per exercise.
- Rest for twenty seconds before starting a new exercise.
- Follow with a second rotation using a different set of exercises that work the same muscles.

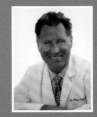
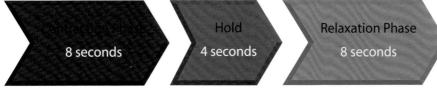

Contraction Phase
8 seconds

Hold
4 seconds

Relaxation Phase
8 seconds

One Exercise Repetition. Each twenty-second repetition consists of a contraction phase, a holding phase, and a relaxation phase. You'll complete five repetitions for each separate exercise.

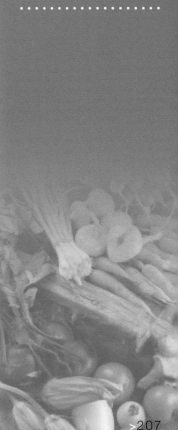

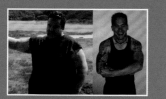

"With 170 pounds gone, I'm half the size I was. I'm alive again!"

DALLAS CARTER
Over one year at optimal health

For years, I prayed that God would help me muster the courage and discipline to take on the challenge of changing my lifestyle in order to better my health and increase my confidence and self-esteem. Simply put, my weight was out of control at 350+ pounds, with no end in sight. I had numerous medical problems (which I never told anyone about, even my family) and my doctor pretty much told me that at this rate I wouldn't have a very long life.

Then my daughter was born, and I knew it was time to change. Through working with a coach, I lost 170 pounds. It's amazing how my life has changed.

Now I'm on a mission—not only to continually improve my health and promote health to my family members, but to improve the health of the entire state of Hawaii! ∎

Results vary. Typical weight loss is 2-5 lbs per week for the first 2 weeks and 1-2 lbs per week thereafter.

Stretching: Five minutes

Spend five minutes stretching the muscle groups you've just worked to improve flexibility, increase your range of motion, and prevent soreness by encouraging your muscles to break down lactic acid (any soreness you do experience will decrease as your muscles get stronger and become reconditioned).

So there you have the EAT Resistance Program—thirty minutes of strength training to create a healthy musculoskeletal system and help you use more energy by:

- Boosting the calorie-burning capacity of all your NEAT and EAT activities
- Increasing your Basal Metabolic Rate (BMR) by adding muscle mass
- Burning energy even after your workout is done as your muscles replenish oxygen

Starting Your Program: Your First Day

Before you begin your first day, review the five exercises you'll be performing. You'll find a detailed explanation and illustrations in the appendix.

Take it slow as you get comfortable with resistance training. For the first week, limit yourself to one rotation to give yourself time to master the five beginning exercises. Beginning in week two, add a second rotation to your routine, consisting of five different exercises that work the same muscle groups.

As with the EAT Walking Program, be sure to monitor your progress by entering each workout's data into a log. You'll find sample logs for upper body and lower body rotations on the next page and in the appendix (also located in the companion workbook and on the Web site at www.habitsofhealth.net). Remember, for the first week limit yourself to one rotation.

To use the log:

- Write down the specific exercise you're doing for each muscle group.
- Note whether you're using your body alone without weights (B) or, if you're working with dumbbells, the amount of weight you're using. Refer to the Borg chart on page 200 to calculate your Rate of Perceived Exertion (RPE).

EAT Resistance Program Key Points

- Before you begin, make sure you've got the EAT Walking Program down and have been racking up 20,000 steps per week consistently for at least a month.
- Choose two days each week for your resistance workouts, leaving at least two days between sessions to let your body recover. (I recommend doing the upper body session on Monday and the lower body session on Thursday.)
- Find a spot where you can focus without distraction, and use an exercise mat for support and cushioning. Take it slow—review each new exercise before you try it out; limit yourself to one rotation for the first week; and add new exercises slowly, letting your body become accustomed to the new movement.

EAT RESISTANCE PROGRAM TRAINING LOG: UPPER BODY

Muscle Group	Exercise/Level (level one, level two)	Weight: Body (B) or Pounds (lbs)	Rate of Perceived Exertion (RPE)
Rotation A			
Core			
Chest			
Back			
Shoulders			
Arms			
Rotation B			
Core			
Chest			
Back			
Shoulders			
Arms			

EAT RESISTANCE PROGRAM TRAINING LOG: LOWER BODY

Muscle Group	Exercise/Level (level one, level two)	Weight: Body (B) or Pounds (lbs)	Rate of Perceived Exertion (RPE)
Rotation A			
Core			
Thighs			
Gluteals			
Hamstrings			
Calves			
Rotation B			
Core			
Thighs			
Gluteals			
Hamstrings			
Calves			

Your Complete Habits of Motion System

To create and maintain optimal health, you need to be active every day. My Habits of Motion system is designed to make sure you get enough activity to keep your weight under control while moving you toward optimal health. You'll get most of this healthy activity through the NEAT System and the EAT Walking Program. The EAT Resistance Program takes you the rest of the way

Dr. A Says . . .

Stay fit on vacation by signing up for a walking trip, such as those offered by the Smithsonian Institution, or entering a walking or running event for charity. What better way to keep yourself healthy and do something great for others in need!

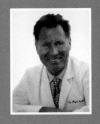

● ● ● ● ● ● ● ● ● ● ● ● ● ● ●

A Typical Week on the Habits of Motion System. By reviewing your activity and total calories burned for a week on the NEAT and EAT systems, you can see how effective these activities are at upping energy expenditure without taking a lot of time from your day.

by helping you maintain your cardiovascular and musculoskeletal systems for the long term. If you want to take it even farther, a fitness trainer can help you create a more advanced program tailored to your goals (I've started using a trainer regularly myself), or you can use the Ultrahealth EAT enhancement system you'll learn about in chapter 24.

Now that you've put the Habits of Motion system together, let's take a look at the program in its entirety. Here's what one week might look like once you're in the swing.

	NEAT System	EAT System	Time spent	Calories burned
Monday	Walked 4 flights Walked to lunch	30 minute EAT upper body	30 minutes	450
Tuesday	Walked 4 flights Cleaned closet	30 minute EAT walk	30 minutes	425
Wednesday	Walked 4 flights Washed car	30 minute EAT walk	30 minutes	375
Thursday	Walked 4 flights Raked lawn Washed dishes	30 minute EAT lower body	30 minutes	450
Friday	Walked 4 flights Walked to lunch	30 minute EAT walk	30 minutes	400
Saturday	Raked lawn Mall shopping Dancing	30 minute EAT walk	30 minutes	650
Sunday	Climbed stadium to upper deck	30 minute EAT walk	30 minutes	400

You can see how well the Habits of Motion system increases your daily calorie expenditure without causing a lot of disruption to your day or schedule.

● ●

You now have the knowledge you need to take control of your energy management system. These Habits of Motion, combined with the Habits of Healthy Eating you've already learned, will have a dramatic impact on your journey toward healthy weight and optimal health.

We're now going to look at an area of your life that's equally important, but all too often brushed aside in our time-starved world. Yet nothing has the ability to age you faster or extend the quality of your life more than our next essential habit—the Habit of Healthy Sleeping.

Chapter 17

Sleep: Nature's Nurse

"...O sleep, O gentle sleep,
Nature's soft nurse, how have I frighted thee"
　　　　–William Shakespeare, *Henry IV, Part II*

"Sleep that knits up the ravell'd sleeve of care
The death of each day's life, sore labour's bath
Balm of hurt minds, great nature's second course
Chief nourisher in life's feast,—"
　　　　–William Shakespeare, *Macbeth*

Over 400 years ago, Shakespeare penned those statements on the profound importance of sleep—both for its recuperative powers and the prominent role it plays in our lives. Yet that notion itself remained asleep for the three and a half centuries that followed.

In fact, until the middle of the twentieth century, most scientists believed sleep to be an inactive state of little or no value—just something to do once the sun was down, in a holdover from our caveman roots. Even today, most of us consider sleep something of an inconvenient luxury, one that gets in the way of our work, television viewing, and Internet surfing. We may love it, but we somehow manage to do without.

Only in the last few years have science and medicine begun to understand that without enough high-quality sleep, our health and our lives unravel. Just look at the prevalence of sleep disorders in our society—people whose demanding schedules prevent them from getting to bed, others who lie awake for hours hoping for one good night's rest. This lack of restorative sleep is leading many of us into a non-sick state prematurely and, like unhealthy eating and lack of movement, degrading our health.

Are You Getting Enough Sleep?

In this chapter, we'll evaluate the health of your sleep, discuss the implications of poor sleeping, and create a new set of habits to support a lifetime of healthy, restorative, and, above all, cozy sleep for you and your family.

So, first things first—are you getting enough sleep? Answer the following questions to find out.

Do you. . .

• Wake up tired in the morning?
• Need a nap in the afternoon?
• Fall asleep watching TV?

One Child's Sleep: The Beginning of Modern Sleep Science
In 1951, an inquisitive graduate student at the University of Chicago named Eugene Aserinsky hooked his own son to a brain wave monitor to observe his sleep. As the boy lay motionless, eyes darting side to side, Aserinsky noticed spikes of brain activity, an observation that led him to coin the term *REM (rapid eye movement)* sleep. His research, which first identified sleep's roughly ninety-minute cycles, initiated today's scientific study of sleep.

How Much Sleep is Enough? The general consensus is that women require six to seven hours and men seven to eight for optimal health—but it's essential that those hours include rotations through several healthy cycles of REM and non-REM stages.

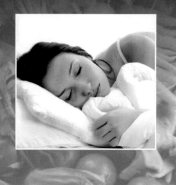

- Have frequent small accidents at home, or large ones on the road?
- Have trouble focusing on the job?
- Find yourself sleepy after lunch?
- Have trouble figuring the correct change from a purchase?
- Feel irritable or depressed most of the time?
- Feel like you're not getting anything done?
- Drink alcohol to get to sleep?
- Drink several cups of coffee or energy drinks to stay awake?
- Have difficulty falling asleep?
- Have difficulty staying asleep?

If you answered yes to more than three of these questions, you're probably not getting the kind of sleep you need to support health. But don't worry—the Habits of Healthy Sleep are going to help change all that, and not a moment too soon!

From Non-Sick to Sick: The Slippery Slope of Sleeplessness

Why are 90 percent of us languishing in a state of unhealth—a limbo between the 5 percent who are outright sick and the 5 percent who are optimally healthy? Along with poor diet and inactivity, poor sleep is a major contributor.

Lack of sleep affects our body in a number of negative ways that go far beyond such common disturbances as mental blurriness, decreased productivity, and impaired relationships. In fact, a growing body of evidence links poor sleep habits to increased inflammation, a higher risk of cardiovascular incidence—and even obesity. Let's look at a few of these sleep-related problems.

Sleep and Weight Gain. Getting too little sleep disturbs appetite regulation, giving sleep deficiency the potential to be a major factor in obesity. Researchers at England's Warwick School of Medicine who studied 28,000 adults and 15,000 children found that getting less sleep almost doubled the risk of obesity, even in children as young as five. Why? When you're sleep-deprived, your body secretes excess ghrelin, a hormone that increases appetite, and less leptin, a

Lack of Sleep Worse for Women, Studies Show

Sleeplessness is no picnic for anyone, but it takes a particular toll on women, a recent study shows. Researchers at Duke University who studied 210 healthy men and women found that while sleep quality was comparable for both genders, the women exhibited greater psychological stress, depression, hostility, and anger, as well as higher levels of substances that increase heart disease risk, including insulin, CRP (C-reactive protein), and interleukin 6.

That's not all—a large study of 71,000 female nurses found that women who sleep only five hours or less a night are 45 percent more likely to have heart problems, and that even those who sleep six hours a night have a 20 percent higher risk.

substance that tells you to stop eating. In addition, lack of sleep prevents your body from replacing dopamine and serotonin, two brain chemicals that bring comfort and satisfaction. As a result, you begin to crave sugar and energy-dense, nutritionally polluted foods—not exactly supportive of healthy eating!

Sleep and Immunity. Your immune system needs sleep in order to repair, recharge, and do the maintenance necessary to keep out intruders. That means that skimping on sleep can make you more susceptible to disease. In fact, getting fewer than six hours can raise your risk of viral infection by 50 percent.

Sleep, Inflammation, and Your Heart. Researchers are discovering that lack of sleep can raise your blood levels of inflammatory activators including CRP (C-reactive protein), a substance that increases the risk of cardiovascular disease and a marker we will watch very closely to assess your health status. In addition to heart disease, this constant inflammation can lead to cancer, premature aging, and other negative consequences. Evidence is also building that connects sleep deprivation to a nightly rise in blood pressure that lasts through the day and raises risk for heart attack and stroke.

Other Sleep-Related Health Issues. Too little sleep—defined as less than seven hours a night—may cause anxiety symptoms, moodiness, depression, and overuse of alcohol, says a 2006 Institute of Medicine report, and the ill effects build as sleep loss accumulates. How big a problem are we talking about? Between 50 and 70 million people in the U.S. alone may be affected.

So What Exactly Is Sleep, Anyway?

Sleep is your body's way of restoring organ function, stabilizing chemical imbalance, refreshing areas of the brain that control mood and behavior, and

**Sleep Apnea
and Obesity:
A Vicious Cycle**
Sleep apnea—a sleep disorder characterized by snoring and airway obstruction that results in ten-second-or-longer periods of non-breathing during sleep—is caused by excess weight, primarily fatty tissue in the neck. Because it interrupts the sleep cycle, sleep apnea can actually spur further weight gain, which then exacerbates the sleep apnea—a vicious cycle of increasing weight and deteriorating sleep.

• • • • • • • • • • • • • • • • •

**The Stages of Sleep:
One Sleep Cycle.** It may seem like nothing's happening while you sleep, but your brain is actually going through a series of important stages that make up a complete sleep cycle. We typically experience four to six ninety-minute cycles a night

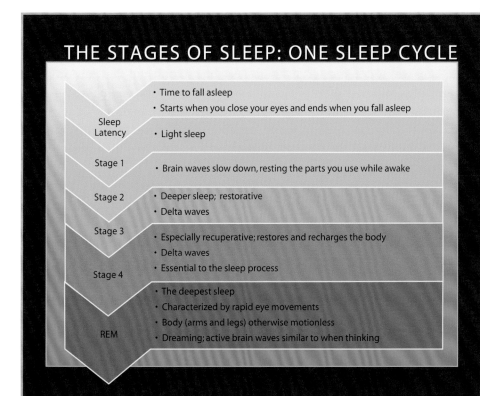

THE STAGES OF SLEEP: ONE SLEEP CYCLE

Sleep Latency
• Time to fall asleep
• Starts when you close your eyes and ends when you fall asleep

Stage 1
• Light sleep

Stage 2
• Brain waves slow down, resting the parts you use while awake

Stage 3
• Deeper sleep; restorative
• Delta waves

Stage 4
• Especially recuperative; restores and recharges the body
• Delta waves
• Essential to the sleep process

REM
• The deepest sleep
• Characterized by rapid eye movements
• Body (arms and legs) otherwise motionless
• Dreaming; active brain waves similar to when thinking

Sleep deprivation, a form of psychological torture, is often considered worse than going without food or water. It rapidly erodes emotions and self-confidence, resulting in erratic behavior.

If you're sleepy, you probably aren't sleeping enough, or sleeping well enough—in other words, like most things, it comes down to your habits!

improving performance. During sleep, your brain replenishes spent nutrients and repairs its circuitry, rearranging your experiences much like a computer rearranges data. After all, during waking hours your brain is too busy processing information to shut down, defrag, and download all the experiences of the day.

And while sleep may seem like one long state of unconsciousness, your brain is actually moving repeatedly through a series of stages the entire time. Together, these various sleep stages make up one cycle that's about ninety minutes long and ends with REM sleep, a stage that's necessary for healthy restoration. We typically experience four to six cycles a night.

As this repetitive cycling goes on during the night, we enter into REM sleep more frequently, and by early morning most of our healthy sleep should be REM. But REM sleep is very sensitive to interruption. Conditions such as sleep apnea prevent deep sleep and activate the immune system, and as a result sufferers don't feel rested no matter how long they stay in bed. They're constantly tired, need naps, go to bed early—and overeat.

Why We Get Sleepy

Humans are designed for sleep. In fact, it's our default mode. And that all starts with our biological clock.

Perhaps you've heard the phrase *the third eye.* This actually refers to the pineal gland, a pea-size organ located in the center of the brain just behind the eyes, which has the ability to sense light. In fact, it's the only endocrine organ to have direct access to the outside world.

The pineal gland releases a substance you've probably heard of—melatonin—which naturally makes you drowsy between midnight and 7:00 a.m. This powerful neurotransmitter sets you up for sleep by cooling your body temperature, lowering your metabolic rate, and moving you into the sleep latency stage. When we're young, our bodies produce lots of melatonin—which explains why toddlers can run at full speed one second and suddenly drop like a sack of potatoes, or why college students find it so easy to sleep through their morning classes. But unfortunately, melatonin levels begin dropping as we age, and by the time we're sixty, we've lost about 80 percent. Just think of older people, who always seem to get up at the crack of dawn—their melatonin is depleted by morning.

Other neurotransmitters, like GABA (gamma-amino butyric acid) and adenosine, also play a part in slowing down brain activity and inhibiting the body processes associated with wakefulness. Because we're diurnal animals, sleepiness naturally occurs as our circadian clock winds down for the night and our body starts secreting sleep chemicals. And, in the simplest terms, when your brain's "awake" chemicals are more active than its "sleep" chemicals, the result is insomnia. Caffeine increases the level of those awake chemicals; melatonin, GABA, and other substances counteract them.

That system worked beautifully for our ancestors 10,000 years ago. It even works for us when we're relaxing at the end of a week's vacation. But what about the rest of the time?

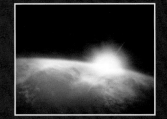

Sleepless on Planet Earth

If 70 percent of us are struggling with sleep, there must be a reason. And as with so many of our struggles—sorry to beat this old drum again!—it comes down to that disconnect between our biological design and the technologically driven world we live in.

Each year, our world seems to get more complicated, more stressful, and more difficult to keep pace with. Terrorism, crime, global warming—there's no shortage of things to worry about, and that takes a toll. Combine that with demanding schedules, computers, music, TV, bright lights, tens of thousands of logos and images each day, and our natural biological rhythm just gets buried by sensory overload.

We try to keep up with all this data by stimulating ourselves with coffee, colas, and chocolate, but these only complicate the picture. Because caffeine has a half-life of six hours, your afternoon Starbucks is still racing through your system at 10:00 p.m., when you should be calling it a night. Your melatonin is releasing, but that vente latte is keeping your awake chemicals high, and your third eye is twitching! So your sleep cycle gets delayed while you watch a couple of hours of late night TV. Or maybe you try to numb yourself to sleep with a glass of something alcoholic. But even if this does the trick, your body soon metabolizes the alcohol, goes into arousal—and you wake up in the middle of the night.

Needless to say, these scenarios are less than conducive to optimal health. Like most other drugs, caffeine, alcohol, and sleep aids may temporarily alleviate symptoms. But those symptoms are there for a reason—to tell you that something's wrong with your body. When we sleep well, we naturally wake up refreshed, without the need for medications, or even an alarm clock. So what are our symptoms trying to tell us, and what can we do about them?

- **Excess weight.** Lie on your back, and you can't breathe well; roll over onto your stomach, and the abdominal pressure constricts your diaphragm, making it difficult to take big breaths. No matter how much time an overweight person spends in bed, he just can't seem to catch up on sleep, leading to more fatigue, and—you guessed it—further weight gain.
- **Pain or discomfort.** Headache, backache, cramps—all can keep you from getting a good night's sleep. You may not even notice the pain during the day,

> Why is it that young people can sleep under almost any circumstances while older people wake at the crack of dawn? Because our body secretes less melatonin—a natural sleep-inducing substance—as we age.

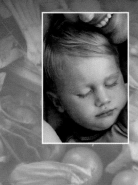

Our Caffeine Society

Caffeine is arguably the most robust and popular self-administered drug known to man, with almost 90 percent of North Americans consuming some form of it regularly.

Most people aren't harmed by moderate doses of caffeine—say 200 to 300 milligrams, or about two to three cups of brewed coffee a day. But it should be consumed in the morning hours to give the drug time to clear. Remember, with a half-life of six hours, caffeine lingers in your body all day—and into the night if you've had an afternoon pick-me-up. (For a list of the caffeine content in common products, see the appendix.)

Just like habits of
healthy eating and
movement, good sleep
habits are within your
control and require your
active participation and
commitment.

when responsibilities and tasks keep you busy. But at night, there's nothing else to distract you as discomfort stimulates your brain. If an over-the-counter anti-inflammatory doesn't do the trick, ask your doctor for help.

- **Allergies.** You know how hard it is to sleep when you have a cold? Allergies create the same type of congestion and headache. If allergies are preventing you from sleeping, see your doctor for relief.

Along with these common disorders, other symptoms can affect your sleep and may signify an underlying condition. If you experience any of the following, check with your doctor:

- Loud snoring
- Trouble breathing (for example, gasping for breath)
- Restless legs
- Heartburn
- Bad dreams
- Frequent urination
- Depression
- Anxiety

The Habits of Healthy Sleep

When you were twenty, you probably didn't think much about sleep. You had plenty of melatonin coursing through your body, and whether you were at a rock concert or crashing on a friend's floor, sleep just came naturally.

Times have changed, and what worked for you then probably isn't working now. In fact, your current rituals and habits may be in direct conflict with healthy sleep. That's why you need to become an active participant in creating healthy sleep habits, just as you've worked to create habits of healthy eating and movement. After all, your melatonin level isn't getting any higher. There's never been a better time to adopt strategies to get you through your first 100 years in great shape!

Let's begin with a simple assessment of the quality and quantity of your sleep.

Sleep Assessment

Part One: Quantity
How Much Sleep Do You Get?

First, answer the following questions:

- What time do you turn off the light to go to bed? _____
- How long does it take you to fall asleep? _____
- How often do you wake up during the night? _____
- How long do you stay awake each time? _____
- What time do you wake up in the morning? _____

To find out how many hours of actual sleep you're getting:

1. Calculate your sleep window (the amount of time between lights out and waking up): _____

2. Subtract the amount of time you spend in bed that you're not actually sleeping (the time you spend falling asleep or lying awake in the night): _____

3. The result is your actual sleep time: _____

Remember, men should be getting seven to eight hours a night, women six to seven. How does your result stack up?

Part Two: Quality
How Restful Is Your Sleep?

Answer the questions below every day for one week, entering your responses in the sleep log located in the appendix. The results will help you figure out which behaviors are affecting your sleep.

1. What time did you get into bed last night?
2. What time did you get out of bed in the morning?
3. What hours did you actually sleep?
4. Did you take a nap? For how long?
5. Did you consume alcohol? How much, and at what time?
6. Did you exercise? How long, and at what time?
7. Did you drink coffee or other caffeinated beverages? How much, and at what time?
8. What hours did you watch television?
9. Did you take any medications? At what time?

Steps to Healthy Sleep

Now that you've got a baseline from the sleep assessment, let's work on improving the quantity and quality of your sleep. We'll start by finding out how your brain is programmed so we can help return it to its default mode—sleep.

Step 1: Find Your Chronotype

Are you a lark or an owl? Your *chronotype* reflects whether you wake up early and are active and alert in the first part of the day, or prefer to stay up late and are most alert in the evening. Most people aren't wholly one or the other, but somewhere in between.

If most of your sleep occurs at the wrong time of day for your chronotype, it's harder to get the rest you need. Optimally, two circadian markers—maximum amount of melatonin and minimum core body temperature—should occur after the middle of your sleep hours, but before you wake up.

Scientists have found that morning people's melatonin declines rapidly after it peaks, which may account for their ability to get up early. It declines more slowly in night owls. As far as body temperature, morning types reach

Owl or Lark? Age Can Make a Difference. Our sleep patterns tend to change as we age. For a young person, a preferred bedtime of 11:30 p.m. may mean they're a morning person, but a person over forty with that same bedtime is probably more of a night owl.

Don't alter your bedtime (or wake time) even on the weekends. If you find that you need extra sleep on the weekend, it means you're not getting enough quality sleep during the week.

their minimum temperature about 4:00 a.m., and evening types at 6:00 a.m.—closer to the time they usually have to get up.

While morning types and evening types both seem to need about the same amount of sleep, knowing which one you are will help you determine which habits and behaviors suit your needs and are therefore more likely to succeed. If you're a lark, you might want to get to bed earlier, complete your task list in the evening, and exercise in the morning (actually, this is the ideal time). If you're a night owl, see if you can rearrange your work schedule so you can arrive and leave work later.

Step 2: Set a Bedtime

Whichever type you are, there's a good chance you have to get up for work in the morning, so in order to set your bedtime you should first decide what time you need to get up. Count back from that time seven hours (for a woman) or eight hours (for a man). That's when you should be *asleep*. Your *bedtime*—the point at which all lights (and other electronic devices) are off—marks the beginning of the sleep latency period, or falling-asleep time.

It doesn't really matter if your bedtime is 9:00 p.m. or 1:00 a.m. What's important is establishing a uniform pattern that sets a rhythm and puts your pineal gland back in charge.

Remember that the optimum sleep length—seven hours for women, eight for men—is just a guideline. You need to find out what's optimal for you. A good time to do this is on vacation, when you've left behind the hustle and bustle of your everyday routine (yes, that includes the kids) and can say good-bye to the alarm clock for a while.

You should reach a point when you're going to bed at the same time each night and waking up the same time each day feeling rested. That's the optimal sleep length for you. Even cutting back by one hour can decrease your alertness by 35 percent and move you to a non-sick state.

You'll know you've hit it right when you wake up just before the alarm clock was set to go off!

Step 3: Set Your Routine

Today's chaotic schedules mean that, for the most part, we sleep only when our inability to function forces us to. But with a little planning, you can change the behaviors that are sabotaging your sleep. In fact, from the moment you wake up, you can start preparing to sleep better that very night.

During the day:

- **Get out of bed.** Once you wake up, get up. Limit your in-bed activities to sleeping and lovemaking to avoid sending the wrong signals to your brain.

- **Limit caffeine.** You don't have to give up coffee or caffeinated tea—just savor them in the morning. Once noon rolls around, limit or avoid anything caffeinated, and make sure you have absolutely no caffeine within three hours of sleep time. (For a list of the caffeine content in common products, see the appendix.)

- **Eat responsibly.** *Avoid eating within three hours of sleeping.* If you really need something before bed, try a small glass of skim milk or chamomile tea. For optimal sleep, eliminate high-glycemic foods throughout the day, and avoid large, energy-dense, or fatty meals in the evening (a small fueling or portion-controlled meal replacement is fine).

- **Say no to naps.** Children need more sleep than they can get in a night, but for adults, napping is a recipe for sleep disruption, especially if you doze off for longer than an hour. If you're so tired that you need to nap, avoid high-glycemic and fatty foods at lunch and schedule your sleep time a little earlier. (That being said, a short, five-minute power nap won't hurt—as long as your boss doesn't catch you!)

In the evening:

The evening is your time, and it's important to plan for it wisely. As you head home from work, make a mental note of any tasks or activities that need to be done. For instance, plan to complete your EAT exercises and any other activities that make you break into a sweat at least two hours before bed, and even earlier if it seems to interrupt your latency. Here are some guidelines to help you prepare for what I like to call *sleepy time*—the half hour before lights out.

- **Decrease stimulation.** Since the pineal gland is light sensitive, it's a good idea to lower your home's ambient light several hours before bed. Turning on a bright light to look for something you need the next day can startle your "third eye." Thirty minutes before you plan to hit the pillow, shut off the TV (including the news), stop e-mailing and surfing the Internet, and turn off any loud music. Disturbing images and work e-mails can lead to repetitive thoughts when you're trying to drift off to sleep.

- **Eliminate cell phone use.** Recent research indicates that radiation from your phone may actually stimulate your brain and interrupt sleep. A study at Wayne State University concluded that people who used their cell phones in the evening took longer to fall asleep and experienced more headaches. If you must talk on your cell phone in the evening, use a headset and turn it off at least two hours before you plan to fall asleep.

- **Minimize liquid intake.** Getting up to go to the bathroom is a common sleep disruption. If you find this happening to you, avoid drinking anything two hours before bed and make sure to empty your bladder just before turning in.

- **Avoid exercise within two hours of bedtime.** Any other time of day, exercise is a good thing, helping increase the body's natural chemicals that induce sleep. But it's too stimulating right before sleep. And make sure you're not sacrificing sleep time for exercise by getting up too early. Giving up some TV time instead leaves you with room in your schedule for exercise and no negative consequences!

Start Your Day Right: Say Goodbye to the Alarm Clock and Hello to the Dawn Simulator
Being startled into alertness by your alarm clock doesn't exactly set you up for a balanced, stress-free day, does it? To minimize this a.m. trauma, try a dawn simulator, a light that increases in intensity gradually at a time you pre-set. As the light falls on your eyes, your brain gets the message to reduce melatonin, preparing your body to wake up naturally. They're readily available online (visit www.habitsofhealth.net for resources).

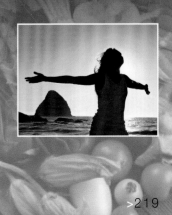

**Prepare for Tomorrow,
Sleep Easy Tonight**
Put your mind to rest
before bed by making
a to-do list of tasks
and priorities for the
next day. You'll go to
sleep confident that you
won't forget something
important once your
busy day gets going
(or wake up in the night
worrying about it). Just
be sure to make up
your list early enough in
the evening so you're
not thinking about
tomorrow's concerns
right before bed.

- **Take your medications.** If pain or allergies keep you up, make sure you take any medications *an hour before bed* so they have time to reach effectiveness. A hot bath can help pain relievers such as ibuprofen get to those sore muscles quicker. Of course, check with your doctor before taking any medication.

- **Avoid alcohol within ninety minutes of bedtime.** Alcohol is actually a stimulant and can suppress normal sleep patterns. When used to induce sleep, it can cause you to wake up in an arousal state and make healthy sleep difficult to come by. If you're finding it hard to get to sleep, you may even want to try skipping the drink with dinner.

- **Resolve family issues.** Arguments with your spouse, logistical concerns about getting the kids to school, to-do lists for the next day—all these issues should be resolved before sleepy time. Never go to bed mad!

Sleepy Time

This is your time to leave the rest of the world behind! By developing your own personal sleep ritual—one that stays the same each night—you create a conditioned response that tells your body, your brain, and everyone else that you're going off duty. You send the message that, just like a closed ticket window, you and your neurons are simply no longer available (unless the house is on fire, that is!).

1. **Preparing your bedroom.** Aim to make your bedroom as visually calming, mentally relaxing, and stress free as possible (see box, page 221, Creating an Environment for Sleep). That means that pets, children, and other critters should be in their proper places—usually their own beds. (I love my lab, but he's a bed hog and on a different biological clock than mine.) And if your significant other snores or has restless legs, get them to the doctor. You'll be helping them out *and* increasing your chances of a good night's sleep.

2. **Preparing yourself.** Take some time in the bathroom to wash your face, floss, and brush your teeth. If you have time, take a hot bath or shower—research indicates that as your temperature comes down, your body gets sleepy. Then head into some comfy, loose-fitting PJs that don't overheat you—flannel in the winter and cotton in the summer usually does the trick—and maybe even a pair of socks to dilate the blood vessels in your feet and help you relax.

3. **Getting into bed.** Once you're in bed and ready to get sleepy, keep things calm. Some people like to meditate, do breathing exercises, or even a little yoga. (For more information, see the sections on stress reduction in chapters 19 and 25.) You may choose to read a relaxing book (set a time limit), cuddle with your partner, or relax with a scalp, neck, shoulder, or foot massage—or whatever else comes up. Or just turn off the light and share a goodnight kiss. You can even count sheep! The most important thing is to just let go and let your body drift off naturally, without forcing or obsessing. . . just release. . . sweet dreams!

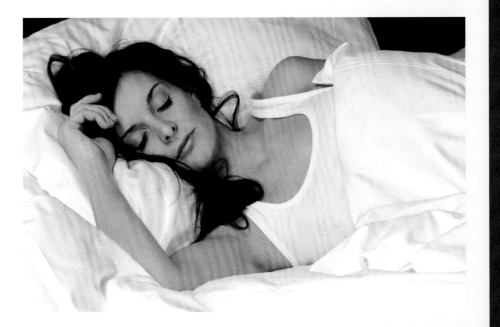

Still Can't Sleep? If you can't get to sleep after twenty minutes, don't lie in bed getting frustrated! Get up and do something else. Go for a walk around the house, take a bath, or read a relaxing book—then reboot and try again. And even if you're tired the next day, get up at the scheduled time. A day or so of being tired may be all you need to get a good night's rest next time and get back in the habit of healthy, deep, restful sleep.

Creating an Environment for Sleep

Make your bedroom a comfortable, sleep-inducing cocoon! Here are some tips:

- **Color.** Choose a color that soothes you to encourage sleep. Soft pastels such as light blue, green, pink, lavender, yellow, and ivory are calming colors, but so are rich, warm, dark colors such as medium to dark green, chocolate brown, or any rich tans.

- **Light.** Put your lights on a dimmer and use the lowest setting. Avoid fluorescent bulbs in the bedroom. Scented candles are fine as long as you remember to blow them out before you get too sleepy. Once the lights are out, make sure your room is completely dark, free of moonlight, streetlights, or glowing clocks and other electrical devices—especially the TV. If necessary, invest in blackout curtains, blinds, or shutters.

- **Scent.** Try aromatherapy scents like chamomile, jasmine, lavender, neroli, rose, sandalwood, or sweet marjoram. Add essential oils to a dispenser or a hot bath, or just put a few drops on a handkerchief and slip it into your pillowcase.

- **Your bed.** Take your time choosing a mattress that's the right level of firmness for you. Make sure your spine is aligned neutrally with your pillow—not too high or too low.

- **Your temperature.** Make sure your bed doesn't get too hot or too cold during the night. Far-infrared quilts, sheets, and pillows can help keep your body temperature neutral. Avoid electric blankets, which can interfere with sleep.

- **Ventilation.** Cool the room to 68 degrees or lower, and maintain adequate ventilation.

- **Clutter.** Put things away before you make your pre-bedtime bathroom stop, so you're ready to relax once you hit the pillow.

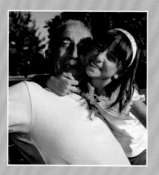

Proper Support:
The Keystone
to Optimal Health.
You've learned how to
take charge of the three
most important health-
related areas of your life:
eating, motion, and sleep.
What holds them
together is
your support
network.

Healthy
Eating

Support

Healthy
Motion

Healthy
Sleep

Chapter 18

Building Your Support System

The Keystone to Optimal Health

Your life is now in motion! Until now, some of your choices may have supported health and many probably didn't. However, that changed once you made the fundamental choice of optimal health.

You now have a comprehensive plan to take control of the three most important areas that determine health: healthy eating, a healthy activity level, and healthy sleep. Mastering this triad is the bedrock of the Habits of Health. But in order to lay the foundation for a lifetime of optimal health, these new habits need to be studied, absorbed, and internalized until they no longer require any conscious effort on your part.

This chapter is going to help you do just that. I know that change is sometimes difficult, but I've discovered a way to make it a little more doable. Research indicates that people who use a support system are more likely to succeed in making positive changes and to maintain these changes over time. In fact, I believe this so strongly that if I could pop right out of these pages and look you in the eye, I would say to you as your coach: *Building a support system is the single most important thing you can do to incorporate and maintain the Habits of Health.*

It's the difference between *thinking* about becoming healthier and actually *doing* it, as I've learned through the thousands of people I've coached and mentored over the years. By following the simple path I've outlined, you can change your health and your life forever, and in a relatively short amount of time. These principles of health are straightforward—*but you have to apply them.*

Your support system starts with me as your coach and this book as your guide. From there, you can build a broader network of support that's tailored to your wants and needs. To help you out, I'm going to give you a variety of options that have the potential to make incorporating your new healthy behaviors easier, quicker, less confusing, and even more fun. In addition to the suggestions in this book, you can find more information at the Web site, www.habitsofhealth.net.

Mastering the Habits of Health

Are you at optimal health right now? If not, how can you go about mastering the Habits of Health? Well, it starts with acknowledging that you actually do need help!

Just as you're an expert in your particular field, I'm an expert in creating health—but as your coach, I can only help you if you're willing to learn and willing to change. First you need to know just what your responsibilities are, and you need to choose a plan of support that works for you. You also need to become a student. Remember, you're never too old or too smart to learn! Times are changing fast today, and if we want to create health and make it last, we need an open mind and a desire to grow. In the words of futurist Eric Hoffer: "In times of change, learners inherit the earth, while the learned find themselves beautifully equipped to deal with a world that no longer exists."

Learning through Baby Steps

The path to optimal health is a daily journey of small choices that pay big dividends. It's an uphill path, but well worth the effort. And it's available to anyone who's willing to get on it and *stay on it*. That's a lot easier when you have a solid support system and are willing to ask for help.

You'll find that each step, each small success, builds momentum. If you immerse yourself in the process, you'll be rewarded with health that grows stronger and stronger. And who knows? As you improve, you might even want to help others—which in turn will help you reinforce and live out your decision and commitment to your own optimal health goals.

Let's look at three methods that will help you master the Habits of Health.

Studying. Get excited about the new you that's unfolding, and get busy learning. This includes attending trainings, using online resources, and reading sources such as this book and the companion guide, and watching the new *Dr. A's Habits of Health Video Series* on DVD. For more information, visit www.habitsofhealth.net.

Doing. Here's where the rubber hits the road. Knowledge only goes so far—to make lasting change, you actually have to eat low-glycemic foods, not just identify them, and actually give up that dinnertime cup of coffee that's keeping you awake at night. A coach can be particularly helpful here. Remember, health is not a spectator sport!

Modeling. The people we hold up as role models can have a profound effect on our lives. Let's put that to the test. Write down the names of your five closest friends (they don't have to live close by, as long as you communicate with them regularly). Now write down where and what they eat, what they do for fun, how they sleep, how much they weigh, and what their current health is like. Why? Because the people we're close to and emulate are what we become, particularly if they're the same sex.

In my own work, I've taken this concept of modeling and helped turn it into a support system that's available to you, including a plan, a coach, and an entire health-oriented environment. It's called a *bionetwork*, and you'll find out more about it on page 226. It's a great way to combat the overload of information that's out there on diets, exercise, nutritional supplements, and so forth—much of which is confusing and misdirected. Whatever type of support system you choose needs to give you the power to stay on your path in the face of all that confusion.

Support Systems

What kind of support system works best? There are different choices that work for everyone, ranging from working on your own (if you have the discipline!), to sharing the experience with others in a group setting, to utilizing the guidance

Want Better Health? Health creation professionals help people utilize the relatively new science of health creation by teaching key behavioral, physiologic, and lifestyle changes. Through instruction and motivation, health creation experts help those who've made the fundamental choice of optimal health reach and maintain the highest degree of health possible.

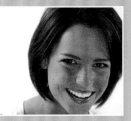

Studying the Habits of Health doesn't mean anything if you don't *do* them. Fortunately, modeling the optimally healthy people you admire can help motivate you to stay on course.

If you're going it alone (and even if you're not) there are a number of reputable online resources in addition to my Web site that can give you great ideas for low-glycemic eating and healthy activities, some with advanced tracking tools that will help guide you and support your health. You'll find links for these on my Web site at www.habitsofhealth.net

of a professional coach, to a comprehensive support system that combines aspects of all of the above.

You on Your Own

For some of you, working on your own with a user-friendly, sensible system like Dr. A's Habits of Health is enough. Because I've written this text with the same conversational style and methods I use when I'm coaching, in essence you have the benefit of my support when you use this book, the companion guide, the new *Dr. A's Habits of Health Video Series* on DVD, and my Web site (www.habitsofhealth.net). If you can overcome the logistical issues of today's complex lifestyle and have plenty of discipline, you can succeed with these sources alone.

However, I'm from the school of thought that you can never get enough help, so I highly recommend you consider exploring additional means of support.

You in a Group

Whether it's a friend, co-worker, family members, or a larger, more organized group, working with others can make all the difference. When two or more people share similar goals and values, people create synergy. So, along with encouraging each other, you'll have someone to walk with, dine with, and build healthy habits with.

- **Friends, family, or informal group settings.** Not only is sharing the Habits of Health with family and friends socially satisfying, it increases accountability and creates an entire environment of health. And wouldn't you rather help change your friends' habits than have to think about changing your friends?
- **Formal settings.** Evidence suggests that group meetings can be a more effective way to lose weight than doing it on your own. Some medical facilities offer clinically based behavioral groups that spur weight loss and health maintenance by combining group dynamics with a professional counselor. Commercial programs also offer opportunities to attend group meetings for support, discussion, and even assignments such as food diaries. However, studies show that the drop-out rate for these types of groups is high due to busy schedules and travel considerations. If you do choose a group and stay with it, though, you may well benefit from the extra accountability you'll have through e-mail, phone, and face-to-face contact with others.
- **Online.** Internet-based programs have advanced tremendously. Today's sites are generally highly interactive, and the privacy and convenience they offer may make them more attractive than ongoing sessions with a counselor. In fact, one leading researcher, Dr. Jean Harvey-Berino, has concluded that, contrary to her findings as recently as 2002, a Web site with dynamic, socially supportive, interactive features is just as effective as behavioral counseling.*

As the medical director of Medifast®, I've worked closely in the creation of the Medifast/Take Shape for Life™ online community and have witnessed this community assist thousands in reaching their goals. (For more information on using an online support system, see the resource list on page 370.)

*Micco, N., et al., "Minimal In-Person Support as an Adjunct to Internet Obesity Treatment," *Annals of Behavioral Medicine* 33 (1): 49–56.

In the end, I believe that having someone to work with and provide a personal touch is the most powerful form of support there is. For weight loss, it's invaluable. And for that, you need a coach.

You with a Coach

Having your own professional one-on-one coach can be very effective. Personal health coaching is a growing specialty because it fills a huge demand for personal instruction. In fact, I believe in personal coaching so much that we have created an entire network of health coaches who model the Habits of Health and are trained to teach them.

Your coach helps you stay accountable by holding up the mirror to make sure you're clear and honest about your current reality and progress. Working together, you and your coach can devise a customized plan that focuses on the healthy habits you need to work on the most, at an appropriate pace. And if you have the services of a certified trainer, you can also get instruction on how to exercise properly.

What's the downside? Some clinical and commercial coaches can be expensive and take up too much time. After all, it only works if you keep going—and trekking to a group meeting or a clinical facility every week for the rest of your life may not be the answer for you. So when you select a coach, make sure that you find one that fits your personality and budget, and that you'll utilize for the long term. The logistics will only work if their services are convenient to your lifestyle.

My recommendation? If you have difficulty starting or need some help staying on track until your new Habits of Health have become automatic, a personal coach may be your answer.

A Social Network

A recent study in the *New England Journal of Medicine* validated a social phenomenon that I've observed for years while working with people struggling with their weight and health.* In it, researchers followed an interconnected network of over 12,000 subjects and determined conclusively that people who associate with overweight people become obese themselves—even if they're not geographically close. And while the study focused on a group of individuals who have placed themselves in an unhealthy environment and are practicing the Habits of Disease, the converse idea—the notion of healthy people working together collectively—is intriguing as well. By modifying someone's social structure and spreading positive health behaviors, we can harness obesity. *By associating with people who are healthy and thin, we too can develop those attributes.*

This idea of a support system is becoming more widely recognized by experts around the world as a potential solution to our obesity epidemic. And it's a solution I've been using to help people create health in their lives for years!

Do Internet-Based Weight-Loss Programs Work? These popular sites offer privacy and convenience that traditional weight-loss programs can't. If you're Internet savvy, they can be an effective tool, especially when combined with a personal coach. In fact, I believe that access to a caring person—whether actual or virtual; by e-mail, phone, or face-to-face—will eventually be proven the best way to create and maintain long-term Habits of Health.

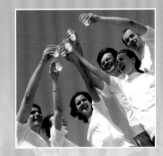

*Christakis, N. A., et al., "The Spread of Obesity in a Large Social Network over 32 Years," *New England Journal of Medicine* 357 (July 26, 2007): 370–379.

>225

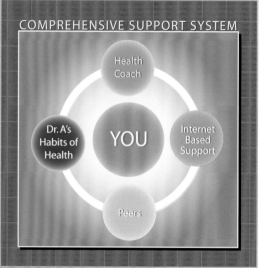

COMPREHENSIVE SUPPORT SYSTEM

Health Coach

Dr. A's Habits of Health

YOU

Internet Based Support

Peers

Modeling Works!
Studies show that by associating with others who have the qualities you desire—optimal health, for example—you're more likely to develop those qualities yourself.

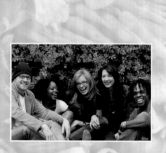

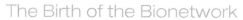

The Birth of the Bionetwork

In the 1990s, growing increasingly frustrated as I watched my patients succumb to the ravages of less-than-healthy lifestyles, I began exploring the concept of social structures and networks to support change. That research into group dynamics led me to create the bionetwork—a system of like-minded health care professionals and certified laypeople working together to help others change their health.

In 2001, I met Brad MacDonald, the CEO of Medifast, and together we co-founded the first commercial application of the bionetwork, Take Shape for Life. Medifast, the brand recommended by over 20,000 doctors since 1980, provided a perfect partner for us to help build a health network. Since its inception, we've been able to build a comprehensive support system—one that's convenient, inexpensive, effective, and available to anyone who wants to enjoy better health. It includes a team of properly trained health coaches and health care professionals who provide a comprehensive approach to helping people create health through personalized coaching and an environment that fosters optimal health.

The take-home message for you? Associate with people who've made the decision to create health in their own life! It can be as simple as hanging out with a few healthy friends. But if you're interested in a firmer foundation, we can connect you with a whole group of people who, like you, are making the decision to get healthy.

For more information about Take Shape for Life, visit www.habitsofhealth.net or www.tsfl.com.

A Final Word

One of the leading cultural anthropologists of our time, a woman named Inga Treitler, recently evaluated a group of individuals who had mastered successful weight loss by losing at least sixty pounds and keeping it off for at least five years. Although they had lost weight in many different ways, these long-term success stories had one thing in common—they had all changed the way they live their lives. They made a 180-degree change in orientation, in the way they experience the world! In fact, Treitler describes this phenomenon as a "rite of passage." For some, this meant leaving their old jobs to become coaches, teachers, and mentors. They in essence went from being passive to active participants in their own lives.

As you know, this book is a compilation of the lessons I've learned from people who've been successful at losing weight and reaching optimal health. By studying their successes—and the failures of others—the Habits of Health provides a path that many are following in order to reach and maintain optimal health. Many of these very same people who are living the Habits of Health are now helping others, which, as Treitler observed, is also helping them maintain optimal health. Working together, staying connected through an environment that inspires and creates long-term success, is a great way to give yourself the gift of comprehensive support and a lifetime of personal health and fulfillment.

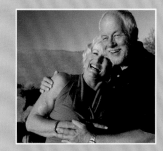

Phase III
Optimizing Your Health
Thriving for Life

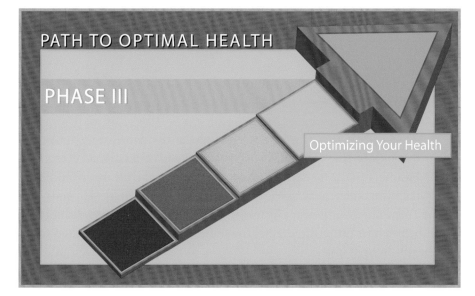

PATH TO OPTIMAL HEALTH

PHASE III

Optimizing Your Health

Up to this point, we've focused on the three major physical elements that set the stage for a healthy weight and optimal health—healthy eating, an active lifestyle, and restorative sleep. We've also talked about building a support system to help you maintain success. But these essential Habits of Health are really just the foundation of your continuing progress toward ever better health and a more vibrant life. You're now ready to make your final ascent toward optimal health.

To set the framework for Phase III, let's return once again to our energy management diagram.

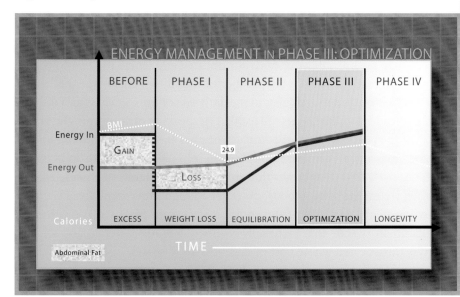

ENERGY MANAGEMENT IN PHASE III: OPTIMIZATION

	BEFORE	PHASE I	PHASE II	PHASE III	PHASE IV
Energy In					
	GAIN		24.9		
Energy Out		Loss			
Calories	EXCESS	WEIGHT LOSS	EQUILIBRATION	OPTIMIZATION	LONGEVITY

TIME

Abdominal Fat

Energy Management in Phase III: Optimization. In Phase III, you continue to add movement and muscle by increasing your energy output (green line) while also increasing your energy intake (red line). As you build muscle and reduce fat, your BMI may actually increase slightly. This means that your body composition is approaching a healthy state, complete with lean muscle, which is heavier than fat.

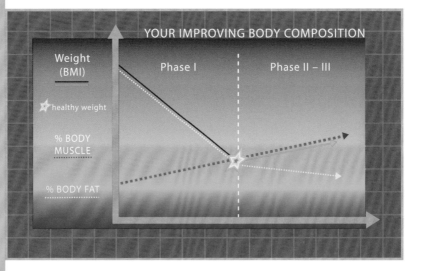

YOUR IMPROVING BODY COMPOSITION

Weight (BMI)

Phase I

Phase II – III

healthy weight

% BODY MUSCLE

% BODY FAT

Your Improving Body Composition.
In Phase I, we focused on reducing your weight and getting rid of dangerous abdominal fat fairly rapidly (dotted yellow line) until you reached your healthy weight (star). Because you're getting leaner, and muscle weighs more than fat, you may experience a slight increase in weight (green line) as you enter Phase III.

As you recall, in Phase I we created an imbalance—more energy out than energy in—by lowering your intake of calories so you could unload excess visceral (abdominal) fat. Once you reached a healthy weight, we moved to Phase II, in which you added healthy foods to balance out your energy expenditure. We then continued our journey by teaching you a progressive movement plan, which helped you offset the slightly lower metabolic rate that resulted from your healthy weight loss.

You're now eating a balanced diet of low-glycemic carbohydrates, muscle-stimulating proteins, and healthy fats. You're continuing to add movement and weight resistance training through the EAT System, which is helping you increase your percentage of muscle mass—a key determinant of optimal health. (Because muscle is denser than fat, you may actually gain a little weight as your muscle increases.)

In Phase III, you'll continue to balance your energy in and energy out through your healthy eating plan and active motion schedule. You'll continue to add movement and build muscle, and you may be particularly excited to note that your total energy intake will increase as well.

As you add muscle and shed fat through your new Habits of Health, your body composition is starting to resemble that of a healthy person. In fact, the leaner you become, the healthier you become. By shedding fat and gaining muscle, you're positioning your body for optimal efficiency. You're also regaining the good graces of one of your most critical body systems—one that may have turned on you and moved over to the dark side of non-sickness and disease before you adopted the Habits of Health. I'm speaking of your immune system.

In the past few years, medical science has begun to learn more about the many ways a hyperactive immune system robs us of our health and takes years off our lives. And what causes this imbalance? The Habits of Disease, of course! When we eat the wrong foods, don't get enough movement, live in unhealthy environments, and suffer from constant stress, our body reacts by creating an inflammatory state that eventually erodes our brains, arteries, and joints, and paves the way to a whole host of degenerative diseases. In fact, researchers are currently investigating the impact that a hyperactive immune system may have on such conditions as Alzheimer's, arthritis, heart disease, autoimmune diseases, cancer, and the entire aging process. That's why we're going to focus on eliminating inflammation from your body by adopting the Habits of Health you've already learned, as well as several more you'll discover in the next few chapters.

Continuing to lower your body fat and add muscle is one of the best tools available to beat inflammation. The combination of exercise and lean muscle mass provides a powerful one-two punch to a hyperactive immune system. Take a look at the diagram below. Note the dramatic decrease in the biological marker of inflammation known as C-reactive protein (CRP), represented by the dotted red line, as visceral fat goes down and movement goes up. It's a strategy you'll be using again and again to keep inflammation in check.

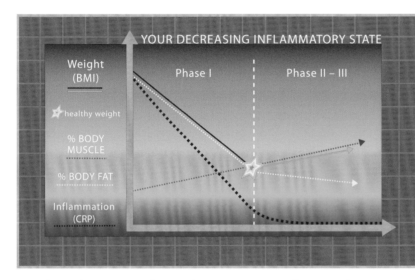

Your Decreasing Inflammatory State. As you reduced body fat in Phase I, your level of inflammation, measured by the amount of CRP in your blood (dotted red line), started to go down. Now that you're becoming leaner and continuing to add muscle mass, you're doing even more to keep dangerous inflammation in check.

These next three chapters are designed to equip you with a complete anti-inflammatory strategy that—along with your healthy diet, increased activity level, and lower body fat—will help you knock out the remaining unhealthy elements that are holding you back from a longer, healthier life. Let's take a look at how these new techniques will prepare you for the final stage of your journey to optimal health.

Chapter 19 examines how the daily assault of our environment overstimulates your immune system, turning your own body against you. You'll find out how to protect yourself from this onslaught and restore optimal balance through cutting-edge ideas that are simple to implement.

Chapter 20 looks at additional methods you can use to optimize your performance from the inside, including nutritional supplements adjusted to your particular needs and your age. No matter where you are on your life's journey, there are ways to help you look and stay younger!

Chapter 21 explores how you interact with your world and how that interaction affects your emotional well-being. As you'll see, your brain has a powerful influence over your health, and in order to optimize your physical being you need to minimize stress. We'll work on that by helping you figure out what it is you really want out of life and how to better align yourself with these important goals.

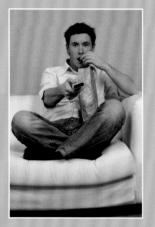

Chapter 19

. . . .

Inflammation: Dousing the Flame

The negative effects of an overactive immune system aren't felt overnight. But over time, if we keep our immune system on constant alert through bad habits such as eating unhealthy foods, avoiding exercise, and neglecting our sleep, our bodies will begin to age and break down prematurely.

For most of us, inflammation probably conjures up images of a swollen sore throat that keeps us in bed all weekend gargling salt water, or the red, pus-filled lump that swells around a cut. In cases like these, our immune system jumps into appropriate action, sends in white blood cells, bombards the invading bacteria. . . and we're back to normal in a few days.

So, what does all that have to do with optimal health?

The immune system—our own personal 24/7 on-call emergency service— has an incredible ability to seek out intruders such as bacteria, viruses, and parasites. In fact, it's the most complex system in the body, not only defending us but remembering every battle it's ever fought in order to recognize repeat threats and avoid wasting time on harmless ones. Its purpose is to restore balance to an unbalanced body, and once it's done its job it should settle down into its normal, vigilant state to await the next crisis.

Unfortunately, that's not always what happens. As medical science is beginning to discover, this benevolent protector has a darker side that can all too easily turn on its master—if we make the Habits of Disease our way of life.

When you eat donuts and coffee for breakfast, a fatty cheeseburger for lunch, and a bowl of ice cream before bed; when you carry extra fat around your middle, smoke cigarettes, and refuse to get off the couch—your immune system goes on alert. Not on an all-out attack that gets your attention, like the throbbing that accompanies a sprained ankle or the fever that means you're coming down with the flu. Instead, it trickles inflammatory molecules into your blood in quantities so small they can only be detected through a special test. Unnoticed, these inflammatory biochemicals work their sinister effect against your blood vessels, joints, brain, and other critical systems. It may start with stiff, painful joints, or tired-looking skin, or something far more menacing—like cancer, stroke, or Alzheimer's disease.

Our hostile environment stimulates our immune system every day through thousands of little exposures, and the resulting damage to our health and longevity can be staggering. In fact, we're only beginning to understand the magnitude of the effect that a chronically elevated immune system has on our body. But this much is known: the continual production of inflammatory markers is relentlessly aging our organs, and us, prematurely. In fact, it's quite likely that human longevity could stretch to 150 years or more—but only if we can get our immune systems under control.

Inflammation—A Key Player in Heart Disease

Until just a few years ago, the medical community focused on cholesterol and triglycerides as the main culprits in heart disease. But it turns out that's not the whole story. Now, thanks to a landmark study at the Harvard School of Public Health, we know that chronic inflammation—specifically the presence of C-reactive protein, an inflammatory marker—plays a major role in the development of heart disease.*

*Pai, J. K., et al., "Inflammatory Markers and the Risk of Coronary Heart Disease in Men and Women," *New England Journal of Medicine* 351 (December 16, 2004): 2599–2610.

The Silent Enemy

Most of us only pay attention to inflammation when it's acute. But we now know that chronic, low-grade inflammation attacks our health and plays a central role in degenerative diseases and aging. Just look at the chart below to see the many ways a hyperactive immune system can affect your body. These are just a few of the more obvious results of long-term exposure to a hyperactive immune system—the things that happen once you actually get sick. But the negative effects begin long before these disease states express themselves.

It begins when the immune system becomes overstimulated, perhaps by something you breathe, eat, drink, see, feel, hear, or think—even something as benign as sitting on the couch for too long. Carrying those extra pounds around the middle is a major contributor. Whether precipitated by the need to fight dangerous bacteria or the onslaught of a Big Gulp loaded with high-fructose corn syrup, the result is the same. Inflammatory molecules begin circulating at high levels in your blood—killing the enemy, yes—but at the same time having some serious consequences on innocent bystanders,

THE SILENT ENEMY

Cardiovascular system	high cholesterol/triglycerides, high blood pressure, atrial fibrillation, abdominal aortic aneurysm, stroke, sudden death
Respiratory system	asthma, nasal polyps, sinus infections
Kidneys	glomerulonephritis, nephrotic syndrome, nephritic syndrome, acute or chronic renal failure
Gastrointestinal system	ulcerative colitis, Crohn's disease, inflammatory bowel disease, obesity
Immune system	atopic dermatitis, rheumatoid arthritis, multiple sclerosis, psoriasis, allergies
Brain	Alzheimer's, mood disorders, depression, schizophrenia
Eyes	macular degeneration
Endocrine system	diabetes, nonalcoholic fatty liver disease
Other	breast, colon, and prostate cancers

The Silent Enemy: Conditions Caused by Inflammatory State (Elevated CRP). Chronic, low-grade inflammation attacks our health and plays a central role in degenerative diseases and aging, and can cause diseases such as these.

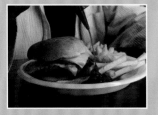

including your heart, blood vessels, brain, pancreas, kidneys, and other blood-rich organs, which begin a series of small civil wars against you.

The good news is that you have an antidote to these insurgencies—the Habits of Health. And to top it off, I'm going to teach you a whole new set of habits to help turn your immune system back into the protector it's meant to be. Let's start by looking at how your immune system operates: what puts the bad guys in motion and just how they cause so much trouble.

Free Radicals and Oxidative Stress

In a controlled state, the oxygen in your body fuels health. But when those oxygen molecules are disrupted—forming what you've probably heard described as *free radicals*—they can kill cells, damage your DNA, and cause you to age prematurely.

Actually, in short-lived, local release, these oxygen radicals aren't harmful. Produced through a process called *oxidative stress,* they're actually used by the immune system to protect you by killing dangerous invaders. Under normal circumstances, your body has a tremendous ability to scavenge and control oxygen radicals once their job is done, and in the next chapter we'll discuss foods and supplements that can help your body do just that. But if oxidative stress and inflammation are allowed to continue, a dangerous cycle is set into motion, with inflammation creating more oxidative stress and more oxidative stress fueling the inflammatory process. As you can see from the illustration below, the Habits of Disease have a profound effect on that cycle.

Habits of Disease That Cause Inflammation. Inflammation is spurred by internal factors, external factors, and the foods we eat. These Habits of Disease increase oxidative stress, causing our body to create oxygen radicals that, when left unchecked, produce chronic inflammation and cause further oxidative stress—a vicious cycle that slowly erodes our health and brings about disease.

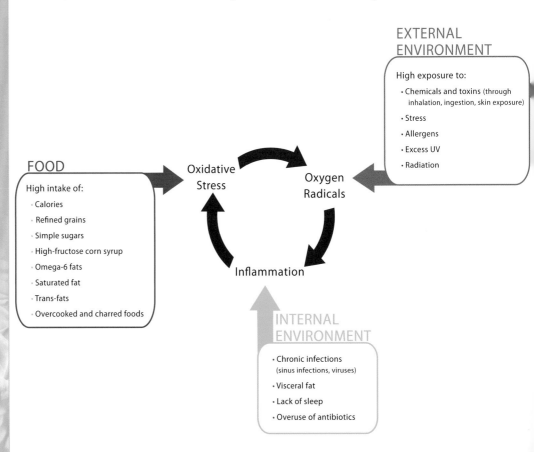

EXTERNAL ENVIRONMENT

High exposure to:
- Chemicals and toxins (through inhalation, ingestion, skin exposure)
- Stress
- Allergens
- Excess UV
- Radiation

FOOD

High intake of:
- Calories
- Refined grains
- Simple sugars
- High-fructose corn syrup
- Omega-6 fats
- Saturated fat
- Trans-fats
- Overcooked and charred foods

Oxidative Stress

Oxygen Radicals

Inflammation

INTERNAL ENVIRONMENT

- Chronic infections (sinus infections, viruses)
- Visceral fat
- Lack of sleep
- Overuse of antibiotics

Internal Environment

Exposing our bodies again and again to the Habits of Disease and the environment that supports them eventually erodes our health. Like a boulder slowly becoming worn down in a mountain stream, that erosive effect doesn't happen overnight. But over time, it leaves us with a battered body, premature aging, and a shortened life. Our blood vessels and organs actually wear out, leaving us vulnerable to attack. You may have experienced a taste of this when you've been run down and more susceptible to infection. Your immune system is just too fatigued to strike back.

So how do we get rid of this dangerous inflammatory state? By creating a microenvironment of health, both through the Habits of Health you've already learned and through some new ones you're about to discover.

Are You At Risk?

There's actually a way to measure your level of immune activation, using the C-reactive protein (CRP) test. Elevated CRP, which occurs when inflammation is present in the body, is highly predictive of cardiovascular disease. In fact, elevated CRP can boost your heart attack risk by 300 percent, even if cholesterol levels are normal. It can also predict your risk of other inflammatory diseases, such as arthritis and cancer.

While anything under 3 mg/L is considered a normal CRP, our goal is to get you down to under 1 mg/L through healthy diet, exercise, and by looking closely at three important contributors to inflammation—the food we eat, our environment, and our stress level.

Food and Inflammation

Food provides us with critical nutrients that keep us healthy and help us grow, but many types of foods also contain toxins that harm or even poison our bodies.

The typical Western diet is full of processed, high-glycemic carbohydrates and saturated animal fats, both of which are extremely inflammatory. In fact, many of the elements that make up these foods actually provide more toxins than nutrients.

Processed food. An astounding percentage of the average Western diet—over 90 percent—is now made up of processed foods. The high level of chemicals in processed foods stimulates the immune system, which senses those chemicals as foreign intruders and attacks. Conversely, you can lower your state of inflammation by eating healthy, unprocessed whole foods. If, due to time constraints, you absolutely must eat processed foods, try to choose those with the fewest chemical ingredients.

Carbohydrates. Processed, high-glycemic carbohydrates contribute to inflammation. But the good news is that the healthy, low-glycemic foods we've discussed in the chapters on diet can actually help reduce it. To help your body

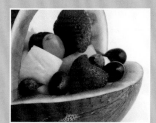

Ask your doctor about testing your CRP level. You should be tested at least every five years using a *high-sensitivity C-reactive protein assay (hs-CRP)*, which can help determine your risk of heart disease and other inflammation-related conditions. (If you choose to progress to a state of Ultrahealth, which you'll learn about in chapters 22–26, you'll want to be tested even more frequently to better monitor your progress.)

scavenge free radicals and quell inflammation, increase your consumption of the following:

- Low-glycemic foods
- Fruits and vegetables, especially those that are red, orange, or yellow
- Carotenoids (found in papaya, tangerine, yellow peppers, pumpkin, winter squash, sweet potato, carrots, apricot, cantaloupe)
- Vitamin C (found in citrus fruits, tomatoes, berries, peppers, sweet potato, broccoli, cauliflower, asparagus, dark green leafy vegetables)
- Quercetin (found in blueberries, blackberries, dark cherries, grapefruit, onions, apples)

Fats. Fats can have amazing anti-inflammatory properties—as long as they're the right type of fats. The following chart will give you a quick guide, but on the whole it's best to stick with monounsaturated and some polyunsaturated fats whenever possible.

Anti-inflammatory and Inflammatory Fats.
A healthy, anti-inflammatory diet should contain primarily monounsaturated and, to a lesser extent, polyunsaturated fats. Saturated fats and trans-fats are inflammatory and should be avoided.

ANTI-INFLAMMATORY FATS	
Monounsaturated Fats	• olive oil • canola oil • peanut oil • almonds • avocados
Polyunsaturated Fats	• vegetable oils (corn, soybean, safflower, cottonseed) • fish

INFLAMMATORY FATS	
Saturated Fats	• whole milk • red meat • butter • coconut oil • cheese
Trans-fats	• partially hydrogenated vegetable oils • most margarines • baked goods • vegetable shortening • commercially prepared french fries and onion rings

Nix the Barbie!
Overcooking, and especially charring, food on the grill creates extremely dangerous compounds called advanced glycation end products (AGEs) that are potent inflammatory agents and can actually increase your level of LDL—the bad cholesterol. Steam, bake, or boil your foods instead.

Let's break this list down a bit more to give you a better sense of the benefits of these important foods.

Monounsaturated fats have proven health benefits that include reducing cholesterol, inflammation, and cardiovascular risk. Olive oil is perhaps the most important and useful of these fats, with its own unique antioxidant properties, including a large dose of oleocanthal—a powerful agent that works like ibuprofen and similar over-the-counter medications to reduce inflammation and pain.

Polyunsaturated fats occur in two main types of fats—omega-3 and omega-6—both of which contain essential fatty acids. However, Western diets tend to include too much omega-6. To keep inflammation in balance, it's important to maintain a ratio of no more than 4:1 (omega-6 to omega-3), though a 1:1 ratio is ideal!

Anti-inflammatory Omega-3

Oils: flaxseed, canola, walnut, olive
Fish: mackerel, sardines, herring, salmon, bluefish, cod, crab, scallops, tuna, lobster
Nuts/Seeds: flaxseed, walnuts, pecans
Grains/Beans: soybeans, tofu
Greens: spinach, kale, collard greens

Inflammatory Omega-6

Oils: corn, cottonseed, safflower, sesame
Margarine
Prepackaged foods or foods with a long shelf-life

In addition, you should avoid reusing all vegetable oils, as they rapidly become breeding grounds for hydrogenated byproducts and oxygen radicals. Even food that is cooked in trans-fat-free vegetable oil becomes saturated on repeat cooking!

Which Oils Are Best? Which Should You Avoid?

A healthy, anti-inflammatory diet should include the following three oils:
- Canola: The least saturated oil, high in vitamin E
- Olive: Highest in oleocanthal, a powerful anti-inflammatory that works like ibuprofen to reduce pain and swelling
- Flaxseed: Rich in omega-3 and low in omega-6

Steer clear of the following:
- Trans-fats: An extremely inflammatory fat
- Fatty meats, especially overcooked or charred foods: Can increase inflammation through the breakdown of protein and fats

Anti-inflammatory Omega-3 and Inflammatory Omega-6 Fats. Omega-3 fats are an essential part of a healthy, anti-inflammatory diet. However, most Western diets are too high in omega-6. Be sure to keep your ratio of omega-6 to omega-3 less than 4:1 (a ratio of 1:1 is ideal).

Fight Inflammation while You Eat! According to research from the U.S. Department of Agriculture, eating antioxidant-rich foods can help ward off inflammation by blunting the oxidative stress produced by a meal high in carbohydrates, proteins, and fats.* So when it comes to antioxidants, timing is everything!

*Prior, R. L., et al., "Plasma Antioxidant Capacity Changes Following a Meal as a Measure of the Ability of a Food to Alter In Vivo Antioxidant Status," *Journal of the American College of Nutrition* 26 (2): 170–181.

Want to learn some great anti-inflammatory recipes and find out more about the relationship between food and inflammation? Check out *Anti-Inflammatory Foods for Health,* by Barbara Rowe, MPH, RD, LD, CNSD, and Lisa M. Davis, PhD, PA-C, CNS, LDN (Fair Winds Press, 2008).

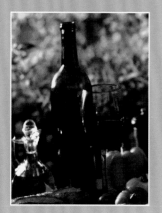

Other anti-inflammatory foods. Who said fighting inflammation has to be all about depriving yourself? Here's a list of some specialty foods with unique properties that can help you quell the fire of inflammation, including some favorites that you might enjoy adding to your diet!

- Herbs: Many herbs are great for countering inflammation, including ginger, rosemary, turmeric (and its component, curcumin), oregano, cayenne, cloves, nutmeg, feverfew, and boswellia.
- Teas: Teas contain catechins, a powerful anti-inflammatory and antioxidant. White tea contains the most, followed by green tea, and then black tea. Try to drink two to three cups per day to begin receiving the benefits.
- Chocolate: Chocolate also contains catechins, and well as polyphenols, another antioxidant. Choose dark chocolate (at least 70% cocoa), which contains ten times the antioxidants found in milk chocolate.
- Wine: You've probably heard of the French paradox. Despite a diet high in saturated fats, the French have lower rates of heart disease than many other Western nations. Why? Because they enjoy wine in moderation. Moderate amounts of alcohol (one drink a day for women, one to two for men) lowers inflammation and the risk of heart disease and type 2 diabetes. Red wine in particular is a potent antioxidant and anti-inflammatory and has even been shown to extend life in animal studies. (For more information on red wine and longevity, see chapter 26.)

Your Environment and Inflammation

Like the foods we eat, the world around us can affect our immune system. But by paying attention and making the necessary changes in the way we live, we can decrease our exposure to potential immune activators.

The air you breathe. Sure, we'd like to lower the amount of smog and pollution in the environment. But did you know that our greatest air pollution risk is actually inside our very own homes and offices?

The development of more energy-efficient houses and buildings, combined

---

Keep Inflammation in Check with These Handy Diet Tips

- Maintain a healthy weight by lowering your daily calorie consumption.
- Eat good fats (omega-3, monounsaturated fats).
- Avoid bad fats (trans-fats, saturated fats, animal fats, excess omega-6).
- Avoid overcooking and charring foods.
- Eat more fruits and vegetables, especially low-glycemic vegetables and antioxidant-rich colored vegetables.
- Eat more fiber through whole grains.
- Avoid sugar, highly refined carbohydrates, and high-fructose corn syrup.
- Cook with anti-inflammatory herbs and spices.
- Incorporate modest amounts of antioxidant-rich supplements and foods such as red wine, dark chocolate, and green tea.

> **Beware These Toxins in the Home!**
>
> While many of us already filter our water and air, other sources of toxins in the home may not be so obvious.
>
> - **Your lawn.** Pesticides and herbicides contain toxic substances that can be absorbed through the skin. Don't walk barefoot on your lawn, and remove your shoes before going in; better yet, manage your lawn organically.
> - **Your closets.** Plastic covers and dry cleaning bags contain a dangerous substance called perchloroethylene, which has been shown to cause dizziness, confusion, inflammation, and even cancer. Keep it out of your house and off of your body by machine-washing clothes instead of dry cleaning, or by choosing a dry cleaner who uses less toxic substances such as carbon dioxide or wet dry-cleaning processes. To find a professional near you, check out www.nodryclean.com or www.findco2.com.

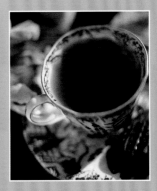

with a greater use of synthetics, has resulted in a new medical condition called *sick building syndrome.* Even brief exposure to volatile organic compounds such as radon, chloroform, and styrene can raise your CRP level. How do you know if you're affected? If you suffer from headaches, fatigue, or respiratory symptoms that are relieved when you're away from home or work—on vacation, for example—but that come back immediately on your return, you may want to get tested (or get a new job!). A simple CRP screen can help determine if you're being exposed to an inflammatory environment.

Other toxins include bacteria, molds, mites, and biological toxins in the air, including the very dangerous Stachy toxic mold. Treatment begins by identifying the source of the toxins if possible and removing them from your environment. Air filters may help, as well as increasing ventilation by opening windows and doors, especially in new buildings. (For more information on air filters, visit my Web site at www.habitsofhealth.net.)

I highly recommend that you use a HEPA (high-efficiency particulate air) filter, either through a whole-house system or in individual rooms. Also available on vacuum cleaners, HEPA filters are capable of filtering even tiny particles as small as one micron. Yes, these filters can be expensive, but remember that every particle they filter out of the air you breathe would otherwise be inhaled into your lungs and make its way into your blood—leaving your overburdened immune system with the task of locating, identifying, and disposing of each and every particle, and inhibiting your ability to move toward optimal health.

Your water supply. It's hard to look at the news these days without hearing about another contaminant found in our tap water. Painkillers, hormones, pesticides, household cleaners, all are potent inflammatory agents—not to mention the plasticizers, dioxin, and heavy metals that have been linked to autoimmune diseases. More and more people are turning to bottled and filtered water to avoid substances like these. But deciding which type is best can be confusing.

Dr. A Says . . .

Help ward off skin cancer by eating a diet high in omega-3, polyphenols (such as in green tea), and carotenoids (like beta-carotene), all of which have been shown to prevent melanoma. Of course, remember to wear your sunscreen too!

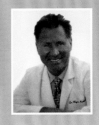

If you have children—
Remember that bottled
waters do not contain
fluoride, and reverse
osmosis (RO) systems
remove fluoride from
tap water. If you use
these sources for your
water, talk to your
dentist about fluoride
tablets or other sources
of fluoride for children
whose teeth are still
developing.

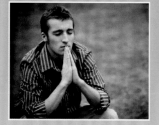

Bottled water comes from a variety of sources, usually indicated on the packaging. Artesian well water taps into an aquifer under the earth's surface, which helps protect the water from contamination. Mineral water comes from an underground source that contains natural minerals and trace elements. Spring water is sourced from underground springs that flow naturally to the earth's surface. Other bottled water sources include well water and even plain old municipal water that's been specially treated before bottling. Any of these sources can provide clean, safe water—just make sure that whichever brand you choose has been properly inspected.

Filtered water, available through a home filtration system, is a good option that's typically more cost-effective than bottled water. According to the Brita company, their widely available home filter system can produce water for eighteen cents a gallon, compared to a dollar or more for an 8- to 12-ounce bottled water. Home filtration systems generally attach to the faucet, filtering water as it comes through the tap. Systems like Brita and PUR also use containers that have the filter built right into them.

According to the Water Quality Association, consumers can feel confident about the quality of water provided by brand-name home filtration systems. However, it's important to maintain the filters according to the manufacturer's instructions in order to avoid build-up of bacteria and other contaminants. In addition, you should be aware that these systems do not eliminate volatile organic compounds. For the purest water available through a home system, choose a reverse osmosis (RO) system, though these tend to be more expensive than systems that use regular filters. For more information on water filters, visit my Web site at www.habitsofhealth.net.

Noise, noise, noise. Loud sounds from traffic, construction, even high-volume music in your ear buds can overactivate your immune system, as can noisy distractions when you're trying to concentrate. Soft, inexpensive foam earplugs are one solution, or even better, invest in a good pair of noise-cancelling headphones.

But sounds aren't all bad. Music can actually be a therapeutic way to lower stress, reduce inflammation, and calm the immune system. In fact, when you sing, play an instrument, or even just listen to music, you lower your level of immune-activating cytokines and increase your level of relaxing endorphins—the body's natural morphine.

X-rays and other radiological techniques. While the dose of radiation from X-rays is extremely low, it makes sense to avoid excess or unnecessary radiological diagnostic tests and to use a lead shield during dental X-rays and other tests that focus on specific areas of the body.

Excess antibiotics. Using antibiotics unnecessarily can disturb intestinal flora, allowing opportunistic bacteria to invade and spur inflammation.

Multiple sex partners and other high-risk behaviors. These increase your risk of contracting acute or chronic infections that cause inflammation.

> **Beat Stress and Curb Inflammation**
> **with These Healthy Behaviors**
>
> - **Get a massage.** Nothing works like human touch to promote feelings of well-being.
> - **Do some yoga.** You'll learn to breathe deep, stretch unused muscles, and even find a little inner peace. For more information, see the section on stress reduction in chapter 25.
> - **Take a warm bath.** Soothe your muscles and your mind by taking some time for yourself.
> - **Make your home cozy and inspiring.** Turn on soft music, put up some beautiful art, plant a garden, create a spot for meditation, hang wind chimes, or build a waterfall or reflection pond.

Stress and Inflammation

Stress. It's a part of life for all of us in today's world. In chapter 21, we'll spend considerable time discussing the importance of organizing your life around what really matters to you—an act that can go a long way toward lowering your daily stress level and keeping inflammation at bay. But what can you do about stress right now, while you're working on getting your life in order?

De-stress your job. The phone rings of the hook, you've got too much to do, you don't get along with your boss, layoffs are pending. There are so many ways our jobs create stress and activate our immune systems.

One major cause of on-the-job stress is simply poor communication, whether it's a lack of opportunity to express your concerns and frustrations or too little information about what's expected of you. Maybe you have too much responsibility and too little authority, or you're worried that you're not competent enough to maintain your position. You might even feel overwhelmed by success in the form of a recent promotion that's loaded you with more work than ever.

If you feel underappreciated at work, unfulfilled in your career, or unsupported by colleagues, your stress level—and your immune system stimulation—is likely to go way up. What can you do about it? Meet with your supervisor and ask questions about your performance, how you fit in, what you can do better, and what chances there are for promotion. Concrete information about your current reality and future opportunities will help you decide whether your job is really right for you—before you waste a moment more of your life or squander your precious health.

Exercise. We've already discussed how a lack of activity can directly raise your inflammatory state. The flip side is that getting sufficient exercise is probably the single most effective way to *lower* your inflammatory state, counteract stress, and decrease your CRP level. The chapters on movement should give you plenty of ideas on incorporating healthy amounts of exercise into your daily life.

Another Source of Inflammation: Ultraviolet (UV) Radiation
As anyone who's had a sunburn knows, excess UVA and UVB rays can damage and inflame our skin. In fact, this oxidative stress is not unlike what happens to an apple slice left exposed to the air. Luckily, those free radicals respond readily to the antioxidants found in many lotions, which, when used frequently in combination with a sunscreen that blocks UVA and UVB, can help protect you and your children, who are particularly vulnerable. For more information, visit my Web site at www.habitsofhealth.net.

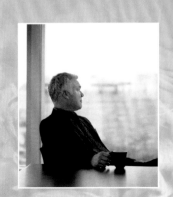

Don't Forget to Disconnect! Whether you're a high-earning executive or working from home, be sure to unplug from work and make time for yourself. Turn off the phone, power down the Blackberry, shut off the computer, and relax.

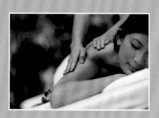

Get out and about. One of the best ways to decrease stress is to spend time with people we enjoy. Whether it's other new moms, dog lovers, fishing buddies, or siblings, just knowing you're not alone can go a long way toward helping you cope with stress.

Make sure you're spending plenty of time with people who, like you, are interested in improving their lives. Conversely, avoid relationships that bring on stress and codependent behaviors. Being around people who love life is not only rewarding, it's great therapy.

Go natural. I'm convinced that we all need to get out in nature and get in touch with our 10,000-year-old design. Whether it's a walk on the beach, letting the waves flow over your ankles as you bathe in the sun; a rented cabin in the country, where the nights are filled with croaking frogs, crickets, and a sky blanketed with stars; or a hike in the pristine air of a high-alpine region—nothing is more important than leaving behind the madness of our high-tech world to spend some time simply absorbing all that connects us and puts us in synchronicity with life.

Treat your body. Anything from a light massage to deep structural therapy can help you relax and restore balance to your musculoskeletal system when you're stressed, stiff, or just worn out. And it even helps lower CRP and inflammation! Here are a few options:

- *Western massage,* also known as Swedish massage, is the traditional kneading, friction, and tapping, characterized by long strokes.
- *Myofascial release* is designed to relax your connective tissues, and can also improve your range of motion and reduce tension. For more information, visit www.myofascialrelease.com.
- *Rolfing* realigns the body by manipulating the connective tissue, and can be quite intense. For more information, visit www.theiasi.org or www.rolf.org.
- *Acupressure* is similar to acupuncture, but without the needles. Instead, acupressure therapists use their fingers to create pressure and improve the flow of energy, or chi. For more information, visit www.acupressure.com.
- *Thai yoga massage* combines elements of shiatsu, acupuncture, and yoga to align energy meridians. It improves range of motion and flexibility, and because it's also meditative it's especially useful for relieving stress. For more information, visit www.thai-massage.org.

Laugh. Laughter has been shown to reduce stress, decrease CRP, and lower unhealthy hormone levels. Watch a funny movie, tell jokes, and find time to laugh with friends and family. Or next time you feel stressed, just try rustling up a great big smile. While it may feel forced at first, smiling by its very nature reduces bad feelings.

Focus on the positive. It's easy to slip into a negative self-image. But why say something bad about yourself that you wouldn't even dream of saying about someone else? Turn that internal dialogue into a running commentary on all the reasons you have to be grateful.

Stop, challenge, and choose. We all have to deal with day-to-day problems. Learning to focus on the outcome you want can help defuse a potentially stress-filled situation.

Here's a simple Habit of Health that I use in my own life and have taught to my children, my wife, my clients, and my patients. When a situation creates stress and negative feelings, try the following exercise.

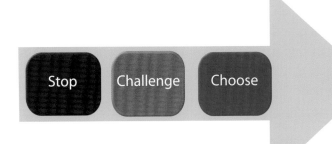

1. *Stop before responding.* We live in a reactive world. All too often, our first response is to lash out at whatever or whoever has created a situation we find less than ideal.

2. *Challenge why you feel the way you do.* It's easy to make assumptions or take things personally. By challenging what we're thinking or feeling, we can disengage the reactive, emotional parts of our brain and engage our logic center.

3. *Choose your ideal outcome.* Looking at the long term helps you put what's happening right now in perspective. Choosing the outcome you really want puts you in control and turns off stress.

Breathe deeply. You can't live without it—and it's one of the most powerful stress reducers there is. Each day, we breathe almost 20,000 times, exchanging carbon dioxide, a byproduct of metabolism, for life-giving oxygen. Yet we almost never think about this act that has such a profound effect on our emotional state and well-being—and vice versa.

From panic attacks caused by blowing off too much carbon dioxide to common stress that tenses our muscles and restricts our breathing, our emotions and breathing are closely intertwined. When our breathing is restricted, our normal pulmonary function becomes impaired and our heart rate can be affected, both of which can activate the immune system and negatively affect your health and longevity.

Optimal breathing. Yoga masters understand that slow, controlled breathing can create a stress-free state of harmony and health. When we're under stress, we tend to breathe more rapidly than usual, using mostly our chest muscles. Yogic breathing, on the other hand, expands the diaphragm, causing the abdomen to extend outward. This more desirable type of breathing releases stress and ramps down the immune system.

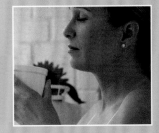

A Habit of Health:
Defusing stress before it gets out of hand

When you're faced with a stressful situation, *stop* (pause before you respond), *challenge* (are you reacting logically or out of emotion?), and *choose* (what outcome do you really want?).

**Can Deep Breathing
Help Heart Patients
Recover Faster?**
According to a recent
study,* patients who
practiced complete
yogic breathing (slow,
deep, abdominal
breathing) for one hour
a day had higher levels
of blood oxygen and
performed better on
exercise tests in just
one month.

*Bernardi, L., et al., "Effect
of Breathing Rate on
Oxygen Saturation and
Exercise Performance in
Chronic Heart Failure,"
The Lancet 351 (May 2,
1998): 1308–1311.

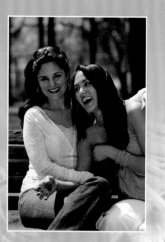

> ### *Which Kind of Breather Are You?*
>
> When we're stressed, we tend to breathe with our chest muscles. Abdominal breathing, on the other hand, is associated with a relaxed state.
>
> **Try this exercise:** Stand quietly with one hand on your chest and the other on your abdomen. Take some slow, deep breaths, paying attention to the movement of your hands. If the hand on your chest is most active and your chest is moving upward, you're a chest breather. If your belly is moving outward while your chest remains relatively still, you're an abdominal breather.

Much like your sleep cycle, the rhythm of your breathing plays a major role in your health. A good goal is to try to breathe primarily from your diaphragm at a rate of around six to twelve times per minute.

The best way to slow down your breath and promote healthy breathing is to prolong your exhalation. Ideally, the ratio of inhalation to exhalation should be around 1:2. In other words, you should exhale for about twice as long as you inhale. That can take some practice! We're so used to carrying our stress, and gulping and gasping through our hyperactive days. But once you begin to make slow, deep, abdominal breathing a conscious part of your life, you'll be able to apply it in times of stress—for instance, when you're practicing Stop-Challenge-Choose in response to a difficult circumstance. Deep breathing is also a great way to prepare for sleep. Eventually, it will become a Habit of Health that will take you closer to your goal of optimal health.

• •

Stress, poor eating habits, lack of exercise, and a toxic environment contribute to a hyperactive immune system that creates a dangerous internal environment of inflammation, taking a toll on your life over time. But by avoiding behaviors and conditions that stimulate your immune system and by actively developing habits that limit stress and lessen inflammation, you can position yourself for a lifetime of optimal health. With the right knowledge and tools—the Habits of Health—you can beat this modern scourge and live not only longer, but better.

Chapter 20

The Best You Can Be

Optimizing Your Life at Any Age

As you make your final ascent to optimal health, there are a few more tools in our arsenal that can help keep you in the best possible condition at any age—and even extend your life.

Take a look at the illustration below, The Optimal Health Journey. The red line represents the lifeline of those who remain passive to the daily insults of our obesigenic world. Their optimal health quickly becomes a state of non-sickness—overweight, elevated CRP (inflammation), insomnia—which decays to disease over time. Medications may bring about some limited improvement by decreasing the symptoms, but these folks never really regain their health.

Contrast that with the graduate of the Habits of Health (blue line), who continues to enjoy optimal health for life. But notice something interesting—in order for our graduate to reach and maintain optimal health, he or she must continue to adjust to the changing conditions of aging and environment to remain in the optimal health zone.

The upshot? Optimal health isn't static. It looks different at age twenty than at age eighty, and it requires vigilance and adjustment to the changes your body undergoes as you mature. We're now going to spend some time looking at your body's changing needs to help you learn how to adapt as you follow your path to better and more vibrant health.

**Half of America
Now on Meds**
For the first time in history, more than half of all insured Americans are taking prescription medications regularly for chronic health problems such as high blood pressure and cholesterol—problems often linked to heart disease, obesity, and diabetes. (Medco Health Solutions, *2008 Drug Trend Report*.)

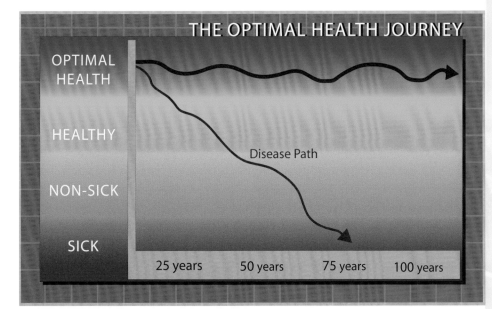

THE OPTIMAL HEALTH JOURNEY

OPTIMAL HEALTH

HEALTHY

Disease Path

NON-SICK

SICK

25 years   50 years   75 years   100 years

The Optimal Health Journey. The red line represents the path that many people take—a premature decline into non-sickness and sickness. The blue line represents the path of optimal health—a steady journey of vibrant living into your 100s and beyond. But staying in this state takes vigilance and adaptation as you age and your body's needs change.

243

Nutrients aren't like medications. While medications are foreign intruders that work temporarily in acute situations (and often cause side effects), nutrients are already present in our body. By supplementing them in just the right amount, you're simply helping your body reach its optimal efficiency. In fact, nutrients are the very fuel of optimal health!

When it comes to the new specialty of health creation, nutrients, not medications, are key.

Reaching the Summit

Up to this point, we've utilized your body's inherent capacity to heal itself. That's been accomplished through healthy eating and nutrition, increased daily movement, better sleep habits, and the removal of toxins from your internal and external environments.

Now we're going to *augment* these normal physiological processes with some valuable tools that can take you even farther up the summit of optimal health—namely, vitamins, minerals, and other critical nutrients for enhanced vitality.

Understand that nutrients are very different from the medications that today's medical delivery system relies on to treat disease. While medications work rapidly and effectively in acute situations when a body process needs to be blocked temporarily, they're actually foreign intruders that aren't otherwise present in the body. Over time, most medications become problematic—first, because they interrupt normal body function, and second, because they cause a large number of secondary side effects. *So while medications have their uses, creating health isn't one of them.*

Nutrients, on the other hand, are great facilitators. They may take a bit more time to create an effect, but since they're already present in the body, they're extremely safe. Nutrients can help you create a thriving, healthy life and augment the health of every cell and organ in your body. They're the very fuel of optimal health.

I'm actually a bit embarrassed to admit that my understanding of the significance of nutrients in health and disease treatment didn't come from my medical education. The nutritional focus in medical school and my postgraduate training was on little more than replacing the nutrients that patients lost as a result of particular diseases such as pernicious anemia, scurvy, and iron deficiency. Nutrients played little more than this minor role as replacement therapy.

It wasn't until years later, when I began to use nutritional intervention in critically ill patients, that I came to understand the pivotal function that nutrients play in creating health. I'm now convinced that in the not-too-distant future, the role of medications will be relegated to secondary status, treating cases that resist our primary tools of nutritional and behavioral intervention. When it comes to the new specialty of health creation—the domain of nutrients—medications have no role.

Nutrient Restoration:
Reversing the Effects of a Deficient Diet

Today's modern farming techniques have caused our foods to become nutrient deficient. Sadly, that's a reality—not just some crazy premise cooked up by vitamin manufacturers.

Inorganic fertilizers, susceptible crops laden with pesticides, over-farmed soils lacking iodine, zinc, and selenium—all contribute to producing foods that are nutritionally inadequate. Combine that with vegetables treated with sulfites (to give the appearance of freshness), and you can see that the foods available in our markets have become inferior products.

Then there are nutritionally degraded processed foods, which now make up over 90 percent of a typical Western diet, and the canning, cooking, microwaving, and reheating that leaves us with serious micronutrient deficiencies. In addition, we rely heavily on refined grains, sugar, and barely enriched cereals that lack the normal complex array of vitamins, minerals, and other nutrients essential for optimal health. What it all adds up to is this: the food we're eating is seriously depleted—and so are we.

In fact, less than half of a typical modern diet—mostly fast foods and sodas filled with high-fructose corn syrup—has any nutritional value whatsoever. As a result, our bodies begin to crave more food, hoping that the next bite will provide the fuels and nutrients we need.

Making up for these deficiencies is critical if we are to reestablish our equilibrium and our health. The Habits of Health go a long way toward this, but to create optimal health, we need to look toward supplements.

Nutrient Augmentation: Upward to Optimal Health

Taking some extra nutrients to make up for a deficient diet is an important part of health maintenance, but in fact nutrients can do much more—by providing us with a premium fuel that can actually enhance cellular and organ function.

Scientist Linus Pauling coined the term *orthomolecular* to describe the process of providing optimal amounts of the substances already present in the body, a concept that's been embraced by a number of innovative physicians, including the legendary Dr. Robert Atkins, who pioneered the role of vita-nutrients in health.

One particular group of nutrients we'll be paying close attention to are the antioxidants. As we discussed in the previous chapter, antioxidants play a central role in health optimization by shielding us from the attacks of dangerous free radicals that can damage our cells. In addition to the inflammation-beating diet tips you've already learned—consuming deep green and brightly colored vegetables, for example, as well as green tea, certain spices, and even red wine—I'll now add to your arsenal with fish oils, vitamins, and other supplements that are chock full of antioxidants.

Pesticides, preservatives, depleted soils, processed foods— all add up to a diet that's nutritionally inadequate. Today's typical diet simply can't build or sustain optimal health.

Antioxidants—Your Daily Dose of Protection

Antioxidants protect our cells from the damage caused by free radicals— the dangerous byproducts of a hyperactive immune system, brought on by today's Habits of Disease. Try to consume between 3,000 and 5,000 ORAC units (oxygen radical absorbance capacity) each day, through a combination of healthy foods such as green and colored vegetables and green tea and supplements such as fish oil, vitamins C and E, carotenoids, zinc, selenium, and glutathionine.

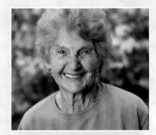

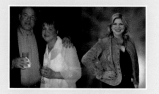

"The freedom to live a full, happy, and healthy life."

JOAN MUELLER
Two years at optimal health

My mother died of a heart attack one week before her fiftieth birthday, having had her first at only 33. I didn't want to go down that same path. But I knew that many habits I'd learned from her—overeating, eating fatty foods, avoiding exercise, and doing for others before myself—set me up to follow in her footsteps.

Thankfully, I met Dr. Andersen and began applying the Habits of Health. No more yo-yo dieting for me! I lost 40 pounds using Take Shape for Life™, and I learned to keep it off. I'm now at a healthy weight that I can maintain for the rest of my life. The Habits of Health have given me the freedom to live a full, happy, and healthy life. Food no longer has control of me! I still eat what I enjoy in moderation, but my weight remains constant, and I look and feel fantastic. Where I once merely hoped to live past fifty, I now fully expect that the habits I've learned and apply on a daily basis will give me longevity far beyond what I'd ever thought was possible for me. ■

Results vary. Typical weight loss is 2–5 lbs per week for the first 2 weeks and 1–2 lbs per week thereafter.

Do Supplements Work as Well as Whole Foods?

You've probably read that the best way to get the proper nutrients is through healthy whole foods. That's absolutely right! Filling your plate with fresh fruits, vegetables, and unrefined grains that contain all the complexities of nature is the best way to create optimal health. Unfortunately, hectic schedules, high costs, and limited availability sometimes prevent us from having healthy foods at our fingertips. That's why the prudent, informed use of complete, complex supplements—especially antioxidants—is a smart idea. PCMRs are fortified with strong vitamin and mineral premixes, and provide an additional means of obtaining supplementation.

To get the most out of your supplements, just make sure they're from a reliable source—and for extra assurance that you're getting full functionality, choose combined forms (such as B complex) rather than isolated versions.

Renewing and Optimizing through Nutrients: Your Personal Guide

The guidelines that follow will help you add supplements to your daily diet in the ideal amounts to support optimal health. You'll also learn how to maximize your antioxidant production to avoid immune stimulation and prevent damage to skin and organs, and learn the first steps of your lifelong anti-aging strategy.

Fish Oils

The omega-3 oils in fish provide numerous health benefits. To name just a few, they boost heart health by controlling arrhythmia; decrease sudden death; lower blood pressure; decrease cancer risk, especially breast and colon cancers; and decrease immune activation and autoimmune diseases. In addition, the DHA in fish protects the brain and retina. On top of this, a recent study confirmed that fish oil supplements combined with regular exercise help reduce body fat and improve cardiovascular and metabolic health.

While eating fish regularly is a good way to gain these benefits, there's a growing shortage of safe fish on the world market. That's why I've become a big advocate of supplementing your diet with 1–3 grams of pharmaceutical-grade fish oil daily. Be sure to choose oil that's been tested and from which all heavy metals have been removed, such as the enteric-coated oil I helped design for Medifast®. For more information, see the resource list on page 370.

Vitamins

The term *vitamins* refers to certain organic compounds that we need in tiny amounts as nutrients but that we can't synthesize in sufficient quantities by ourselves and therefore must obtain through our diet. This category doesn't include other essential nutrients such as dietary minerals, essential fatty acids, essential amino acids, or the large number of other nutrients that promote health but are required less often.

Vitamins serve a number of functions, acting as hormones (as in vitamin D), antioxidants (vitamin E), growth regulators for tissue and cells (vitamin A), and precursors for enzymes involved in metabolism (vitamin B complex).

Vitamin A

The original infection-fighting vitamin, vitamin A ranks right up there with vitamin C and zinc as a powerful immune booster. Used topically (on the skin), it helps heal wounds and keep skin healthy. It can also stabilize blood sugar in diabetics.

Take about 5,000 IU of vitamin A every day. (You can get it from cod liver, but I myself would pass on that!)

Multivitamins

Multivitamin mixtures generally provide vitamins A through E as well as vitamin K. Studies have shown that multivitamins can lower CRP and boost the immune system. They also prevent major deficiencies, particularly in people whose nutrition is depleted as a result of consuming highly processed diets low in fruits and vegetables. Despite these recommendations as to their effectiveness, only about two in every five people take multivitamins daily.

Carotenoids

This group of powerful antioxidants protects the heart and helps shield you from cancer. They're present in a variety of natural foods including kale, squash, tomatoes, broccoli, and spinach, and should be consumed as a group for the most benefit.

- *Beta-carotene* in its synthetic form is not as effective as its natural form, but you can supplement with 10,000–15,000 IU derived from algae such as Dunaliella salina.
- *Lutein* and *zeaxanthin* help protect the retina from stress oxidation as a result of excess sunlight. They're available in kale, collard greens, spinach, and other leafy green vegetables, or you can take 40 mcg of lutein a day.
- *Lycopenes,* probably the strongest and most underrated carotenoid, decrease inflammation, lower immune hyperactivity, and are particularly protective against breast, lung, endometrial, and prostate cancers. They're found in cooked tomatoes or can be taken as supplements of 20–40 mg per day.

Vitamin D

Vitamin D isn't really a vitamin, but a hormone. Essential for optimal bone health, it facilitates our absorption of calcium and vitamin D_3, and directs minerals to our bones to increase their density.

Vitamin D can be produced by exposure to sunlight. Twenty minutes of sun on your face and legs each day should provide an adequate amount, but note that sunblock prevents the production of vitamin D. Alternatively, you can supplement with 400 IU per day, increasing up to 1,000 IU as you get older. Of the five different forms of vitamin D, cholecalciferol (D_3) is probably the most effective. Vitamin D is also found in yogurt, dairy products, soy milk, and fatty fish such as salmon.

Despite the fact that multivitamins have been proven extremely effective for health, only two in five people actually take them.

IU = international unit

mg = milligram

mcg = microgram

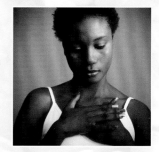

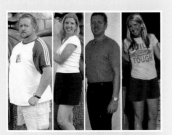

Inositol

This natural vitamin can help you burn fat, sleep better, and relax. Consuming more whole grains, meats, and milk will help, but on occasions when you need to relax and fall asleep naturally, you can take 500–1,000 mg before bedtime.

Biotin

Often part of the B complex vitamins, biotin is essential for skin and hair health, and looks quite promising for use as a glucose metabolism facilitator in diabetes. In higher doses, it's been helpful in reversing diabetic neuropathy. Because you can easily increase your intake by eating soybeans and brewer's yeast, supplementation usually isn't necessary. If you do choose to supplement your dietary intake, take an additional 100–300 mcg per day. People experiencing hair loss, especially during weight loss, may be helped by 5–15 mg in divided doses. For use in diabetes, please see your diabetic specialist or your primary care physician.

Bioflavonoids

The benefits of this group of powerful antioxidants, once known as vitamin P, are enhanced when combined with vitamin C. Here are some of the most important of their over four thousand members.

- *Quercetin* is a powerful anti-inflammatory, antioxidant, and antihistamine that also protects our blood vessels against LDL. It includes citrus compounds and is found in apples, onions, broccoli, and tea. As a supplement, take 500 mg per day on an empty stomach.
- *Pycnogenol*, part of a group of powerful antioxidants called proanthocyanidins, are anti-inflammatory substances that boost the immune system, help repair and strengthen capillaries, and can help rejuvenate the elastic recoil of your arteries. Take 50–300 mg per day as pycnogenol or grape seed extract.

Minerals

Minerals originate in the earth and can't be made by living organisms. Plants obtain minerals from the soil, and most of the minerals in our diet come directly from plants or indirectly from animal sources. Because the mineral content in soil varies geographically, the type and amount of minerals in the plants we eat also varies, as do the minerals in our water. Here are some key contributors to our health from this important nutrient group.

Calcium

Calcium's role in providing the substance of our bones and teeth and facilitating muscle contraction is undeniable. It's even been shown in recent studies to facilitate weight loss! In short, we need calcium.

Despite what the milk industry says, there are far better ways to get calcium than through milk products, which are great for babies but should be consumed in moderation or not at all by adults. The good news is that there are many other terrific sources of calcium, including pink salmon, almonds, Brazil nuts, mustard greens, bok choy, pinto beans, cooked spinach, and sardines.

If you have osteoporosis, are at high risk for colon cancer, or just want to make sure you're getting enough calcium, you can supplement with either calcium hydroxyapatite or calcium citrate. Men should take around 1,200 mg and women 1,500. You can test the solubility of the type of calcium you choose by putting it in a couple of ounces of vinegar. It should be totally dissolved within thirty minutes.

Magnesium

Magnesium is the heart's most important mineral, and, like calcium, it's essential for bone and muscle health. It also plays a key role in nerve conduction, lessens inflammation, and enhances immune function, particularly in people who are stressed or who have diabetes or gastrointestinal problems. Magnesium deficiency has been linked to high blood pressure, migraines, osteoporosis, diabetes, cancer, heart arrhythmias, and asthma. This was a major problem in the ICU where I worked, and in fact, it's probably the most common mineral deficiency, affecting 10 to 15 percent of the population, especially the elderly in nursing homes. I found that the addition of magnesium dramatically improved my patients.

You can boost your magnesium level by eating more green leafy vegetables, nuts, whole grains, and legumes such as soybeans, beans, and peas. To supplement, take 200–400 mg per day of magnesium glycinate or aminoacid chelates. If you experience diarrhea or stomach cramping, discontinue use, and avoid magnesium supplements entirely if your kidney function is poor.

Selenium

I believe that everyone should increase their intake of this potent antioxidant for its terrific cancer-fighting, heart-protecting, anti-inflammatory qualities. Unless you happen to live in a part of the world with selenium-rich soil, you should supplement with 200 mcg per day of sodium selenite, selenmethionine, or, as long as you're not prone to yeast infections, yeast-derived selenium. Or just eat two Brazil nuts, which contain about the same amount. Taking selenium with vitamin E appears to enhance both their benefits.

Zinc

Zinc is essential for the healthy functioning of all our cells. Its role in immunity has received a lot of popular attention recently, thanks to its widespread use in throat lozenges for the common cold. Zinc is particularly important for reproductive health and should be replaced regularly in men who are very sexually active. Older people, who commonly have difficulty absorbing zinc, should supplement as well.

Zinc deficiency is likely to become more common as our soil becomes depleted and as animal-protein consumption decreases. Hair loss, diarrhea, fatigue, and slow healing of wounds can all signal a zinc deficiency.

Zinc is found in peas, beans, legumes (especially soybeans), beef, poultry, and, yes, oysters. I recommend you take 15–25 mg of zinc per day. If you can't taste it on your tongue, increase the dose until you do. A word of caution, however: because zinc competes with other minerals, especially copper, manganese, and iron, do not exceed 200 mg per day.

Test the effectiveness of your calcium supplement by putting it in vinegar. It should be totally dissolved within thirty minutes.

Try an old-fashioned Epsom salt bath for some extra magnesium. Pour a warm, relaxing bath and add some Epsom salts—your body will draw out the magnesium it needs.

Always check with your
doctor before taking
an iron supplement. It
is possible to have too
much iron in your body.

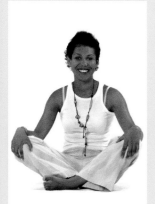

Iron

This building block of the blood is vital to our health. Women with heavy menstrual cycles can lose as much as 30 mg of iron per cycle, resulting in iron-deficiency anemia. Interestingly, women who are struggling to lose weight may have an iron deficiency as well. Other causes include the regular use of aspirin or NSAIDs (non-steroidal anti-inflammatory drugs) for arthritis, which can bring about bleeding, and a non-meat diet that's high in carbohydrate and fiber.

Yet while some people have too little iron, others have too much. Excess iron can create dangerous oxidative radicals that attack your blood vessels and body like rust. Too much iron is dangerous to your heart, can stimulate cancer formation, and has been implicated in Parkinson's disease. To be safe, don't take any iron supplement without first having your blood tested by your doctor.

If you do find that you have an iron deficiency, eating red meat can help—though that's not exactly a Habit of Health! It's probably a better idea to just take 5 mg in the form of ferritin capsules several times a day until the deficiency is resolved. Women of childbearing years who are menstruating should probably supplement as well. To help with iron absorption, particularly if you have an underactive thyroid, take iron with vitamin C and 20,000 units of vitamin A. Once your deficiency is under control, continuing to supplement with vitamin C will actually help you extract more iron from your food.

Copper

Copper is important in several metabolic pathways, and its balance is critical for a healthy immune system. With today's growing consumption of processed foods and high-fructose corn syrup, copper deficiencies are increasing. But as with iron, you can have too much copper, particularly if you drink tap water from copper pipes. Excess copper has been linked to anxiety, migraines, depression, schizophrenia, and macular degeneration.

Copper can be obtained through foods such as soy products, nuts, and seeds. Alternatively, check with your doctor about supplementing with 2–3 mg per day of copper sebacate.

Manganese

Although we need just a minute amount of this mineral, it's essential for growth, peak cognitive performance, reproduction, and metabolism, particularly as our diets of refined flour and sugar and the depletion of our soil work their negative effects on our hearts, brains, and ability to manage our blood sugar and cholesterol.

Manganese can be replaced by eating more soy and animal products. If you choose to supplement, maintain a balance of one part manganese to two to six parts zinc, and add vitamin C as well.

Iodine

The addition of iodine to commercial salt has virtually eliminated the deficiency of this mineral, which is vital for healthy thyroid function. There's no need to supplement if you use salt or have a diet rich in seafood or kelp. For those on salt-restricted diets, a daily supplement of 10–150 mcg is more than sufficient, as high amounts of iodine can be toxic.

Vanadium

This relatively new player is showing great potential in helping to improve glucose metabolism in diabetics and in lowering LDL cholesterol and triglycerides. A small amount may facilitate normal cholesterol and glucose metabolism, though diabetics should consult their doctor before supplementing, as proper dosage has not yet been determined.

Chromium

While vanadium's part in glucose metabolism is still being investigated, chromium is known to play a central role in both glucose metabolism and body fat. In fact, it's actually been found to help reverse fat accumulation. Regarding glucose, it's been shown that a chromium deficiency can cause you to crave sugar, further depleting your stores. Almost 90 percent of people in the U.S. are chromium deficient. Chromium also affects heart disease, high blood pressure, and the aging process, and can inhibit the release of immune-activating cytokines that stimulate the inflammatory state.

Chromium is found in brewer's yeast, eggs, chicken, apples, bananas, and spinach, or you can supplement by taking 200–600 mcg per day. Note that some people develop mild insomnia when they begin taking chromium supplements. Also, if you're a diabetic, it's critical that you and your doctor watch your blood sugar closely, as your levels will drop with the addition of chromium.

> The vast majority of Americans are chromium deficient, a condition that can cause sugar cravings. Conversely, getting enough chromium can actually help reverse fat accumulation!

Molybdenum

This trace element acts as a scavenger, purifying the body of toxic compounds, and as such, it's a great friend of the immune system. It can help clear the mental fog of sulfite allergies and aldehydes from yeast infections. If you eat a lot of eggs, sulfite-containing wines, or lots of sugar (a no-no!), you should supplement by taking 200–500 mcg per day. People with a history of gout should avoid molybdenum.

Boron

Important for creating strong bones, boron has also been shown to improve reproductive health in both sexes, including libido in older men. Some people feel that it aids with arthritis as well. Boron is found in vegetables, nuts, seeds, wine, and beer, or you can supplement with 3 mg per day. For hormonal and arthritic benefits, doses as high as 6 mg have been taken long term without side effects.

Amino Acids

Amino acids are the building blocks of our body, and maintaining the right balance is important for health. The best way to achieve the proper amount and balance of amino acids is from animal sources, particularly eggs. That's why it's particularly important to supplement your daily intake of amino acids if your diet is low in animal protein. Here are some of the amino acids that are most important for augmenting health.

Glutathione's role as an anti-aging, anti-cancer agent is second to none! Take it as a supplement or increase your intake of vegetables such as broccoli, cabbage, cauliflower, bok choy, and brussels sprouts.

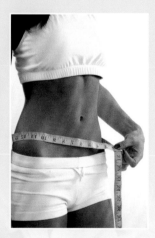

Arginine

In one of the greatest discoveries of recent time, nitric oxide was shown to help modulate blood flow, vessel relaxation, and immune function. The ability of arginine to modulate nitric oxide has allowed us to harness this powerful health agent. Arginine also protects muscle mass, improves the immune system, and even helps with male erectile dysfunction.

You can supplement with 1–4 grams per day without side effects. Take arginine with broad antioxidant protection including CoQ_{10} and alpha lipoic acid to avoid free radical formation. If you have a virus such as herpes, you'll also need to supplement with lysine to avoid stimulating the virus. If you're interested in taking arginine to improve the capacity of specific organs, consult your doctor.

Glutathione

One of our most important antioxidants, with a role in cancer prevention and anti-aging that's second to none, glutathione is actually a protein made up of three separate amino acids. It's a wonderful detoxifier and has a powerful ability to slow immune activation, making it a potent anti-inflammatory.

To raise the level of this powerful optimal health protein in your body, increase your consumption of cauliflower, cabbage, bok choy, Brussels sprouts, and broccoli. As a supplement, it must be dissolved in your mouth to be effective. Take it in a reduced form of 100–200 mg daily, or combine it with L-carnitine, and you can take 1–2 grams safely. To boost its effect, take N-acetyl cysteine (NAC) as well, which also decreases inflammatory response.

L-carnitine

L-carnitine is known as the fat burner for its ability to facilitate the conversion of fat into fuel, a process that provides almost two-thirds of the heart's energy. It can also lower CRP and decrease immune activation. Since its whole food source is fatty meats, I recommend you supplement instead, with 500–1,000 mg per day. Another form, acetyl L-carnitine, which acts as a super carnitine, has the added benefit of protecting brain cells against aging, and in fact it may be helpful for Alzheimer's. Heavy exercise increases your level of acetyl L-carnitine, but you should also supplement by taking 500–1,000 mg per day, along with an equal amount of L-carnitine.

Other Important Nutrients

Coenzyme Q_{10} (ubquinone)

This vitamin-like substance, naturally present in most human cells, is responsible for the production of the body's own energy. In fact, 95 percent of the human body's energy requirement is converted from the food we eat with the aid of CoQ_{10}. It helps optimize your heart and immune system, is a powerful anti-cancer agent, and is absolutely critical for optimal health. Like L-carnitine, it can also facilitate the conversion of fat to an energy source. Our level of CoQ_{10} decreases after age forty and as a result of taking statin drugs.

Since whole food sources are excessively fatty, it's best taken as a supplement. It does tend to be expensive, but if you use a hydro-soluble (dissolving in water) form, you'll receive benefits from just 100–200 mg per day.

Alpha Lipoic Acid

This universal antioxidant is important both as a protector and for its ability to enhance glutathione, CoQ_{10}, and vitamins E and C. It also helps prevent and reverse diabetic neuropathy, fights insulin resistance, and reduces immune activation in autoimmune disorders and degenerative brain disease—and it's recently been shown to double the life of mice in combination with the drug selegiline! I suggest you take 100–300 mg per day. Diabetics should be aware that it can lower the need for medications.

Phosphatidylserine

This important brain food acts as a lubricant to keep brain cells fluid and flexible, and can actually help increase receptor sites. It also slows mental aging and decreases stress response and cortisol release. Take it in the morning to awaken the brain. It requires supplementation; I recommend 200 mg per day for one month and 100 mg per day thereafter for brain optimization.

Fiber

In the chapters on diet, we discussed the importance of fiber in lowering cholesterol and blood sugar, creating satiety (fullness), and improving intestinal health. But there's even more to this important nutrient—a high intake of fiber directly decreases the inflammatory state.

Much of today's increase in heart disease, diabetes, and degenerative diseases and cancer can be attributed to the development and profusion of refined grains and sugar. Adding fiber to your diet can immediately improve your intestinal flora by giving beneficial bacteria such as lactobacilli and

CoQ_{10} is critical for optimal health. While it can be expensive, you only need a small amount of the water-soluble type to get the benefits.

Fiber does so much! Along with being a great anti-inflammatory agent, it can lower cholesterol and blood sugar, improve intestinal health, and make you feel fuller.

Açaí: The Super-Berry

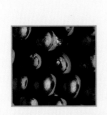

Açaí (ah-*sigh*-ee), the high-energy berry of an Amazonian palm tree, is a veritable powerhouse of antioxidants, amino acids, and essential fatty acids. Available in many whole food and health stores, açaí has a vibrant flavor of chocolate and berries. While it can be taken in juice form, you're much better off consuming it as pulp to reap the full benefits of the following:

- High levels of antioxidants (thirty times the anthocyanins in red wine).
- Monounsaturated (healthy) fats, dietary fiber, and phytosterols for cardiovascular and digestive health. Açaí's fatty acid content resembles that of olive oil and is rich in monounsaturated oleic acid, an important partner to omega-3 fish oils in promoting cellular health and longevity.
- Essential amino acid complex and valuable trace minerals for muscle contraction and regeneration.

bifidobacterium abundant food. These healthy intestinal dwellers flourish on the fiber that we can't digest, enabling them to overcrowd and wipe out dangerous bacteria.

Fiber also slows down the absorption of glucose, which helps control blood sugar and allows more time for the process of offloading cholesterol. And by preventing toxins from entering the bloodstream, fiber takes a burden off of the immune system, making it a powerful tool for optimal health.

Let's take another look at the two types of fiber.

- *Soluble fiber* slows the breakdown of complex carbohydrates and helps reduce blood sugar. It dissolves in water, forming a gel-like mass that binds cholesterol in the stool. If you eat enough, it can actually help lower blood cholesterol. Good sources of soluble fiber include vegetables, legumes, fruits, and grains such as rye, barley, and oats.

- *Insoluble fiber* does not dissolve in water and is not absorbed or digested by the body. Because it's filling, it reduces hunger. It also helps keep your gastrointestinal tract clean and aids in regular bowel movements by pulling water into the colon. Good sources of insoluble fiber include brown rice, whole wheat breads, cereals, seeds, fruit skins, vegetables, and my favorite food—legumes!

The foods listed above average around 3 grams of fiber per cup. Men need at least 38 grams of fiber per day, and women at least 25. As a general rule, you should try to eat 20 grams of fiber per thousand calories. While this should be doable under the Habits of Health, which encourage you to eat significant amounts of vegetables and fruits, it doesn't hurt to supplement! The following fiber supplements are sugar-free:

- Methylcellulose (Citrucel)
- Guar gum (Benefiber)
- Psyllium husks (Konsyl)
- Pectin (Medifast)

Probiotics

On occasion, we may find ourselves forced into a period of unhealthy eating or extra stress, or need an antibiotic for acute infection. These stressors can wreak havoc on our intestinal flora and cause gastrointestinal distress in the form of gas, cramping, bloating, and diarrhea. Some people may find that their existing sinus, ear, and respiratory problems or food allergies are exacerbated as well.

At times like these, the addition of friendly bacteria in the form of probiotics can help you reestablish a healthy intestinal tract and recover optimal health. Probiotics can also help reduce CRP and immune hyperactivity, and assist in the manufacture of such nutrients as biotin, folic acid, and vitamin K.

To supplement, look for a high-quality brand with at least four million bacteria per dose, including the following:

- *Acidophilus* to help augment the immune system and inhibit growth of candida and E. coli.

At times when your system is stressed or you haven't been eating right, probiotics can help you get back in balance.

> *Prebiotics and Probiotics: Different Animals*
> Probiotics aren't the same thing as prebiotics. While ***probiotics*** add helpful bacteria to your digestive system, ***prebiotics*** contain nondigestible food ingredients that selectively stimulate the growth and activity of beneficial micro-organisms that are already in your colon. When probiotics and prebiotics are mixed together, they form yet another type of substance—a ***synbiotic.***

- *Bifidobacterium,* our most abundant and important bacteria, which lowers cholesterol, digests lactose, and helps with the manufacture of B vitamins.
- *Bulgaricus,* a powerful immunity enhancer.

Probiotics are enhanced by the addition of FOS (fructooligosaccharide), a sugar that's not absorbed by the body. As a prebiotic, FOS has been shown to help lower sugar and cholesterol and alleviate constipation and diarrhea.

Phytonutrients

Phytonutrients are produced by plants to protect them from infection, disease, and oxidation. They often give plants their vibrant colors, and have been shown to help protect humans as well. Here are a few important ones you should know about.

- *Polyphenols* are powerful antioxidants that have anti-cancer properties as well. They're found in extra virgin olive oil, dark chocolate, fruit skins, green and white tea, and red wine.
- *Resveratrol* is a potent antioxidant that can help us live longer (more on that in chapter 26). It's found in the skins and stems of grapes, and in higher concentration in red wine. You can supplement with around 50–200 mg per day, or just open up a good cabernet and have a daily glass!
- *Genistein*, an isoflavone found in soy, can provide both antioxidant and anti-inflammatory protection with a resulting decrease in immune activation.
- *Curcumin* is a spice derived from the turmeric root, which is used commonly in curry dishes. It's an anti-inflammatory that can help autoimmune diseases as well. Use the powder in cooking or take 250 mgs per day, divided into three doses every eight hours.

Medications

Aspirin

Aspirin (acetylsalicylic acid) is the only medication I include with nutrients. It has a wonderful ability to block the immune system's production of cytokines and CRP, and in small doses is a weapon against immune hyperactivity. It's well known for its antiplatelet, or anticlotting, effect, which makes it an important ally for anyone at risk for cardiovascular disease due to family history or Habits of Disease such as smoking, excess abdominal fat, high LDL, low HDL,

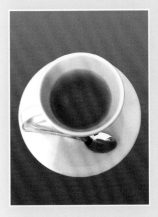

Many of these powerful antioxidants can be enjoyed in the form of tea, dark chocolate, and red wine!

> ### An Aspirin a Day. . .
>
> A daily low dose of aspirin has important health benefits, but like any drug it can cause side effects. Generally, I believe the benefits—in particular a 35 percent reduction in heart attacks in men over 35 and women over 40—outweigh the slight risk. Just be sure to check with your primary care physician before beginning daily aspirin therapy. Here are a few more recommendations:
>
> - Men over age 35 and women over age 40 should take 162 mg of aspirin a day.
> - Aspirin therapy is not advised for people who are allergic to aspirin (only about 1 in 2,000) or anyone who drinks more than three alcoholic beverages a day.
> - Discontinue use if you have any gastric side effects or bleeding. Additionally, bleeding while shaving or flossing may indicate that you need to reduce the amount of aspirin you're taking or stop entirely.

inactivity, and high triglycerides. It's also helpful for those at risk due to diabetes or aging. Additionally, recent studies show that aspirin affects colon cancer and polyp formation by preventing the ability of cancers to create a blood supply for growth.

I consider aspirin a safe and inexpensive weapon in the health arsenal. I myself take the recommended dose of 162 mg in the morning, with a glass of warm water to help it dissolve and minimize gastric irritation (see box, above, An Aspirin a Day. . .). To achieve the right dose, slit a whole aspirin in half, take two baby aspirin, or take a specially formulated, enteric-coated low-dose aspirin by a maker such as Bayer.

Where Do You Go from Here?

We've just covered a lot of ground! Now, obviously, if you took each and every one of these recommendations for supplementation, you'd have no time or money left for anything else. So our goal is to identify areas where you have specific deficiencies or special needs and to focus on adjusting your current intake to reach an optimum level. I'll also highlight some key areas where nutrition augmentation can help you reach and maintain optimal health.

One simple way to pinpoint areas of deficiency is to take a look at your current health assessment from chapter 5 and note any areas where you had negative or low scores, paying particular attention to your lipid evaluation, nutritional evaluation, current diseases and medications, and family history of disease. Another way to get more information is to ask your doctor for an hs-CRP test (high-sensitivity C-reactive protein), which can help determine your risk of heart disease and other inflammation-related conditions.

Once you've identified your areas of deficiency and current health challenges, you'll be able to create an individualized, targeted plan that not only brings you into better balance but actually augments your health for optimal

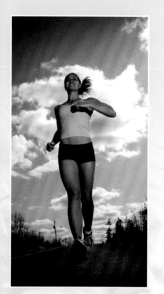

living. To do that, we'll look first at some general guidelines from the U.S. government, then at some more specific recommendations of my own that you can use to guide your choices.

U.S. Government Recommendations

U.S. government recommendations are used on commercial food and nutritional products to give consumers a general idea of the amount of daily nutrients they should obtain and the amount that each product provides. But bear in mind that these are general guidelines only and not tailored to your specific needs.

Let's take a look at some of these recommendations. First, you'll need to learn a few terms. RDI (reference daily intake) calculates the recommended amount of vitamins and minerals. DRV (daily reference value) calculates the recommended amount of energy-producing nutrients (fat, carbohydrates, protein, and fiber). For the purposes of food and product labels, the U.S. government calculates DRV as a percentage of a 2,000 calorie diet. This means that your own recommended amount may be higher or lower, depending on the number of calories you eat in a day. Here are the percentages the U.S. government uses to calculate their DRV, versus the percentages we've set as our goals for healthy weight maintenance and optimal health.

The U.S. government recommendations that are published on food labels only go so far. Because they're just general guidelines, they're not tailored to your specific needs.

Food Group	U. S. Government Recommendation	Our Goal
Fat	30% of calories	Less than 25%
Saturated fat	10% of calories	Less than 5%
Carbohydrate	60% of calories	45–60%
Protein	10% of calories	15–25%
Fiber	11.5 g per 1,000 kcal	20 g per 1,000 kcal

U.S. Government DRV (Daily Reference Values) for Energy-Producing Nutrients (Fat, Carbohydrates, Protein, and Fiber). These are the amounts of nutrients that the U.S. government recommends you obtain daily, based on a diet of 2,000 calories per day.

Food Component	DRV
fat	65 grams (g)
saturated fat	fatty acids 20 g
cholesterol	300 milligrams (mg)
total carbohydrate	300 g
fiber	25 g
sodium	2,400 mg
potassium	3,500 mg
protein (adult)	50 g

· · · · · · · · · · · · · · · ·

**U.S. Government RDI
(Recommended Daily
Intake) for Vitamins
and Minerals.**
These are the amounts
of vitamins and minerals
that the U.S. government
recommends you
obtain daily.

Nutrient	Amount
vitamin A	5,000 International Units (IU)
vitamin C	60 milligrams (mg)
thiamin	1.5 mg
riboflavin	1.7 mg
niacin	20 mg
calcium	1.0 gram (g)
iron	18 mg
vitamin D	400 IU
vitamin E	30 IU
vitamin B6	2.0 mg
folic acid	0.4 mg
vitamin B12	6 micrograms (mcg)
phosphorus	1.0 g
iodine	150 mcg
magnesium	400 mg
zinc	15 mg
copper	2 mg
biotin	0.3 mg
pantothenic acid	10 mg

RDI? DRV? Just What Are These Letters on My Food Label?

The various terms used in U.S. government nutritional guidelines can be confusing. Here's a quick synopsis:

RDA (Recommended Dietary Allowance): A set of estimated nutrient allowances established by the National Academy of Sciences. It is updated periodically to reflect current scientific knowledge.

DRV (Daily Reference Value): A set of dietary references that applies to fat, saturated fat, cholesterol, carbohydrate, protein, fiber, sodium, and potassium.

RDI (Reference Daily Intake): A set of dietary references for essential vitamins and minerals and, in selected groups, protein. It replaces the term *U.S. RDA (Recommended Dietary Allowance).*

DV (Daily Value): A relatively new term that attempts to simplify the guidelines by combining both DRV and RDI.

Dr. A's Supplement Guidelines

Now let's take a look at some guidelines that are based on *you*—not just some calculated deficiency model!

Step 1: Add Fish Oil

Make one of the following a part of your daily routine:

- 4 ounces of fatty fish three times a week (e.g., salmon, mackeral, sardines)
- 3–6 walnuts a day
- 1–3 grams of omega derived from a cold-water arctic fish, with EPA and DHA, taken thirty minutes before meals (sprinkle flaxseed on your breakfast as well)

Step 2: Take a Daily Multivitamin

If you're not already taking a multivitamin, start today with a one-a-day multivitamin specifically designed for your sex and age. Make sure it's a high-quality bioavailable vitamin, not one from a wax matrix (some companies use a petroleum-based process that interferes with proper vitamin and mineral absorption).

Step 3: Add B Complex Vitamins

The B complex vitamins work as a team. Unless you have specific needs, it's usually best to take them in the form of a high-potency B complex formula. If these aren't included in your one-a-day multivitamin, add them as needed to reach the following daily doses.

Vitamin	Full name	Amount per day
B1	Thiamine	25 mg
B2	Riboflavin	25 mg
B3*	Niacin	30 mg
B5	Pantothenic acid	100–300 mg
B6	Pyridoxine	4–50 mg
	Folic acid	400 mcg
B12**	Cyanocobalamin	100–400 mcg
	Biotin	100–300 mcg

* If you're at high risk for heart disease, talk to your doctor about increasing this amount.
** 100 mcg/day until age 40, 200 mcg/day from age 40 to 60, and 400 mcg/day after age 60. *Take only in combination with other B vitamins, not on its own.*

CHAPTER 20
THE BEST YOU CAN BE: OPTIMIZING YOUR LIFE AT ANY AGE

Remember, if you're pregnant or breastfeeding, limit your intake of fish to once a week.

Step 4: Augment with Other Key Vitamins

Add any necessary vitamins and minerals that aren't part of your multivitamin and B complex.

Vitamin	Amount per day
A	5,000 IU
C*	1,000 mg
D	400–1,000 IU
E (mixed tocopherols)*	100–400 IU
K	20–100 mcg

*These two powerful antioxidants can compete with the anti-inflammatory effects of statin drugs. If you take statins, check with your doctor and decrease vitamin C to 200 mg/day and vitamin E to 100 IU/day.

Step 5: Add Antioxidant Power

To enhance vitamin C's antioxidant capacity, combine it with one or both of the following:

- *Quercetin.* Found in apples, onions, broccoli, and tea; includes citrus compounds. Take 500 mg per day on an empty stomach.
- *Pycnogenol.* Part of a group of powerful antioxidants called proanthocyanidins. Take 50–300 mg per day as pycnogenol or grape seed extract.

For further antioxidant support, try these:

- *Lutein.* Obtain from kale, collard greens, spinach, and other green leafy vegetables, or take 40 mcg per day.
- *Lycopenes.* Found in high levels in cooked tomatoes. Eat ½ cup tomato sauce per week (500 mcg) or take 10–20 mg per day as a supplement.

Step 6: Add Key Minerals

Take the following daily dose of these important minerals:

- *Calcium.* Women take 1,500 mg, men take 1,200 mg.
- *Magnesium.* Supplement with 200–400 mg or take a warm Epsom salts bath.
- *Selenium.* Take 200 mcg as sodium selenite, selenmethionine, or, if you're not prone to yeast infections, yeast-derived selenium, or eat two Brazil nuts. Take with vitamin E for enhanced effectiveness.
- *Zinc.* Take 15–25 mg of zinc per day. If you can't taste it on your tongue, increase the dose until you do. *Caution: Zinc competes with other minerals, especially copper, manganese, and iron. Don't exceed 200 mg per day.*

Step 7: Take an Anti-inflammatory Package

Inflammation is an area that often goes unnoticed by both patients and doctors, but as you've discovered throughout Phase III, dousing the inflammatory flame is a major part of our core strategic plan to optimize your health.

Dr. A Says . . .

Red fruits and vegetables like tomatoes and watermelon are full of lycopene, an important antioxidant that may help protect against cardiovascular disease and certain types of cancer. And cooking those tomatoes actually increases their lycopene content!

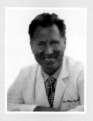

As we discussed in chapter 19, a good way to determine your current level of inflammation is with an hs-CRP (high-sensitivity C-reactive protein) test. Here are some guidelines to follow once you know the results of that test.

- *If your hs-CRP is over 3*, we need to adopt an aggressive plan to lower it. Begin by reviewing the information in chapter 19 and applying all possible techniques to reduce your immune activators. In addition to the Habits of Health, you should start on the following: at least 2 grams a day of vitamin C; 800 IU of mixed vitamin E; a mega B complex; 3 grams of fish oil; 1,000 units of vitamin D; chromium, magnesium, selenium, and zinc supplements; and increase your fiber to more than 40 grams per day.
- *If your hs-CRP is 1–3*, evaluate your risk factors, and in addition to applying the Habits of Health make sure you're taking a multivitamin and fish oil.
- *If your hs-CRP is less than 1*, your immune system is in great shape! While this is a fine goal, you can actually do even better. In fact, our ultimate goal over time is to lower your hs-CRP to less than 0.5—a great marker that you've optimized your chances for long-term health!

Step 8: Bonus Round

Ask your doctor about these other key nutrients that can help you reach and maintain optimal health.

- *Alpha lipoic acid.* Take 100–300 mg per day. (Diabetics note that this may lower your need for medications.)
- *Coenzyme Q$_{10}$.* Yes, it's expensive, but by using a hydro-soluble form you can cut the dose to 100–200 mg per day.
- *Chromium.* Found in brewer's yeast, eggs, chicken, apples, bananas, and spinach, or supplement with 200–600 mcg per day. (May cause mild insomnia. Diabetics should watch blood sugar closely with their doctor, as levels will drop.)
- *Aspirin.* Take 162 mg per day in the morning with warm liquid. *Check with your doctor before beginning aspirin therapy.*
- *Probiotics.* Take a dose that provides 4 billion lactobacillus per day, including acidophilus, bulgaricus, and bifido.

• •

You now have a great outline of the nutritional support you need, not only to correct any deficiencies that have resulted from our modern lifestyle, but to flourish and thrive at your best—now and for many years to come. Add this to the anti-inflammatory practices you learned in the last chapter, and you're nearly ready to take on the world!

But first, let's take a closer look deep inside, where the seeds of health are planted. Not at the *physical* you that we've been optimizing through healthy foods and supplements, but at the *emotional* you, whose ability to deal with stress and find happiness and fulfillment is a key component of the journey to optimal health.

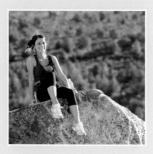

Chapter 21

Creating Well-Being

Taking the Stress out of Life

You haul yourself out of bed, drink a cup of coffee, rush to the car, get to work, turn on your computer, answer your e-mails, do your job, grab a bite to eat, focus all afternoon, drive to the dry cleaners, stop at the grocery store, go home, fix dinner, watch a little TV, and hit the bed to rest a bit before getting up and doing it all again.

So now it's the weekend, and what happens? You get home late Friday night, do chores on Saturday, sleep in on Sunday morning out of pure exhaustion, maybe spend some time at your place of worship, watch some afternoon TV... and just about the time *60 Minutes* comes on you get a sinking feeling in your gut because you know that in less than twelve hours you're going to launch yourself into another chaotic, energy-draining week of work.

Sound familiar?

Despite our material wealth, our generation ranks the quality of our lives *lower* than our parents'—for the first time in history.

Let's get some perspective on our modern lives by getting out the time machine and taking a peek at our caveman ancestors. Ten thousand years ago, those early humans had to work hard every day for food, shelter, and protection. As a result, they were in shape, lean, alert, and robust. But when it was warm, they took time to lie in the tall grass and feel the warmth of the sun. They watched the stars and the moon in wonder. They created art, and left wonderful drawings that depict a simpler time. At night they made spectacular campfires and gathered in groups as they told great stories of the hunt and discussed the eternal mysteries of life. They laughed, and even played instruments for sheer pleasure.

Now contrast that picture with today's overworked, overstressed, overweight, flabby, and sleepless society. We're the first generation ever to actually rank the quality of our lives *lower* than our parents'. *How did this happen?*

OK, here I go again—it comes down to our love affair with technology. We've become used to measuring success by our possessions, our house, our car, our income, our position. And as a result, our preoccupation with having the most RAM, the fastest processor, and the latest flat screen TV, cell phone, and PDA has taken us away from what really matters.

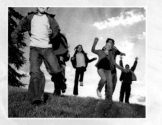

What is that?

Do you know what really matters to you? Sadly, many of us don't have any idea. We look to the Internet, the latest TV commercials, or our neighbor's driveway, as if someone else can answer the question for us.

And what answer do we come up with? For many, it's financial security, or the resources to be able to buy whatever they desire. But if you dig a little deeper and ask *why* they want those things, their answer is more fundamental. They believe that those things will make them feel better, happier, or more secure.

Well, I have an important message for you—first of all, money and material goods won't make you happy if you're unhappy to begin with. And second, in our lives there's no such thing as security.

So, why am I telling you all this? Because I want you to create optimal health for yourself and for the people who matter to you, and as a physician and life coach, I've found that if an individual is not on purpose in their lives, helping them create long-term health is an uphill battle. Conversely, aligning your mind with your heart's desire is a powerful force that can do much to support a lifetime of health.

The truth is, the modern world is a complicated, unsettled, and sometimes threatening place. Thanks to technology, we're more aware than ever of tragedies, political unrest, economic challenges, and climate change all around the globe. The vicissitudes of modern life affect us all—our friends, families, and neighbors may face challenges they want us to fix. If we're not in control of our intent, we can easily get caught in a vortex that feeds on stress and frustration—the vicious cycle of buying more things on credit, needing more vacations, working more hours in the hopes of a promotion. We search desperately for relief, hoping that the sleekest car, the most exotic vacation, or a new position will make us feel better somehow, reduce the stress, or bring more meaning to our existence.

But there's a way to get back in touch with what's really important—to regain a sense of direction and create the life you really want, whatever that may be. You've worked hard to learn new systems for healthy eating, movement, and sleep. Now I'm going to teach you a system to help build your life around what really matters to you.

Even if you're already happy on the whole, these techniques will teach you new ways to reduce stress and make your day-to-day life even more enjoyable. And if you feel you've lost touch with your guiding purpose, the lessons you learn will be just what the doctor ordered. Let's go!

If You Could Live Your Life Over. . .

In the end, what really matters? That's what Richard Leider, author of *The Power of Purpose,* wanted to know. He spent over twenty years interviewing people in the final years of their lives, asking them:

If you could live your life over again, what would you change?

Three universal truths emerged:

- **They would have paid more attention to the big picture.** They spent so much time being busy that life just seemed to pass them by.
- **They would have taken more risks.** They wish they'd found work that was more meaningful to them, and the courage to be better friends, parents, sons, and daughters.

Security is mostly a superstition. It does not exist in nature . . . . Avoiding danger is no safer in the long run than outright exposure. Life is either a daring adventure, or nothing.

—HELEN KELLER

As a physician and life coach, I've found that if someone is lacking a true sense of purpose in their life, creating health is an uphill battle.

In order to create and maintain optimal health, you need to organize your life around what matters most to you.

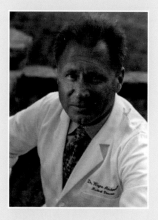

Aligning our life with our sense of purpose should be our top priority, not something that gets swept aside while we put all our energy into the mundane, day-to-day details of life.

• **They would have left a legacy.** They wish they had made more of a difference.

Waiting until the sunset years of life to make these discoveries is just about the most tragic realization I can imagine. Connecting what really matters to the fabric of everyday life should be one of our highest priorities!

The fact is, if you're living for your vacations, you're not going to enjoy a long, optimally healthy life. In fact, finding out what really matters *and acting on it* can make all the difference in the world.

It has for me.

My Own Journey to a Life of Purpose

When I was very young, I lived with my mother and grandparents in a crowded apartment in an asphalt jungle of a city. My father was in the military, assigned overseas, my mother worked for an airline, and my grandfather worked as a beat cop.

One weekend, as a special treat, my grandmother drove me down to Annapolis, Maryland, to see the Naval Academy. I loved to read books about boats and the sea, but to that point my experience with water had been limited to playing in a gushing fire hydrant on a hot summer day.

I fell in love with Annapolis, a historic town surrounded by water and full of boats of all kinds. All the way home, I told my grandmother that someday I would be a ship's captain and live on the water in that wonderful place. I was five years old at the time, and no one in my modest family had even been to college, yet my grandmother helped me set up a piggy bank and I started saving my pennies.

Years passed. As a military brat, I traveled all over the world, including to faraway places like Spain and Japan. And eventually I went to college, medical school, and on to my medical residency.

Upon finishing my fellowship in the newly emerging specialty of critical care—from the nation's top program—I began my practice in the landlocked state of Ohio. I became director of critical care, and soon found the love of my life, my wife, Lori. We were married and built a beautiful house on a creek, which, just to give me my water fix, included a 500-gallon salt-water aquarium. A few years later, we were blessed with our first daughter, Savannah, and three years later Erica came into our lives.

And they lived happily ever after. . .

That should be the end of story, but it's actually only the beginning. For the first fifteen years, I was fully immersed in taking care of my patients, working 100 hours a week, and loving life. But somewhere along the way, stress started creeping in. Jumping out of bed in the morning, eager to start the day, gave way to hassles with HMOs, belligerent doctors, and overworked, stressed-out nurses. I started gaining weight, my sleep deteriorated, and I just wasn't having fun. And to top it off, I was growing more and more frustrated with the little I could do to help people recover from lifestyle-induced diseases, with the knowledge that so many patients were just getting sicker. I wasn't dealing well with stress, and was starting to resent having to spend time away from my family.

So I left my practice behind! Lori and I gave it all up, gathered a few belongings, sold everything else, and with our one- and three-year-old daughters in tow—and amid heavy protests from our friends, family, and colleagues—we moved across the country.

Our goal was to redirect our efforts to help people create health, and in the process to rediscover our own health. In the beginning, we made no money and were forced to live on credit cards in a small rented house, with no one to rely on but ourselves. But then a curious thing happened. Despite the fact that we'd left the trappings of success in our rearview mirror, I started having fun again. My stress level went down considerably, and I began to thoroughly enjoy this simpler, less material life that left me with time to go for rides with my wife and my girls. I even shed those extra pounds and started exercising.

Seven years later, I have an incredible, thriving life. We're financially sound, and I have time to attend every one of my children's parent-teacher conferences, even in the middle of the day (of course, I'm usually the only father there).

One last thing: I now live on the water, with a boat at the end of my dock, less than a half mile from where this story began fifty years earlier—Annapolis, Maryland.

The Quest for Fulfillment

If having the things that modern life provides doesn't complete us, what does? The one ingredient that seems to be missing for most of us is *fulfillment*—a dimension that's critical to our happiness and our health.

Psychiatrist and author Viktor E. Frankl, who wrote his seminal *Man's Search for Meaning* based on observations he made while being held in World War II concentration camps, discusses fulfillment as a separate yet essential component of our lives—one that's determined by internal rather than external measures. Does your life have purpose? Is it going in the right direction? Do you feel complete?

Success is great, and no doubt financial freedom beats being destitute, but the bottom line is that your status and your material things do not define you. As Nietzsche put it, "He who has a *why* to live can bear almost any *how.*"

Now that's not to say that our modern lives, as complicated and unsettling as they may seem, are anything like the horrific experiences that Frankl and his fellow prisoners suffered. But if we can discover what really matters to us and find a way to bring our needs for both *success* and *fulfillment* into alignment, we can elevate ourselves to lives full of order and purpose. And, as an immediate benefit, when our minds and hearts are in alignment this way, our stress begins to vanish. The hassles of everyday life become more tolerable, and that in itself has a direct, positive influence on your immune system and your health. And it starts by looking at the level of fulfillment and sense of purpose in your life as it stands today.

Fulfillment and Success Continuums: Where Are You Right Now?

Are you happy? Are you doing what you really want? Take a look at the illustration on the next page. Where would you say you are on the continuum between depressed and fulfilled?

> Organizing our life around the pursuit of what's most important to us appears to convey a type of immunity, an enhanced tolerance of whatever life dishes out.

Fulfillment-Depression Continuum. Figuring out where you are on this continuum—happy and fulfilled, purposeless and depressed, or (like most of us) somewhere in between—is the first step in creating a life of purpose.

Success-Failure Continuum. How successful would you say you are right now in terms of external, more material factors such as finances, your job, and your standing in the community? Remember, there's nothing wrong with wanting these things as long as you don't pursue them at the expense of your happiness.

At the end of life, when asked what they'd do differently, no one wishes for a bigger house or a better car. It's the things that make us feel fulfilled that matter in the long run.

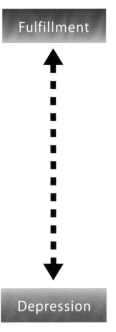

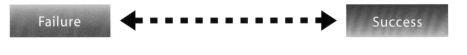

Let's look at the other axis—the success-failure continuum illustrated below. Success is defined primarily by external factors, like financial status, your place in the community, and your job. Are you comfortable with your current house, car, and professional position? What level of achievement would you say you enjoy now, compared to where you'd like to be? After all, having money is better than not having money, as long as it's not at the expense of your happiness.

Now let's put these two parameters together to see how the *internal* (fulfillment-depression) and *external* (success-failure) determinants balance out (see Well-Being Chart, page 269). Looking at your current reality in two dimensions allows you to see if what you're doing with your life is in alignment with what matters most to you.

Which quadrant would you say you're in right now?

Comparing your success track to your degree of fulfillment can be an enlightening exercise. Think back to the elderly subjects in Leider's interviews. When asked what they'd do differently, they all responded with wishes from the fulfillment-depression axis—less focus on the daily grind, more meaningful work and relationships, making a difference. Not one of those people said they wish they'd had a better car, a bigger house, or more money.

What it comes down to is balance in creating a comfortable life arranged around the things that matter most to you—whatever it is that puts you in that upper-right quadrant that signifies abundance.

Once you do, you'll find that when your life is guided by what really matters, the very way you respond to daily life changes. The inconveniences, the complications, the changes, the difficult relationships—when you're immersed in creating the things that are important to you, it suddenly all seems so much more tolerable. Whether you're working toward a new occupation, hobby, or relationship, having a purpose frees your mind from sweating the small stuff. You're too busy going after what really matters!

And even if over time things change, if what you thought mattered most turns out to be something else entirely, what's important is having the flexibil-

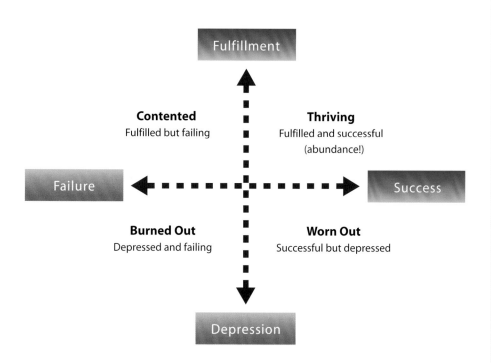

Contented
Fulfilled but failing

Thriving
Fulfilled and successful
(abundance!)

Failure

Success

Burned Out
Depressed and failing

Worn Out
Successful but depressed

Fulfillment

Depression

Well-Being Chart.
Which quadrant are you in now? By putting both axes together, we can get a more objective picture of our current state of well-being and see more clearly whether the way we're living now is aligned with what matters to us most.

A Habit of Health:
Having the flexibility to recognize when change needs to happen and to adjust accordingly

ity to recognize these changes and adjust accordingly. In fact, it's a fundamental Habit of Health. Without that flexibility, stress will return, and in time you'll be back on your old path to non-sickness and disease. That's why being able to identify and reassess your position on the well-being chart is so important. It was for me!

Fresh from my fellowship in critical care, I felt ready to take on the world. In my quest to become the best physician I could be, I threw myself into my work, even staying up all night in the operating room or the intensive care unit. I was single, and driven by the satisfaction my work gave me, so that even at the bedside of a patient whose life hung in the balance, I felt little stress. In fact, the toughest cases only fueled my passion. My finances, my position as chief of the department, and my level of fulfillment all contributed to great health (with a little fatigue at times, perhaps), and my life was *thriving*.

Fast-forward fifteen years. Stressed, with no time to see my family, and experiencing a change in philosophy stemming from my growing desire to help others create health rather than merely react to disease, I had sunk into the "worn out" quadrant of the well-being chart. My physical and mental health were putting me on the path to the very diseases I was treating.

Fortunately, I did something about it. Leaving my practice, taking those risks, seemed scary at the time, but I knew I had to align myself with what was important. And I also knew that what was important wasn't the big house or the respected position—it was my family, and my desire to help create health. Changing my life immediately put me way back up on the fulfillment scale—although on the success continuum I underwent a temporary backslide as Lori and I struggled financially looking for the right vehicle to fuel our passion.

Today, I'm smack dab in the middle of the abundancy quadrant and once again thriving. And you can be, too!

. . . .

**My Well-Being Chart
from 1986 to 2008.**
In my own journey, I've
gone from being successful
and fulfilled, to depressed,
to happy but broke, to
where I am now—thriving!

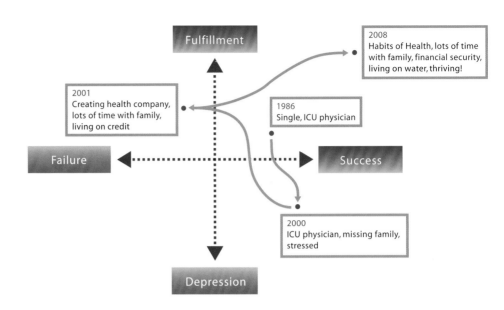

Creating Well-Being: Your First Steps

First, mark where you believe you are on the well-being chart below.

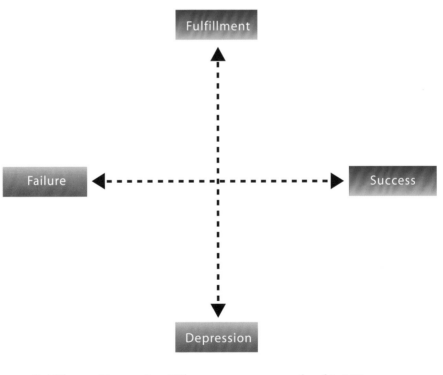

Fulfillment-Depression: Where are you on a scale of 1–10? _____

Success-Failure: Where are you on a scale of 1–10? _____

Now spend some time in a quiet place to think about what really matters to you in terms of your fulfillment and success, and compare that to where you are right now.

Not sure you want to go there? I realize this process is difficult, and may make you uncomfortable. You may be thinking, what if I find out that what

I want is completely different from what I'm doing now? Scary thoughts? You bet.

But finding out the truth is your first step in understanding what you need to do to move forward on your path to optimal health and a thriving life. It's certainly just as important as the glycemic index, the NEAT System, or any of the other components that support your fundamental choice. Remember, that fundamental choice is yours. No one else—not me, not your best friend, and definitely not the star of the latest reality TV show—can decide what makes you happy.

To help you think about organizing your life around your most important desires, let's take another look at the teachings of my dear friend, colleague, and mentor, Robert Fritz. Remember his concept of structural tension, which we discussed in chapters 3 and 4? We used that idea to create a structural tension chart for your health goals, and then to make specific plans and choices based on those goals. You can use this same idea to create a structural tension chart in all the key areas of your life—your relationships, your job, and whatever else it is that makes up success and fulfillment for you. What do you want your life to look like?

Write down your goals, your deepest desires and aspirations, and create a timeline for their achievement. Take another look at the guidelines we used back in chapter 4 (or see the companion workbook for more detail on desires and aspirations), and consider these ideas as well:

- Think about what you want to create, rather than what you want to eliminate.
- Think about what you want to create, rather than what it says about you.
- Simplify in order to get at what really matters.
- Don't be limited by rules or worry how you're going to do it. Explore all the possibilities!

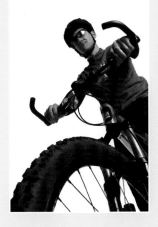

Structural Tension Chart.
A structural tension chart helps you organize your most important goals and create a timeline for achieving those goals. For more information, see chapter 4.

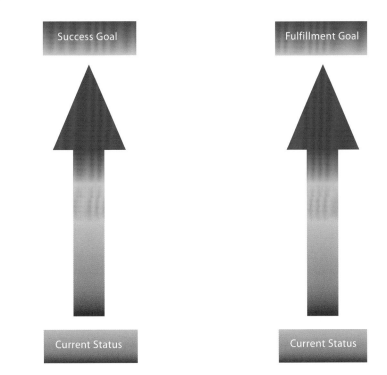

And since most of us have to work, here's a final guideline: *Do what you love or love what you do.* It really is that simple.

This may require you to quit your job, go to school, enter a new line of work, or invent what it is you want to do, or it may simply mean finding new ways to bring meaning to what you're doing right now. But whatever you do, it should bring you passion, spur your interest, and tap into your talents. Remember, this is not a dress rehearsal! Get out and live to the fullest every day, and your body will respond with glee.

I leave you with a quote from author James A. Michener, who wrote so powerfully and movingly of far-off lands like Tahiti and Hawaii:

> *The master in the art of living makes little distinction between his work and his play, his labor and his leisure, his mind and his body, his information and his recreation, his love and his religion. He hardly knows which is which. He simply pursues his vision of excellence at whatever he does, leaving others to decide whether he is working or playing. To him he's always doing both!*

Living a fulfilling life not only satisfies us emotionally, it also has the power to make us more physically vibrant. In fact, without fulfillment, we can't achieve optimal health.

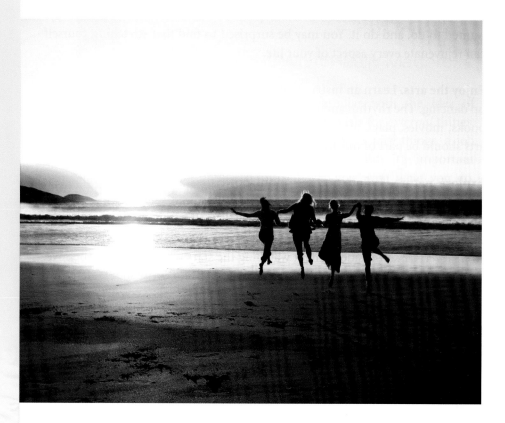

Part Three

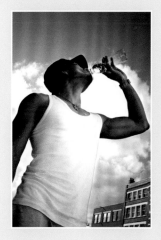

The Path to Longevity

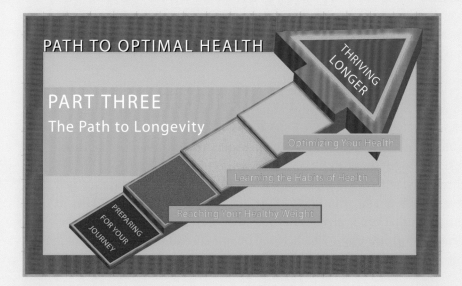

In Part Two, Your Journey to Optimal Health, you undertook a series of phases that taught you the knowledge, skills, and techniques you need to take control of your life and develop behaviors for lasting health. These Habits of Health—designed to be digested in bite-sized pieces at your own pace—are the structure that supports this new world.

Each phase on your journey has followed the next in a logical fashion, based on one unifying principle: using energy management—the relationship between the energy you consume and the energy you use—as a catalyst for health.

Now comes the final piece in the optimal health puzzle: staying as healthy as you can for as long as you can. In Part Three, we'll fine-tune your progress and boost your mileage so you can enjoy lasting optimal health on this new adventure of life.

Phase IV
Thriving Longer
The Principles, Practice, and Future of Longevity

Do thoughts of living a long life conjure up images of lonely nursing home patients slumped in their chairs, or a confused relative who calls you by the name of the cat she had twenty years ago? Or maybe thinking about old age makes you mutter to yourself, "I can't drive at night; I have pain in my knee, hip and back; and the last time I even thought about sex was when Bill Clinton was in the White House!"

But those scenarios describe living in a state of less-than-optimal health—in other words, just surviving—and that's decidedly *not* what we're talking about! Rather, what I want to know is this: if you could live longer in a thriving state while maintaining your optimal health, would you make that choice? My take on longevity is that it only makes sense when you have both long life *and* thriving health. And in fact, the best way to do that is to keep doing the things I've already taught you. Practice the Habits of Health forever! They're your guarantee that you're giving your body the best possible chance to live out your genetic programming—which, based on our current understanding of the aging process, means you could live 100 years or more.

The Three Eras of Medicine

Modern medicine has been a bit slow to enter what some call the third era—the revolution of health. But it's done a great job during the first two eras at eliminating most of the diseases that prevented us from living to 100.

The first era, from the beginning of medicine to the middle of the twentieth century, focused on battling infectious disease and improving infant mortality through the advent of vaccines and antibiotics, better sanitation, and emphasis on hygiene. Once deadly killers such as cholera, typhoid, and polio were eliminated, around the 1950s, we entered the second era of medicine. This era involved wrestling with chronic diseases, especially heart disease, and as a result people are now living longer than ever.

Today, although medicine remains focused on degenerative diseases such as diabetes and cancer, the time has arrived to shift our emphasis to the third era. This groundbreaking movement involves more than just keeping blood pressure, cholesterol, and body mass index out of the disease danger zone. It requires a synergistic partnership between patients and health care professionals to optimize health. The good news is that more physicians and other medical personnel than ever before are joining this revolution, helping to move our medical model forward from one of reaction and repair to a new school of thought focused on creating health. So if you're looking for a partner

Some of us in the medical profession are shifting our emphasis to what's called the *third era of medicine*—a new model that's focused on creating health, not just reacting to disease.

in optimal health and longevity, these third era physicians are the ones you should seek.

Now that medicine has removed the x-factor for longevity by eliminating so many of the diseases that could kill you, you have the advantage. And with the habits you learn in this book, you're well equipped to thrive in medicine's third era!

Our Longevity Plan

To set the stage for your healthy life extension plan, let's revisit our trusty companion, the energy management diagram. You can see that in Phase IV, the longevity phase, your balance of energy in and energy out stays coupled, as it has since we established equilibrium at the end of Phase II. This coupling helps you control your health and is fundamental to extending your new healthy life.

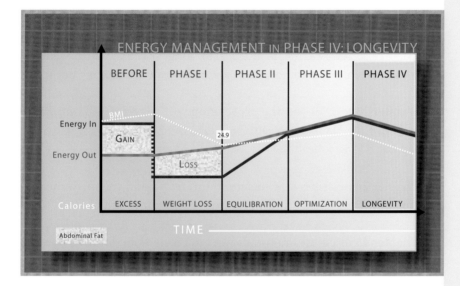

Energy Management in Phase IV: Longevity. Your plan for healthy longevity in Phase IV includes a decrease in calorie intake (red line), with a resulting decrease in body fat (dotted white line).

And what's the overriding principle of that longevity? It's simple—eat less! It's all about reducing your calorie intake and eating healthier food. Sound familiar? It should, because you're already doing it as part of the Habits of Health. We're just going to tweak your energy plan a bit to put you on our thriving life extension plan.

Here's how it works: now that you've reached your optimal health and have reduced your body fat and increased your lean muscle, your body will follow your lead and slow down its rate of cellular aging if you simply reduce your calories by a small amount. This principle—the foundation of almost all current longevity work—is called *calorie restriction (CR)*. A more apt term would be dietary restriction, because what we're really talking about is restricting our intake of high-glycemic carbohydrates and saturated animal fat, along with total calories. Now to some people, that may sound punitive, but that's because the vast majority of those individuals are still in the *before* stage. The chasm between the way they eat now and the way research tells us you need to eat for longevity is huge.

Longevity practices
such as calorie
restriction—modifying
your diet by reducing
the amount of high-
glycemic carbohydrates
and saturated fats,
along with calories—
require only a small
adjustment for those
of us who've already
adopted the Habits
of Health.

For you, though, it's just the next phase of our plan—and when you're ready for it, you'll find that living longer is something you really can do. Now that the Habits of Health are part of your daily life, the adjustments you need to make in order to live longer and healthier are well within your reach. In fact, the very principles and practice of longevity are embedded in the Habits of Health. It's the only scientifically validated, safe method of life extension, and it's on the very cutting edge of the practice of longevity.

But I'm getting ahead of myself. What's important to know right off the bat is that our longevity plan simply takes the daily choices you're making right now for optimal health and refines them a bit. Like the changes you've already made, these are doable, easy baby steps that you can learn and use for the rest of your life—and hopefully that's a good long time to come!

In the next five chapters, we'll explore the principles, practice, and future of longevity, including where science might take us next. But we'll keep our discussion grounded in simple actions you can apply right now as you take control of your future by applying the Habits of Health.

Chapter 22 reviews the principles of longevity, including what the most current scientific research tells us about how we can prolong our lives.

Chapter 23 teaches you the expectations of longevity and outlines our plan to utilize the Habits of Health to create the Habits of Longevity, in order to support a longer, healthier life as a result of optimal health.

Chapter 24 describes how dietary optimization and enhanced movement can create ultimate energy control for extending your health.

Chapter 25 discusses important ways to create brain longevity, an important factor in protecting and enhancing your future.

Chapter 26 describes what it is like to be Ultrahealthy and looks into the future of the science of longevity.

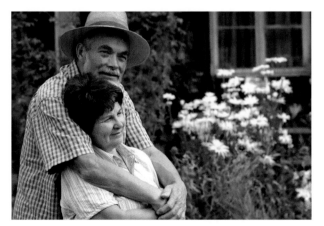

Chapter 22

The Principles of Longevity

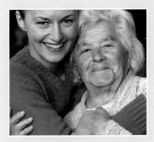

THE FIRST PRINCIPLE OF LONGEVITY

Healthy Weight
Active Individual **>** Overweight
Sedentary Individual

At a recent speech I gave to the International Anti-Aging Society, this was my first slide—and it really says it all. Just take a look at all the healthy people in the world who've reached 100 years of age. Not one of them is obese.

Why? Aging is a cellular process that happens in every one of us, and how long we live is directly related to how well we take care of ourselves and our cells. The good news is that aging is reversible. (Yes, you *can* have a mulligan!) The changes you make starting now can have an effect on your life expectancy in as little as *three months*. And if you start the Habits of Health today, in just three years you'll enjoy the same health you would have if you'd been practicing them your whole life.

So if that's the case, and if you begin your longevity practices right now, just how long can you expect to live?

The Secret of Life Extension

Early science perpetuated a fallacy that our life span is predetermined—that we have some kind of internal clock, and when it strikes midnight, we die.

Now, genetics clearly are important, and do have some influence on how long you're going to live. But studies of identical twins raised in different environments and exposed to different lifestyles have demonstrated that genetics determines only about 20 to 30 percent of your health and longevity. Your own lifestyle and daily behaviors make up the other 70 to 80 percent. So lifestyle really is the dominant factor!

Look at it this way: If you buy a Porsche (the genetic purebred) but don't change the oil or have it serviced properly, it may well be outlasted by a plain old Ford Escort that's been impeccably maintained. You see, it's all about the rate at which our cells age. To continue our automotive metaphor, a car left outside in the toxic acid rain in Cleveland oxidizes quickly, losing its new car

The oldest documented person in recent history is Jeanne Louise Calment, who lived her whole life in Arles, France, and died in 1997 at age 122—just about the maximum human life span. Of course, records are meant to
be broken!

look. Your body can rust out from the same oxidative stress that turns that car into an unrecognizable hunk of orange rust.

So What's My Expiration Date?

Let's start by looking at averages. According to insurance actuarial tables, today's average life expectancy for women is around eighty, and for men around seventy-five.

Of course, that's just the average, meaning that half the population makes it to that age. But by applying the Habits of Health you've already learned, along with the ones I'll be teaching you in these next few chapters, you have the capability to extend your life as much as 35 percent beyond those numbers.

You see, most of us are born in optimal health. It's our modern environment that moves us down the path to non-sickness, beginning as early as our twenties. Why, today we're seeing children as young as ten already suffering the effects of high-fat, high-glycemic diets and inactivity. And as a result, by the time we reach our thirties, our rate of aging accelerates, and actually begins to *double* about every eight years—if we don't take control of our daily choices, that is. Soon enough, we're in poorer health, which leads to disease, which leads to death in our mid- to late seventies. We just rust out!

And of course that's exactly what the actuarial tables predict. Our population is overweight, inactive, living on a diet of processed food—and suffering the degeneration that comes with that lifestyle. We're living at pace with the biological aging of our cells. In other words, our chronological age—how long we've been alive—matches our biological age.

But here's the trick. It doesn't have to be that way. You can actually disconnect your biological aging from your chronological age and live longer, simply by making the decision today to change your path. By adopting the strategies and choices of the Habits of Health, you can achieve better health almost immediately, slow the aging process, and thrive for many more years to come.

In a few years, we'll know if what we're doing today has successfully produced a whole generation of healthy 100-year-olds. My educated guess is that it will. And here's the science to support it.

Longevity Research: The Cutting Edge of Medicine

Why do we age?

To understand that, we first need to look at why we're alive in the first place. And it turns out that it's really not about us—not as individuals, anyhow. It's about us as a species. The celestial committee on design decided to make our ability to pass along genetic material their main concern. So basically, once we reproduce and age out of our reproductive years, we're on our own. That being the case, it becomes important for each of us to understand how to keep the machinery going for ourselves, as individuals.

And for that we need to look deep into our cells, at tiny structures called *telomeres* and *mitochondria*.

Telomeres: The Key to Aging?

Your chromosomes—organized structures inside your cells that contain your genetic information—are like blueprints that tell your body what you look like and determine how your cells function. Every time our cells reproduce, these chromosomes must duplicate themselves.

On the end of each chromosome is a piece called a telomere, which protects the genetic information that's inside, much like a piece of tape placed on the end of a rope stops it from fraying. Each time a cell divides, the telomeres get slightly shorter, until eventually the cell can no longer duplicate. This mechanism is now thought to be the basis of why we age. When we smoke, experience lots of stress, or practice other unhealthy behaviors, our telomeres begin to shorten and stop dividing, and as a result our rate of cellular aging increases. This process is called *senescence*—the aging of a cell to the point where it can no longer replicate itself.

The good news is some of our cells contain an enzyme called *telomerase,* which has the ability to repair these shortened telomeres and keep our chromosomes—and us—healthy. Unfortunately, although most of our cells have the programming for telomerase, many don't actually use it. That's why scientists are currently looking for ways to activate this enzyme and harness its powerful anti-aging capacity. In fact, telomeres represent one of the most exciting areas in longevity and anti-cancer research today.

There's still much to be determined, but what we do know right now is that if you eliminate emotional and oxidative stress and create a rich environment of antioxidant protection, your cells won't need to divide as frequently and will be better able to repair themselves.

Mitochondria: Keep 'Em Happy with Habits of Health

These little powerhouses of our cells are responsible for turning your food into energy so your body can function. But one of the byproducts of this process are oxidative free radicals—dangerous oxidizing agents that spill into the cells and bloodstream, creating inflammation and cellular damage. The DNA in mitochondria can become damaged as well, decreasing their efficiency and accelerating the aging process. These damaged mitochondria—often found in cells that make up the building blocks of our heart, brain, pancreas, and other organs—may even be an accessory to the production of cancer-forming cells.

As we age, our mitochondria become swollen, less efficient, and more likely to contribute to inflammation and disease—in short, the beginning of the end. Luckily, we can do much to improve the efficiency of our mitochondria through exercise and nutrients like CoQ_{10}. And we can slow down the damage by choosing healthy, antioxidant foods that decrease the production of free radicals.

I hope you're starting to see that the core components of living longer are already built into the Habits of Health that you're using right now—not surprising that what gets you healthy keeps you healthy!

An environment that's low in stress and rich in antioxidants will keep your cells healthy and prevent them from dividing as frequently—the key to delaying the aging process.

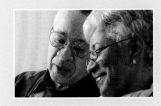

Habits of Health like eating right, exercising, and supplementing your diet with antioxidants help keep your cells healthy. Healthy cells age more slowly and are more resistant to aging—and that means we are, too!

While the term *calorie restriction (CR)* was used early on to describe the field of inquiry into longevity, numerous studies over the past two decades have demonstrated that particular nutrients and methods of restriction are just as important as, and may be more informative than, restricting the total number of calories.

Calorie Restriction (CR): Our Best Bet for a Longer Life?

In the 1930s, researchers restricted the calorie intake of lab rats by about one-third and found that the animals' life spans increased nearly 50 percent. These amazing results—the only proven means of extending life—set in motion a flurry of research. The experiment was repeated on worms, fruit flies, other rodents, even Labrador retrievers, all with similar success. We don't yet know for sure that humans enjoy the same benefits, though studies are encouraging: our life spans are just too long for the data to be complete. But as of now, the science of *calorie restriction* remains the most robust method known for slowing down the aging process.

Actually, calories are only part of the story. A better description would be

---

Mechanisms of Longevity: Recent Research

Hormesis. Hormesis is a biological response in which exposure to a small amount of toxin or other stressor actually creates a positive effect, causing cells to rally in defense. In 2007, Dr. Michael Ristow demonstrated how this works to slow down cellular aging by restricting glucose metabolism in a type of worms, extending their life spans. By slightly increasing oxidative stress initially, the worms ultimately increased their resistance to oxidative stress.*

Insulin signaling. Studies show that if we can turn off the insulin pump and keep insulin levels low, we can increase longevity. The best way to do that? According to research, through exercise, a healthy diet, and keeping lean.

Sir1/Sir2 (sirtuin longevity gene). This longevity gene, discovered in baker's yeast cells, has been shown to extend life span by suppressing DNA instability, and may well underlie the positive effects of calorie restriction. Activated by calorie restriction, the Sir2 enzyme led to a 30 percent life-span extension in yeast. In mammals, the parallel gene is turned on by a calorie-restricted diet, which protects cells from dying under stress.

One exciting development to stem from this research is that resveratrol, a potent antioxidant, can turn this gene on, thus extending the life span of yeast, nematode worms, fruit flies, and mice. Resveratrol has even been shown to extend the life span of vertebrate fish by 59 percent. And where does resveratrol come from? It's found in great concentration in red wine, and likely plays a central role in the French paradox—a phenomenon whereby the French, despite a diet high in saturated fat, enjoy low rates of coronary heart disease.

IGF-I (insulin-like growth factor). Evidence has connected reduced exposure to IGF-I with extended life span in rodents. In humans, elevated IGF-I levels have been linked to a number of age-related diseases that limit longevity, such as cancer. But reduced IGF-I activity has been linked to an increased risk of other diseases, including diabetes and cardiovascular

*Schultz, T., et al., "Glucose Restriction Extends Caenorhabditis elegans Life Span by Inducing Mitochondrial Respiration and Increasing Oxidative Stress," *Cell Metabolism* 6 (4): 280–93.

dietary restriction, because it's really about the type of nutrients we consume, as well as the amount, and how we restrict them.

So how does it all work? In the natural world, the availability of food fluctuates over time. During periods of severe drought or other instances when food is scarce, it's critical for an organism—maybe even for us—to stop reproducing and conserve energy for maintenance and survival. And studies show that this sort of reduction in energy intake triggers cellular activities that actually seem to slow down cellular aging.

There are a number of theories as to the mechanisms at work in this process. You'll find in-depth explanations of these in the box Mechanisms of Longevity: Recent Research. There's a fair amount of scientific information to get through, but I do think it will help you understand just why the Habits of Health are such as effective strategy for life extension!

disease. It's complex, and probably dependent on other factors we've yet to uncover, but clearly IGF-I does play a role in modulating diseases of aging. One attractive hypothesis is that longevity could be maximized by regulating IGF-I levels carefully at various stages of life—perhaps through lower levels during early adulthood and higher levels as we grow older.

Decreased levels of circulating triiodothyronine (T3) and the sympathetic nervous system. Turning down thyroid production turns down our metabolic machinery, reducing the work load for our cells. A resulting decrease in core temperature and BMR decreases mitochondrial production of oxygen radicals. Turning down the sympathetic nervous system decreases stress chemistry as well.

Decreased levels of inflammatory molecules. Calorie restriction can reduce systemic (body-wide) inflammation, protecting us from the deterioration of the immune system that comes with aging.

Decrease degradation of DNA. Calorie restriction may enhance DNA repair, increase the removal of damaged DNA, and lessen the degradation of telomeres.

Free radical and glycation. When lots of energy is available, mitochondria don't operate as efficiently. That means greater production of dangerous oxygen radicals. With calorie restriction, energy is conserved and fewer free radicals are created. And because an organism practicing calorie restriction is leaner, less energy is needed to support its weight, which means less glucose in the bloodstream. Less glucose means there's less sugar to bind with fats and proteins, and that means there's less risk of atherosclerosis. It's also important to decrease beta-amyloid, which interferes with brain function.

Calorie restriction with optimal nutrition. By this I mean lowering your total number of calories not just by eating less food, but by eating nutritionally dense foods so that there's a higher ratio of nutrients to calories—a process that may lead to more ideal and beneficial nutrient levels in the body. Among the benefits: many of these nutrients serve as protective antioxidants, and there are likely to be more antioxidants in the body, since lower food intake means lower levels of free radicals.

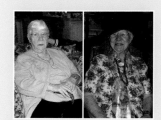

"My family tells me I'm their hero!"

EILEEN MILLER
Enjoying optimal health at almost 90!

I was literally at death's door, having gone through cancer surgery, three strokes, diabetes, and heart failure—but I wasn't ready to give up. My youngest grandson and his wife were going to have twins, and I wanted to be there to give them hugs and kisses. At 237 pounds, I knew I needed to lose some weight. My family had made tremendous changes in their health by adopting Dr. A's Habits of Health and using Take Shape for Life™, so I decided to try it out, too. In just over two years, I've lost 67 pounds, and what's more, I feel terrific for my age. I do volunteer work, socialize with family and friends, and due to the weight loss, my doctor reduced my medications for high blood pressure & type 2 diabetes. My family tells me I'm their hero! ∎

Results vary. Typical weight loss is 2–5 lbs per week for the first 2 weeks and 1–2 lbs per week thereafter.

In this landmark study, subjects who ate a calorie-restricted diet had lower blood pressure, fewer inflammatory markers, and healthier hearts than their counterparts who ate a typical Western diet.

Can Calorie Restriction Really Help Us Live Longer?

I know I got you all excited by telling you we can make your fruit flies live longer—but you're probably wondering, what about us? The answer, based on two major studies, is. . .

Maybe!

Let's look in greater depth at these two important studies and see what conclusions we can draw.

Study 1

Calorie restriction with optimal nutrition may delay primary aging in humans. *

This report provided details of a landmark 2004 research study—the first to show that long-term calorie restriction with optimal nutrition may delay primary aging in humans. The study followed two groups, one that ate a normal Western diet, and one that ate a calorie-restricted but nutrient-dense diet (in other words, a dietary-restricted diet with less saturated fat and more low-glycemic carbohydrates).

Group one: calorie-restricted group
- Calories: approximately 1,671 kcal/day, including 100% recommended daily intake of all nutrients
- Breakdown of diet:
     23% protein
     48% carbohydrate
     28% fat (6% saturated)
- Exercise: twenty minutes, three times a week

Group two: Western diet group
- Calories: approximately 2,445 kcal/day
- Breakdown of diet:
     17% protein
     52% carbohydrate
     31% fat (11% saturated)
- Exercise: none specified

Results: The average body mass index was 19.7 in the calorie-restricted group, as opposed to 27 in the Western diet group. In addition, blood pressure was lower (102/61 vs. 131/83); inflammatory markers based on hs-CRP tests were lower (0.3 mg/dl vs. 1.9 mg/dl); and the calorie-restricted group showed significant improvement in left ventricle relaxation compared to the Western diet group. They simply had younger, more pliable hearts!

My interpretation: Although this trial was limited to a small number of participants, the take-home message is clear—_eating a nutrient-dense diet that's lower in calories, lower in saturated fat, and lower glycemic can decrease blood pressure, improve the performance of the heart, and decrease the level of inflammatory molecules that can cause aging._

*Meyer, T., _Journal of the American College of Cardiology_ 47 (Jan 17, 2006): 398–402; reporting on Fontana, L., et al., "Long-Term Calorie Restriction Is Highly Effective in Reducing the Risk for Artherosclerosis in Humans," _Proceedings of the National Academy of Sciences_ 101 (April 27, 2004): 6659–6653.

And here's something interesting. Note that the subjects in the calorie-restricted group did about the same amount of exercise as we do on our EAT program, ate a very similar ratio of macronutrients as in our healthy eating plan, and reached our goal of getting their hs-CRP below 0.5!

Now, I do realize that the level of calorie restriction and body mass index in this study is lower than what most people are realistically willing to tolerate. But based on my experiences talking with two people in the study, who are also pioneer members of the Calorie Restriction Society, I can report that by balancing healthy nutrition with calorie restriction you can have a thriving lifestyle. In fact, they believe in their way of life so strongly, they've written a book about it.*

Fortunately for those of us who find this degree of calorie restriction challenging, there are other options for creating optimal balance for longevity, as the next study shows.

Study 2

Calorie restriction for six months with and without exercise results in improvement in several markers of longevity.*

In this study, 48 healthy men and women were assigned to one of four groups to study the effects of calorie restriction with or without exercise. The groups were broken down as follows:

- Group 1: control group (weight-maintenance diet)
- Group 2: calorie restriction (25% fewer calories based on baseline energy requirements)
- Group 3: calorie restriction with exercise (12.5% fewer calories plus 12.5% increase in energy expenditure through five-days-per-week sessions, resulting in an average of 569 calories burned per session for men and 403 for women)
- Group 4: low-calorie diet (890 kcal/day until weight was reduced by 15%, followed by weight maintenance)

Results: For six months, researchers tracked these groups' body composition, glucose levels, insulin levels, DNA damage, 24-hour total energy expenditure (TEE), and core body temperature. Here's what they found.

	TEE decrease	Weight loss	Fasting insulin	DNA damage	Core temperature
Control group	0 kcal	-1%	unchanged	unchanged	unchanged
CR 25%	↓ 135 kcal	-10.4%	decreased	decreased	decreased
CR plus exercise	↓ 117 kcal	-10%	decreased	decreased	decreased
Low-calorie diet	↓ 125 kcal	-13.9%	decreased	decreased	unchanged

Even a moderate reduction in calories, when combined with exercise, has a positive effect on markers for longevity such as cellular protection, according to this study in the *Journal of the American Medical Association*.

*Meredith Averill and Paul McGlothin, *The CR Way: Using the Secrets of Calorie Restriction for a Longer, Healthier Life,* HarperCollins: 2008.
** Heilbronn, L. K., et al., *Journal of the American Medical Association* 295 (April 5, 2006): 1539–1548.

Why do some people
live to be 100 while
their friends and
relatives die out in
their seventies and
eighties? Scientists are
studying concentrated
populations of
centenarians around the
world to find out.

The study concluded that, at least in the short term, calorie restriction improves biomarkers of longevity.

My interpretation: The ability of moderate calorie restriction to improve cellular protection and decrease DNA damage is very encouraging, based on this short-term study. Combine that with a mild increase in energy expenditure, and you've got a doable plan for most of us who've followed the Habits of Health!

The Thriving Three-Figures

Studying people who are actually succeeding—people who've beaten the odds and are alive and thriving into their second century—is one of the most fascinating areas of longevity research.

You've probably seen or heard of some of them, perhaps on programs like *The Today Show*. They're special individuals who (through sheer orneriness, perhaps) refuse to let go of this precious thing called life. Somehow, despite the odds, these super-humans retain their mental and physical health. In fact, even at age 92, over 90 percent of them are still functionally independent.

Scientists are obsessed with finding out why the super-old—chronologically speaking, anyway—thrive long after most of their peers have succumbed to the ravages of degenerative diseases. To unlock these secrets, they're studying several groups who seem to drink daily from the fountain of youth.

Since 1976, through the Okinawa Centenarian Study, scientists from the U.S. National Institutes of Health and Japan's Ministry of Health have been studying people aged 100 and over on Okinawa, a Japanese island that nurtures more centenarians than any other place on the planet. They've discovered that, along with getting plenty of physical and mental exercise, these elders have diets that are low fat, low in salt, and high in fiber and antioxidant-rich fruits and vegetables—much like the Habits of Health. They also consume more soy than any other population on earth: between 60 and 129 grams a day, over double the amount consumed by the average Japanese.

And interestingly, they practice their own form of calorie restriction called *hara hachi bu* (eight parts full). In essence, they stop eating when they're 80 percent full, having consumed about 1,800 calories (for the average American, 80 percent would be more like 2,500 calories).

These centenarians exhibit tremendous mental clarity and a very low incidence of dementia, possibly due to a diet high in vitamin E, a protective antioxidant. But perhaps a more likely reason is that they enjoy a strong sense of meaning, purpose, and belonging. When interviewed, they clearly express a high level of fulfillment in their lives. However, researchers have found that if Okinawans leave their island permanently and adopt the diets and behaviors of the new country, within a generation their life span shortens and their heart attack and cancer rates increase dramatically.

Let's turn to Sardinia, another country that supports longevity. Here, too, healthy habits include powerful social networks, active lifestyles, close relationships with extended family and friends, and a strong sense of purpose.

> ### The Three Pathways to Longevity
>
> A study in the *Journals of Gerontology** revealed three separate pathways to breaking 100. Researchers looked at the top ten diseases that kill most of us by age 80 and discovered that among groups of centenarians:
>
> - *Survivors* developed disease before age 80 and yet kept going to age 100. (More women than men [43% vs. 24%] were in this group.)
> - *Delayers* didn't come down with a serious disease until they were over 80. (About 43% of both women and men were in this group.)
> - *Escapers* never developed any diseases at all! (This group had more men than women—32% vs. 15%.)
>
> *Evert, J., et al., "Morbidity Profiles of Centenarians: Survivors, Delayers, and Escapers," *The Journals of Gerontology Series A: Biological Sciences and Medical Sciences* 58 (2003): M232–M237.

And what about the U.S.? The University of Georgia Gerontology Center has found that American centenarians have strong coping skills that may be integral to their longevity. They exhibit dominant personalities—they want it their way! And they're not easily pushed around (just think of the movie *Driving Miss Daisy*). They question information and think issues through before they make decisions (remember our exercise, Stop-Challenge-Choose?). They're practical rather than idealistic, yet they're relaxed. Despite having strong personalities, they remain flexible once they understand the situation. These personality traits lend themselves to high levels of cognition and skill in problem solving and learning, and this in turn creates more blood flow to the brain and continued neural stimulation and growth.

And lastly, these U.S. centenarians enjoy a strong social support system. They're closely connected to their families or to their helpers and confidants, whom they continue to replace as they outlive others. They stay connected to the world through their relationships with younger people.

Of course, genetics does play a role that we can't control. Brothers of centenarians are 17 times and sisters 8.5 times more likely to live to be 100 than those without centenarians in their family of birth. And children of the superold—themselves in their seventies and early eighties—are 60 percent less likely to suffer from heart disease, stroke, or diabetes.

Additionally, scientists are beginning to discover sets of genes that might program for longevity and reduced susceptibility to disease. The Okinawans, for example, appear to have a variant of a gene that provides protection from autoimmune diseases, called the human leukocyte antigen. Other discoveries include genes that may extend life span by shielding the heart from disease.

But even if we do unravel the secret of aging in our genes, there's one thing that's absolutely certain—*if applied consistently, a lifestyle based on the Habits of Health can help extend your life.* And to support that belief, just look to the Seventh-Day Adventists, who, as part of their faith, eat healthy, exercise, and avoid alcohol, caffeine, and tobacco. Despite their diverse genetic background, they live on average eight years longer than their average countryman.

Dr. A Says . . .

The latest scientific research into pathways to longevity confirm what the Habits of Health have been saying all along— exercise, a healthy diet, low body fat, stress reduction, and proper nutritional support all contribute to a long and thriving life!

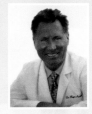

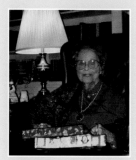

Dee Dee's 98th birthday

The Life of Dee Dee

I couldn't help falling in love with my wife's grandmother, Dee Dee, when I first met her over twenty years ago. She was in her late seventies but had a sparkle in her eye and a love for life. Active in her community, a member of her country club, constantly traveling—she looked like a woman in her fifties. She was always in a great mood, always interested in everything Lori and I were doing, and she had strong advice for us kids about how to have a great marriage (it's working!).

I talked with her recently and found that not much has changed. Sure, she has some arthritis that limits how far she can walk, but when I asked her to what she attributed her ninety-eight years of quality life, she gave me an earful. "Wayne," she said, "I'm dating a man younger than me, and I just had to tell him he wasn't right for me. I avoid confrontation at all costs because it messes up your whole system. But in this case it just wasn't working out, and I had to let him know!"

Dee Dee has a strong connection with her family, including me, and she believes that this deep love is a factor in her longevity. She says she makes it a point to eat well and to exercise her mind daily by reading the newspaper. She especially loves problem solving and makes it part of her daily routine. She knits to stay busy, doesn't like TV, and says she's always happy and relaxed.

Two months ago, on the eve of a special birthday party that the family had planned for her, Dee Dee had a small TIA (a temporary lack of blood supply to part of the brain). She had been up most of the night and wasn't doing well when Lori called to wish her a happy birthday. She told Lori about the incident but said she was fighting through it. When Lori recommended she stay home and rest, she refused, saying, "There is no way I am going to miss my birthday." She went, and she had a ball.

During our conversation, she shared that her pastor told her she's the next parishioner in line to be celebrated as an centenarian. She said she isn't going to disappoint him by missing that.

In the movie *The Shawshank Redemption*, the character played by Morgan Freeman says you either "get busy living or you get busy dying."

Dee Dee is getting busy living. You go, girl! ∎

The Best Possible Time to Be Alive

Why live longer? In short, because there's never been a more exciting time to be alive. We live in a time when you can see the Titanic sink in wide-screen high definition, complete with footage of the actual doomed ship. You can communicate with loved ones anywhere in the world at a moment's notice. You can run your business right from the beach, and have strawberries in the dead of winter. Travel has become safer, whether you're flying in the latest passenger jet or driving in your own car with side airbags, ABS brakes, and an intelligent traffic warning system. And medical technology has virtually eliminated most random killers. So really, there's no reason we can't do it all, at any age.

And there's so much going on! Ray Kurzweil, a science futurist who's made in-depth analyses of the history of technology, believes that our technological growth today is no less than exponential. During the twenty-first century, he says, we'll experience not 100 years of progress, but closer to 20,000. I know I don't want to miss it.

Now it's up to you to do your part—to take control of your health and your life, to harness technology and put it in its proper place as your servant, not your master. All these things are within your grasp and available to help you maximize your healthy time on this earth. And my longevity plan will show you how.

Chapter 23

The Habits of Longevity

Living Longer in Ultrahealth

We're now going to design a plan to help you live longer in optimal health, based on current scientific research, observation, and experience. No matter what shape you're in right now, these Habits of Longevity will slow your aging process. In as little as three months, you'll see measurable changes that directly affect your life expectancy—and in three years your body will have repaired itself to such an extent that physiologically it will be as if you've practiced these habits your whole life.

Our strategy is, first, to make sure you're using all the original Habits of Health that can help slow biological aging. We know that these ensure a longer life. Second, we'll reach out to the very edge of safe science and add new advancements that show the most promise—the Habits of Longevity.

At the core of these habits is a practice I call *dietary optimization (DO),* which uses a combination of vital nutrients and fuel in just the right amount to maximize health and longevity. Dietary optimization is based on the science of nutritional intervention, including current research on calorie restriction. While we don't yet know for sure if calorie restriction can extend the life span of long-lived mammals such as ourselves (conclusive data from studies of rhesus monkeys is still over ten years away), initial reports are extremely encouraging.

There are a number of important factors, however, that we do know for certain. One is that obesity impairs the functioning of most of our organ systems, paving the way to non-sickness, disease, and premature death. In fact, if we don't get the 67 percent of our people who are overweight (including 15 percent of our children) down to a healthy weight, the average life expectancy of our society as a whole will soon drop.

We also know that by making the decision to adopt and practice the Habits of Health you can improve your risk factors for cardiovascular disease and a whole host of other conditions that rob you of vitality and health. And we know that as you reach a healthier weight and adopt a healthier lifestyle, you're more likely to live a longer, healthier life.

Maximum Life Span: Living to Our Potential

So realistically, just how much can you extend your life? The answer depends on two governing principles that determine longevity.

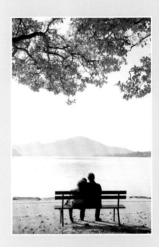

Learning and practicing the Habits of Health is the first step in slowing biological aging. Once you have those under your belt, you're ready to reach out to the very cutting edge of medical science and adopt new practices that show the most promise for extending life span—the Habits of Longevity.

Increasing our
maximum life span
is a bit like breaking
the four-minute mile.
People once said the
human body couldn't
tolerate such intense
demands. But they
were proved wrong,
and today hundreds of
runners have managed
to push themselves
beyond what was
believed to be the limit
of human capability.

The first principle is the limitation of your current design, known as the *principle of primary aging.* In other words, what is the predicted maximum life span of humans—the longest we can possibly live before our parts simply wear out?

That's very different from *life expectancy,* a term that refers to the age at which 50 percent of the population has died. Life expectancy today is 75 years for men and 80 years for women. And while that number has risen dramatically since the early twentieth century, thanks to improved sanitation, medical technology, vaccines and antibiotics, and other advances, many scientists believe that our shelf life—our *maximum life span*—could actually be as high as 150 years.

It's kind of like the four-minute mile. Some people said it couldn't be done, and came up with all sorts of reasons why the human body simply wouldn't tolerate such intense demands. Then, in 1954, along came Roger Bannister to prove them wrong. Since then, our expectations have changed, and several hundred people have run a mile in 3:49 or less.

You may recall from our previous discussion that the longest-living human in recorded history, Jeanne Louise Calment, was 122 years old at the time of her death. She holds the record for the actual maximum life span experienced by a human. But I predict that within a few years science will be able to extend the life of a healthy individual—one who's mastered the Habits of Health—to closer to 150 years.

And to think most of us live only half that amount!

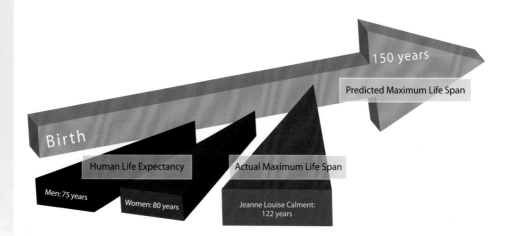

Life Expectancy vs. Predicted Maximum Life Span.
Today's human life expectancy is around 75 years for men and 80 years for women.
The longest any human has actually lived (actual maximum life span) is 122 years.
But many scientists believe that humans could live as long as 150 years (predicted
maximum life span).

> *Want a Longer Life? Give Your Brain a Boost!*
>
> Your brain may not be the first thing you think of when you consider the benefits of diet and exercise. But these essential Habits of Health have an enormous impact on this most critical organ. Just consider the following:
>
> - Habits of Disease such as poor diet, lack of exercise, and too much stress cause a buildup of beta-amyloid, a key component in Alzheimer's.
> - Inflammation and the resulting atherosclerosis can cause brain function to deteriorate by altering blood flow to the brain.
> - Neurotrophins, a substance vital to memory, have been shown to increase through exercise, calorie restriction, and the use of certain spices such as curcumin, and to decrease with stress and inflammation. (For more information, see chapter 20.)
> - Decreasing diastolic blood pressure to below 90 can make a dramatic difference in the onset of brain aging.

Restoring Your Brain through the Habits of Longevity

So why is there such a discrepancy between our life span and Jeanne Louise Calment's?

For the answer we need to look at the second governing principle—the *principle of secondary aging.* This is the process by which the Habits of Disease produce an insidious deterioration of our organ structure and function, resulting in degenerative disease and cellular aging. And sadly, as I've mentioned, this process has begun to accelerate so rapidly that without drastic intervention and lifestyle change, we will soon counter the medical advances of the twentieth century and see our life expectancy as a society sink.

Secondary aging affects all our organ systems, but one that's of particular concern is the brain. Let's face it: living longer in a state of severely limited awareness isn't really in your best interest, or society's. While genetics certainly play an important role in memory loss and Alzheimer's, an unhealthy lifestyle and environment make these afflictions much more likely to occur (see box, above, Want a Longer Life? Give Your Brain a Boost!) Fortunately, the Habits of Longevity can actually reverse decreases in vital brain chemicals.

Why so much discussion on brain aging? Because we want to ensure that your 100-plus-year-old body is well equipped with a fully functioning CPU! That's why in chapter 25, where we look more closely at brain longevity, we'll be spending time focusing on specific strategies you can use to keep your brain humming as you maximize your time on this planet.

Of course, there are no guarantees. But by making the decision to adopt the Habits of Health, you've made the first step. The next step is to really ingrain your new healthy habits for twelve to twenty-four months to ensure that you can maintain and stabilize your new lifestyle. While it may not take you that

> The Habits of Disease cause our cells to age and our organs to deteriorate—including our brain. The Habits of Health help reverse that process.

The Habits of Longevity
are made up of simple
steps that you can
begin taking today.

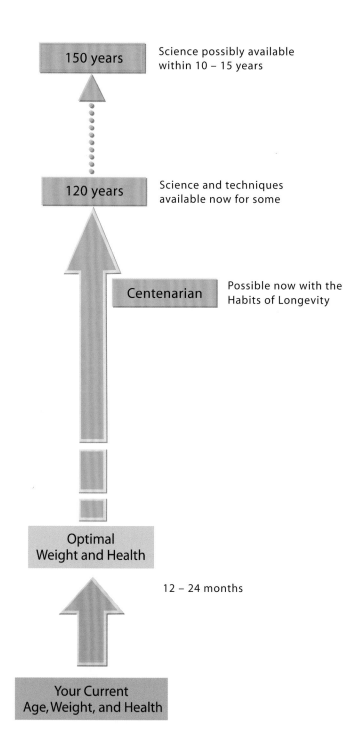

150 years — Science possibly available within 10 – 15 years

120 years — Science and techniques available now for some

Centenarian — Possible now with the Habits of Longevity

Optimal Weight and Health

12 – 24 months

Your Current Age, Weight, and Health

Your Longevity Calendar. Adopting the Habits of Health is the first step. After twelve to twenty-four months, when you've reached optimal health and have added the Habits of Longevity, you may realistically be able to reach 100 years. And as science and technology advances, longer life spans become increasingly possible.

long, it's vital that you're comfortable and have solidified your new optimal health lifestyle before taking that next step.

Once you're ready, add in the Habits of Longevity, maintain your optimal weight and health, and with continued refinement, you could very well live to see the scientific advances that put a 150-year life span within our grasp.

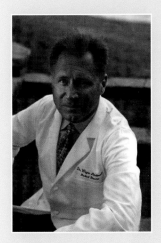

Dr. A's Longevity Plan

Here's my plan for a longer life, broken down into simple steps that you can begin taking today. These steps include a number of basic actions and behaviors that will reduce your likelihood of falling prey to preventable diseases, accidents, and the ravages of an unhealthy lifestyle. They culminate in optimal health—but that's not the end of my longevity plan. In fact, these steps are really a prelude for a lifestyle that can take you even further, to cutting-edge techniques that many scientists and medical researchers believe can extend your life well into the second century. We call it *Ultrahealth™*.

The Habits of Longevity

Step 1: Right Now

- Eliminate tobacco.
- Eliminate all recreational drugs.
- Wear a passenger restraint system any time you're in a car, and purchase a vehicle with front and side airbags as soon as possible.
- Drive the speed limit. (I don't want you dying at age 100 because you're showing off to the twins!)
- Limit your intake of alcoholic beverages to fewer than two drinks a day, and never drink while driving or operating machinery. (For more information on red wine and longevity, see chapter 26.)
- Avoid situations that put you at risk for sexually transmitted diseases, such as having multiple partners.
- Avoid sunburn at all costs.
- Don't exercise on roads used by motor vehicles.

Step 2: Create a Healthy Environment

- Eliminate toxic foods, cleaning supplies, and other poisons such as radon.
- Ensure that your water is clean.
- Ensure that your air is clean.
- Check your smoke detectors to make sure they're working.
- Cover or fence swimming pools.
- Eliminate potential hazards that could cause falls.
- Lock all doors when you're home.
- Lock up firearms.

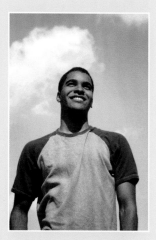

Step 3: Get a Yearly Check-Up

If you didn't see your doctor before you began your weight-loss and movement program, do so now. You're in the process of a whole-body makeover, and it's important to make sure your blood, heart, and general physical health are all in order. Tell your doctor you're taking part in a program that includes healthy diet, regular movement, and better sleep, and see what he says! After he recovers from fainting, have him check the following.

• Record your weight, waist measurement, height, blood pressure, heart rate, and body mass index so you can track your progress. (When you've reached a state of Ultrahealth, go back for another check-up so you can gloat!)
• See if you should lower any of your medications as you lose weight.
• Review the full list of medications you're currently putting in your body. Drug interactions can cause serious side effects, erode our health, and increase the likelihood of falls, motor vehicle accidents, and even cellular aging. And because records aren't always complete—not to mention the fact that many of us have multiple doctors—it's really your responsibility to talk with your primary care physician about lowering or eliminating medications. Remember, prescription medications are one of the top five causes of death!
• Ask for a full lipid profile to assess your cardio-metabolic risk and an hs-CRP test to assess your current inflammatory state (to ensure you're staying in control of your immune system, it's a good idea to continue with follow-up tests for life). If you're 50 or older, a baseline echocardiogram and stress test are in order as well.
• Have appropriate cancer screenings (see box, Your Cancer-Screening Guide for Lifelong Health).
• Make sure you're up to date on your immunizations, including:
  – Pneumovax if you're over 50 (repeat at 65)
  – Tetanus (every ten years)
  – Whooping cough (once for adults)
  – Influenza (yearly)
• Get a baseline TSH to assess thyroid function if you're over 35.
• Have a mineral density scan if you're perimenopausal. Repeat every five years.
• Test sensory systems, including eyes, hearing, and balance. Repeat yearly.

Your Cancer-Screening Guide for Lifelong Health
• *Breast:* self-exam monthly; doctor exam once or twice a year; first mammogram at age 35 to 40, then yearly after 40
• *Cervical:* first pap smear at age 21 or within three years of sexual activity
• *Colon:* first colonoscopy at age 50, then every ten years; hemoccult test every five years
• *Prostate:* digital exam and PSA yearly after age 39
• *Skin:* self-exam regularly for unusual or quick-growing lesions

> *Oral Health and Inflammation: Pathways to Disease*
>
> Gum recession and medication-induced dry mouth—two common complaints as we age—set us up for cavities and gum disease by creating an environment where bacteria can flourish and find plentiful targets. As plaque infects the tissues around the teeth, the gums become swollen and red and slowly begin to pull away, resulting in loose teeth and bad breath. But that's not all. This process also sets up an inflammatory state that can lead to heart disease and diabetes.
>
> The cure? Follow my guidelines for dental health. That's especially important as we age and for diabetics, who are at particular risk for progressive gum disease.

Step 4: Go to Your Dentist

It may surprise you to know that dental health is critical for optimal health and longevity. Keeping your own teeth and maintaining excellent gum and oral health minimizes inflammation and is an important part of our plan.

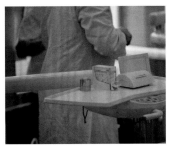

As the nation's first fluoride generation, baby boomers as a whole enjoy extraordinary oral health. However, this may come to a halt as many boomers, now entering their retirement years, come face to face with gum disease. In fact, if recent trends continue, *three out of four boomers will develop gum disease as they age.*

Why? As we get older, we're more prone to certain conditions that put our teeth and gums at peril, including hormonal changes, medical conditions such as diabetes, receding gums that leave roots exposed and vulnerable, and medication-induced dry mouth, which can cause bacteria to proliferate. In addition, the elderly are more likely to have poor dental hygiene and make fewer visits to the dentist.

What can you do about it? For starters:

- Brush at least twice a day with fluoride toothpaste.
- Floss daily.
- Get a yearly check-up from your dentist.
- Have your teeth cleaned twice a year.
- Don't use tobacco products, including cigarettes, chewing tobacco, snuff, pipes, and cigars.
- Drink alcohol in moderation if at all.
- Use lip balm that contains sunscreen.
- Avoid lipsticks that don't contain sunscreen (recent research has shown that the pigment in lipstick can actually intensify UV damage).
- Combat dry mouth and keep your oral cavity moist by taking sips of water or chewing sugar-free gum.

Dental health is often neglected (until it's too late!) but it's an important part of optimal health and longevity. After all, you want to be able to continue to enjoy healthy fresh foods into your 100s!

Step 5: Reach and Maintain Your Healthy Weight

Reaching a healthy weight not only lowers your risk for disease but actually lengthens your life by several years. If you haven't yet begun the healthy meal plan introduced in Phase I, there's no better time!

Step 6: Incorporate the Habits of Health

From learning to eat right, to reaching a healthy weight, to incorporating movement into your daily schedule, to making better sleep a priority—the Habits of Health take you on a complete journey from surviving to thriving.

Step 7: Obtain Optimal Health

No matter what your age, optimizing your health is a fundamental principle of living longer. Not only is it necessary, it just makes sense. After all, if you're going to have a longer life, why not be able to fully enjoy everything this big adventure has to offer?

Now, if you stop right here at this step and focus on being at the height of health for your whole life, you will live longer. But you can do even more. Remember, just as there are no shortcuts to health, there are no shortcuts to longevity. It takes discipline. And just as you made a fundamental choice to be healthy, you can make a fundamental choice to be Ultrahealthy, and take your place among an exciting new generation—the New Centenarians.

Ultrahealth: The Final Step
A Practical Approach to Living Longer

The Ultrahealth system you're about to discover uses principles drawn from the cutting edge of scientific research. Once you've reached a state of optimal health by adopting the Habits of Health, you can use it to go to the next level and attain your maximum life span.

Let's look at the components that determine just who achieves this ultimate state. Basically, your maximum life span is determined by these three factors, in the following proportion:

- Genetic programming (20%–30%)
- Position on the health continuum (70%–80%)
- Luck (< 0.1%)

Genetic Programming

This piece is predetermined (for the moment, anyway). But the good news is that scientists now believe that your genetic programming plays a relatively small role in determining longevity—only about 20 to 30 percent, based on studies of identical twins who were reared in different environments and had different lifestyles.

Genetics—the cards you're dealt in terms of longevity—actually play a much smaller role in determining life span than your lifestyle. And fortunately, lifestyle is a factor you can control!

> *Your Progressive Plan for Ultrahealth*
> 1. Apply the Habits of Health lifestyle.
> 2. Reach and maintain optimal health.
> 3. Add Ultrahealth practices—an additional level of vigilance that focuses on increasing your resilience to aging and disease.

Luck

Luck plays only a tiny role in determining your life span—less than 0.1 percent. You can minimize your chances of falling prey to accidents by adopting steps one and two of the Habits of Longevity, but despite how well you take care of yourself or how exemplary your genetics, if your plane falls out of the sky or you get hit with a golf ball while enjoying a day on the links... well, you might die.

Your Position on the Health Continuum

Adopting a lifestyle that supports optimal health and beyond is by far the biggest factor in longevity, accounting for 70 to 80 percent. That means that the Habits of Health—which are all about moving forward on the health continuum—are a great way to position yourself for a long and healthy life.

In fact, I believe you can add twenty years to your life just by adopting the optimal health lifestyle I've been teaching you. If you're a woman, that means extending your life from 80 years to 100, or from 75 to 95 if you're a man—simply by living the Habits of Health.

What I propose now is a state of health that pushes you to be the very best you can be, a state in which your body operates at optimal efficiency. A state of living a robust and thriving life, eating only the freshest, nutrient-rich foods, lean and strong, with terrific stamina—kind of like our prehistoric ancestors 10,000 years ago (albeit without the saber-toothed tigers!).

It's a state called Ultrahealth, and it's really an augmentation of the Habits of Health lifestyle through dietary optimization, intensified weekly workouts, and a focus on brain health. And it may add another ten to twenty years to your life *beyond* the extra years that optimal health can give you.

The Life Span Continuum. By moving from a state of sickness, to non-sickness, to optimal health, and finally to Ultrahealth, you can add more than 50 percent to your life span and live well into your second century.

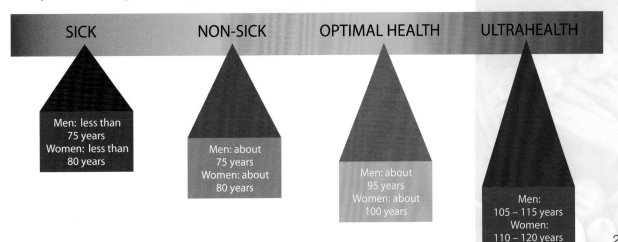

SICK	NON-SICK	OPTIMAL HEALTH	ULTRAHEALTH
Men: less than 75 years Women: less than 80 years	Men: about 75 years Women: about 80 years	Men: about 95 years Women: about 100 years	Men: 105 – 115 years Women: 110 – 120 years

> ### Ultrahealth by the Numbers
>
> The ultimate state of health—one that can take you well into your second century of life—is an entirely new standard for health optimization. Here are the key parameters we're aiming for:
>
> | | |
> |---|---|
> | Systolic blood pressure | 110–95 or less |
> | Diastolic blood pressure | 75–60 or less |
> | Body mass index | 24.9–19.5 (around 20 is ideal; no less than 18.5) |
> | Body fat | 10% for men; 17–23% for women |
> | HDL (good cholesterol) | 50–70 mg/dl |
> | Fasting blood sugar | 75 mg/dl |
> | hs-CRP | 0.5 |

Ultrahealth

Optimal Health

Healthy Weight

The Ultrahealth Plan: Extend and Thrive

Up to this point, you've learned a practical system to integrate all of medical science's *traditional* ways to help us stay healthy and protect against disease. Now, the Ultrahealth plan will take all that and add yet another level of daily choices. Think of it as your postdoctorate degree in health optimization!

This state of Ultrahealth is obtained by making the decision to play full-out with all you have—to organize your life and your daily choices around what's best for your physical, mental, and social well-being.

Now before we go on, let me emphasize: if you haven't learned the Habits of Health and applied them to your daily life, if you haven't reached a healthy weight and aren't currently living an active lifestyle, *you aren't going to be able to apply the Ultrahealth program to your life.*

Why? First, it will simply be too hard for you. It would be like trying to perform jumps on a double black diamond ski run when you haven't even learned how to snowplow on the bunny slopes! And second, it won't work. If you're still eating a tub of ice cream at bedtime, your high-sugar, high-fat intake is creating an inflammatory state that totally negates the Ultrahealth activation of cellular protection and longevity signaling.

If you've already reached and are maintaining optimal health, however, Ultrahealth really won't seem like much of a stretch for you. Let's break it down and see why.

The Ultrahealth plan has three major areas of focus:

• Dietary optimization (DO)
• Movement enhancement
• Brain-health optimization

In the next three chapters, I'll show you specific strategies to enhance your energy management and optimize your brainpower, beginning by focusing on adjusting your dietary intake to improve your body's functioning, reinvigorate you on a cellular level, and set you up with the lowest possible risk for disease as you continue your extended journey through life.

Chapter 24

Ultimate Energy Control

Extending Your Health through Dietary Optimization and Movement

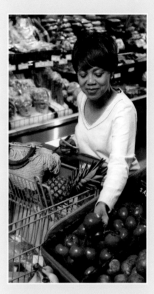

Now that you've learned more about the theory behind life extension and can envision just what's possible, you can begin creating a longer, healthier life for yourself through my concrete, three-part Ultrahealth program. The best part is, this program builds directly on the habits you've already adopted in your journey to optimal health. We're just going to add in some dietary optimization techniques, intensify your movement plan a bit, and teach you some brain-enhancing practices to keep you protected for life.

In Phase III, you reached a balance of energy in and energy out as part of your maintenance plan for optimal health. For your longevity plan, we're going to tweak that slightly by reducing your daily caloric intake by 15 percent. Why? *Because it's been scientifically proven that underfeeding with nutrient-dense foods is more conducive of health and longevity than overfeeding with nutrient-poor, energy-dense food.* (Unfortunately, it's the latter that makes up most diets in Western societies.)

But altering your energy consumption is just one part of our plan. We're also going to focus on eliminating all processed foods so that your diet consists of the freshest whole foods possible.

Be sure to consult your primary care physician before you begin the Ultrahealth program.

When Can I Start the Ultrahealth Longevity Program?

Before starting the Ultrahealth program, I recommend that you reach optimal health and maintain a stable weight and normal lab work (lipid profile, hs-CRP, electrolytes, liver and kidney function, metabolic parameter including blood sugar, and thyroid function if you're over thirty-five) for at least six months, preferably a year. You should also discuss your plan with your primary care physician and, if he agrees that it's safe for you to take part, follow up with visits based on his recommendations. (I usually suggest a visit every three months for the first year and yearly visits after that.)

Warning: Do not allow your BMI (body mass index) to fall lower than 20. Monitor your progress closely with your physician. Any history of eating disorders, immune suppression, or other wasting disorders is an absolute contraindication to this program.

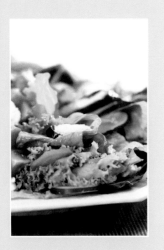

Eating for Ultrahealth: Adjusting Your Daily Intake

First let's calculate your Ultrahealth daily energy intake. To do so, we'll return to the sample patient we used way back in chapter 12 when we determined your healthy eating maintenance plan. Here are her relevant numbers:

- 46-year-old female
- 5 foot, 9 inches (69 inches)
- Utilizing the EAT walking and two-day-a-week weight-training programs
- Body mass index of 24
- 162 pounds (down from 206 pounds)

We'll plug those numbers into the formula for calculating total energy expenditure (TEE), from the same chapter:

$$TEE = BMR + PAL + TEF$$

Let's break that formula down to see how many calories she's currently burning in a day:

1. BMR (basal metabolic rate) = $10 \times$ (weight in pounds $\times 0.455$) + $6.25 \times$ (height in inches $\times 2.54$) $- 5 \times$ (age) $- 161$

$$= 10 \times (164 \times 0.455) + 6.25 (69 \times 2.54) - 5 \times (46) - 161$$
$$= 746 + 1{,}095 - 230 - 161$$
$$= 1{,}450 \text{ calories per day}$$

2. PAL (physical activity level) is the difference between your baseline BMR and your BMR modified for activity (BMR $\times$ Activity Factor). To determine your activity factor, see the Activity Factor Table in chapter 12, page 156. As you'll recall, this modified BMR is called your EEpal.

$$EEpal = BMR \times Activity\ Factor$$
$$= 1{,}450 \text{ calories} \times 1.5 \text{ (active)}$$
$$= 2{,}175 \text{ calories per day}$$

As you can see, her BMR has increased as a result of her level of activity.

3. TEF (thermic effect of food) = EEpal (2,175 kcal) $\times$ 0.1 (that is, 10%)
$$= 217 \text{ calories per day}$$

So by taking the 2,175 calories we calculated by adding in her PAL, and adding the 217 calories she uses to process her food (her TEF), we come up with a total energy requirement of 2,392 calories per day—her TEE.

Currently, this patient is consuming and expending approximately 2,400 calories per day through her new active lifestyle and has remained at a stable BMI (body mass index) of 24 for the past two years. Her blood chemistry is normal, including her glucose and hs-CRP, her lipid profile is within normal range, and she is off the Lipitor. Her thyroid function has never been better, her blood pressure is down to 125/80, and her body fat is 26 percent—all within normal limits. She is enjoying an optimally healthy, energy-filled life and has made the decision to take the next step—to achieve Ultrahealth and seize its potential to extend her new thriving life.

To take that step, she'll need to figure out her adjusted Ultrahealth calorie inake. To do so, she'll start with her optimal health TEE of 2,392 calories per day and use this formula:

Optimal Health TEE × 0.85 = new energy intake per day

Or, for this patient: 2,400 kcal × 0.85 = 2,040 kcal/day of energy intake.

So let's sum up. This woman's *dietary optimization* will include a decrease in daily calories to 2,040 calories. She'll accomplish this by eliminating all processed food and by choosing foods in the dark green section of the food charts in chapter 9. That way, she can be sure she's eating only nutrient-filled, low-glycemic carbohydrates, lean protein, and healthy fats. Here's how her daily eating plan will look:

- 2,040 kcal/day
- No processed foods
- Lowest-glycemic carbohydrates
- Increased soy intake (based on Okinawan longevity studies; see chapter 22)
- Healthy fats, especially olive oil, fish oils, walnuts, and flaxseed
- Every-three-hour eating schedule

Here's a snapshot of a typical daily meal plan for someone consuming about that number of calories under the Ultrahealth program.

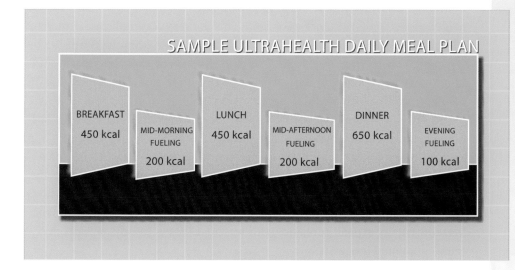

SAMPLE ULTRAHEALTH DAILY MEAL PLAN

| BREAKFAST 450 kcal | MID-MORNING FUELING 200 kcal | LUNCH 450 kcal | MID-AFTERNOON FUELING 200 kcal | DINNER 650 kcal | EVENING FUELING 100 kcal |

Sample Ultrahealth Daily Meal Plan. With the Ultrahealth meal plan, you'll decrease your energy intake slightly from your optimal health level, but you'll still fuel every three hours. Here's an example of how your day's eating might look if you're taking in about 2,000 calories a day.

As you can see, while the calorie level of most of your daily fuelings has increased, I recommend that you keep your evening fueling at 100 calories. I also suggest that if you need to adjust your schedule to eat fewer calories, you steal those from your evening meal.

Note that while the Ultrahealth plan involves reduced caloric intake, it still requires you to fuel every three hours. To make this doable, I recommend you take another look at the fueling strategies in the healthy eating chapters. It's worth noting that Medifast®, as a pioneer and leader in restrictive-calorie diets, provides an excellent method to help you implement a regimen of dietary restriction. Medically formulated portion-controlled meal replacements (PCMRs) are particularly effective in delivering a nutrient-rich, low-calorie diet that also provides plenty of health-supporting soy!

Of course, in addition to eating a full range of nutrient-dense foods, you'll want to make sure you're getting the full range of supplementation outlined in chapter 20. We'll augment that list in the next chapter by adding supplements that enhance your brain capacity and function for lasting health.

Exercise Enhancement: The Other Half of the Equation

Of course, it's not just your energy input that will change under the Ultrahealth system. You'll also be increasing your energy expenditure by 15 percent twice a week, on top of your current EAT walking and resistance program expenditure. Not only will you use more calories, you'll also receive increased cardiovascular benefits from these more intense workouts. Here's the formula you'll use to calculate this increased energy expenditure:

Optimal Health TEE × 0.15 = additional energy expenditure twice a week

Or, for the sample patient above: 2,400 kcal × 0.15 = 360 kcal. That's the number of calories she'll be burning twice a week on top of her already robust EAT walking and resistance program. This can be accomplished either by adding intensity to the two weekly EAT Resistance Program workouts or by switching two of your weekly EAT Walking Program walks for two twenty-minute interval-training sessions (plus ten-minute cool down), depending on your age, ability, and schedule.

In order to assure that your EAT Ultrahealth movements are on the cutting edge of exercise physiology, I've enlisted the help of Greg Freitag, a top exercise physiologist at Johns Hopkins and an expert in the science of exercise. Together, we've designed an enhancement program that's sustainable, provides just the right intensity, and is minimally intrusive to your busy schedule. These additional movements complete our EAT System, enhancing your energy expenditure and cardiovascular fitness to help support maximum functional longevity.

Intensifying Your Workouts: Options for Enhancement

I've developed several options for increasing your energy output. First, let's look at some ways to boost your current resistance workouts. Second, we'll explore interval training, an option you can use to enhance the intensity of two of your thirty-minute walks per week.

Caution: Consult your physician before you begin any exercise program or increase the intensity of your workouts in order to ensure that your blood pressure, lung function, and musculoskeletal systems can handle the increased challenge.

Dr. A Says . . .

Start out slowly by incorporating these enhancements into the EAT resistance routines outlined in chapter 16.

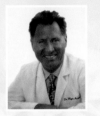

Six Options to Boost Your EAT Resistance Workouts

1. Increase Repetitions

Instead of performing five repetitions of each exercise, perform six to eight, while maintaining the 8-4-8 pattern (contraction-holding-relaxation) as well as your speed.

2. Increase Resistance

Increase the weight or resistance you use in each exercise by 10–15 percent, while maintaining the 8-4-8 pattern and your speed. You can accomplish this by using resistance bands and heavier dumbbells. Make sure your exercise ball is fully inflated to ensure the greatest balance challenge to your core. You'll also want to increase your own focus and effort of contraction.

3. Increase Sets or Rotations

Complete three rotations instead of just two. This will increase your EAT resistance workout time by about one-third, or ten minutes.

4. Decrease Recovery Time

Decrease the amount of time you rest between exercises from twenty seconds to ten seconds. Not only will this increase the demand on your muscle fibers, it will enable you to maintain an elevated heart rate throughout your resistance workout.

5. Increase Your Speed

Increase the speed of each repetition from 8-4-8 (contraction-holding-relaxation) to 4-2-4. You'll generate more force per repetition—which means you should also increase the resistance or amount of weight by 15–25 percent.

6. Maintain Muscular Contraction

Pay closer attention to keeping the contraction in your muscles, not your bones. It's common to "lock out" your joints during an exercise by straightening your elbows in a push-up or your knees in a squat, for example. But this transfers the weight onto your bone structure and away from working muscles, and is not recommended. By avoiding "locking out," you increase tension and maintain a high level of intensity throughout your repetitions.

- High-intensity interval: around 75–90% of your maximum heart rate (MHR), or a rate of perceived exertion (RPE) of around 7–9.

- Low-intensity interval: around 50–60% of your maximum heart rate (MHR), or a rate of perceived exertion (RPE) of around 5–6.

For more information on MHR, see page 197. For more information on the RPE scale, see page 200.

Intensifying Your EAT Walking Workouts through Interval Training

Interval training is an intense, time-efficient way to train your aerobic (cardiovascular) and anaerobic (muscle) energy-burning systems. It's called interval training because it consists of short periods, or intervals, of high-intensity cardiovascular activity followed by short periods of lower-intensity cardiovascular activity. By alternating high- and low-intensity intervals, you intensify the metabolic challenge to your muscles, increasing the amount of calories burned in each twenty-minute session—and that can help prevent injury by keeping exercise time shorter and saving muscles from overuse.

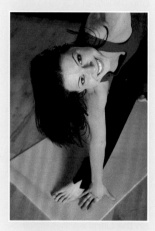

Your Ultrahealth Movement Plan
• NEAT
• EAT Walking
• EAT Resistance
• EAT Enhancement (twice per week, replaces EAT walking or resistance training for that day)

Together, these increased activities provide a robust movement plan that builds optimal cardiovascular, musculoskeletal, and brain health. Combined with the nutrient-dense, calorie-reduced fuelings you'll be getting through dietary optimization, you'll have the tools you need to create an Ultrahealth state and stay in top physical shape into your seventies and eighties.

In fact, there's no reason you can't continue this high level of fitness even into your nineties. Just look at Jack LaLanne, my all-time optimal health hero. At the time of this writing, he's close to becoming one of the first centenarians to live in an Ultrahealthy state—purely by determining to be healthy. LaLanne is currently working with a group of innovative health care professionals to create a supervised program of EAT-type activities specially designed to help senior citizens get fit and stay fit. To find out more about it, visit my Web site at www.habitsofhealth.net.

Maintaining optimal health and fitness for as long as possible is key to supporting the most critical Ultrahealth determinant of all—your brain. By protecting and enhancing the health and well-being of your brain and following the Habits of Longevity, you have a real shot at reaching that three-digit life span. Let's turn our focus to the inner workings of your mind and get you on your way to ultimate health!

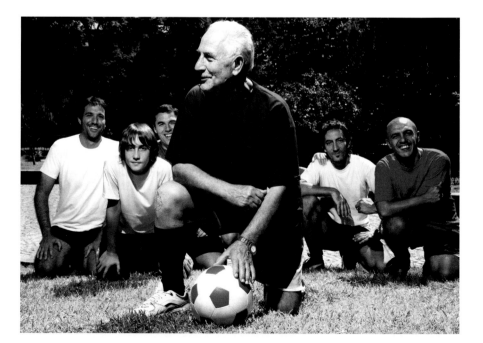

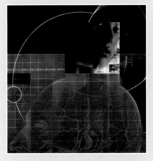

Chapter 25

Brain Longevity

Protecting and Enhancing Your Future

The brain is the source of all health and the master controller of aging. Its most fundamental function is to control all the movement of the body, without which we would quickly go down the path to disease and death. And in fact, the brain is one of the first organs to suffer if our daily movement is impeded. Not to mention that if we don't protect our master controller, we may lose our memory and our ability to think—at which point it really wouldn't make sense to extend our life anyway.

I've singled out the brain for special attention not only because of its central role in health and longevity, but also because it's become particularly vulnerable to injury in our rapidly advancing, technologically driven society. Our Western lifestyle, with its diet high in animal fats and high-glycemic carbohydrates, its lack of exercise, and its excessive stress, is pounding away at our brains as well as our hearts. Fortunately, reaching optimal health through the Habits of Health eliminates most of these negative factors.

Our goal in this chapter is to become laser-focused on the specific habits that will protect and enhance your brain and enable it to continue directing you toward a state of ever-increasing health. Our strategy concentrates on three major areas essential for brain health and longevity:

- Brain exercise (including physical exercise)
- Stress reduction
- Brain food (nutritional enhancement)

Let's start putting those wheels in motion!

The Science of Thinking

As science unravels the secrets of this three-pound CPU on top of your shoulders, we're discovering that the brain has amazing resilience to changing conditions—what the neuroscientists call *plasticity*. Your brain will provide optimal levels of cognition and memory as long as you maintain it under these important conditions:

- Use it.
- Keep enough blood flowing to provide the oxygen it needs to flourish.
- Feed it enough of the right nutrients.

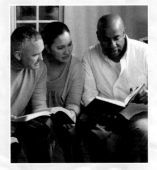

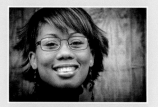

> ### Nomads and Neanderthals:
> ### Survival of the Fittest (Brains, That Is!)
> Our ancestors 10,000 years ago were nomadic. New environments and the need to develop conveyances and survival skills meant that their brains were constantly stimulated. Neanderthals, on the other hand, stayed close to their original territories and caves. As a result, they may have lacked the flexibility and innovation necessary to survive.

In short, keep those brain cells bathed in nutrients, oxygen, and growth factors and protect them from free radicals, and you have a recipe for performing Sudoku into your 100s!

The brain cells we're going to be focusing on are *neurons*—the thinking cells that create and support memory. You have about 100 billion of them, yet they make up only 10 percent of your total brain cells, the remaining 90 percent being composed of support cells that provide housekeeping functions for the neurons.

Neurons have several important components:

- *Axons*—long extensions that work like a TV cable to send messages out to other neurons and, through the spinal cord, to muscle cells
- *Dendrites*—antenna-like extensions that serve as receivers to pull information in
- *Synapses*—neuron-to-neuron connections, with up to 10,000 per neuron

Through these components, each neuron acts as its own separate computer. Based on 100 billion neurons with 10,000 synapses each, that's a total of 100 trillion connections!

This amazing neural network transmits at ten different levels of intensity, each capable of 200 calculations per second. In fact, the number of different brain states your neural network is capable of creating is greater than the total number of atoms in the universe. Think about *that* for a moment. . . (Aha! You just did a brain exercise!)

Memory and learning are dependent on changes in synapses, those neuron-to-neuron connections. And with each change that occurs, the size and health of the two—or 10,000—neurons involved actually increase, making it easier to communicate. This phenomenon is called *long-term potentiation (LTP)*, and it explains why if you stop using certain connections they eventually wither, just like muscles do from lack of exercise.

Which leads us to our first area of enhancement. . .

Brain Exercise

Scientists at Brown University found that when rats were trained to accomplish a new motor skill, their brains changed over the course of the training. The synapses of the brain cells that were used actually grew. Just like doing curls increases the size of your biceps, doing mental exercises repairs damaged pathways and creates new ones, building memory and keeping your brain healthy.

So just what types of exercise can we do to increase our brain health and longevity?

Use It or Lose It: Mental Exercise for Brain Health

Our brains need a workout as much as our bodies do! But it doesn't need to be complicated. In fact, creating brain fitness can be as simple as reading, writing, doing crossword puzzles, hanging out talking to friends, going to meetings, learning how to play a musical instrument, playing video games, or spending the evening dancing.

Anytime you perform an activity that's different from your usual activity, you're creating new neural pathways. Here's an example to try: next time you're at your computer, try moving the mouse with your opposite hand. It will probably feel as awkward as the first time you tried to tie your shoelaces! At the beginning, as your brain builds new pathways, it can be hard to use precise movement, and you'll probably perform tasks more slowly—but if you stick with it, you will improve.

Create new neural pathways by using your opposite hand to perform other daily activities, such as brushing your hair and teeth, combing the dog, sending text messages, dialing a phone number, or try changing the ear you use to talk on the phone.

Work on changing your sensory reality while doing daily chores. Eat dinner without talking, using only visual cues, or close your eyes while washing your hair and getting dressed. Challenge your brain to learn new and novel tasks, especially things you've never done before. Try playing chess or advanced card games, or take up tai chi, yoga, or sculpting. Travel to new places and explore new environments, or if you can't get away, just drive home following a different route, try a new restaurant, shop at a grocery store you've never been to, or check out a museum.

The good news is that whatever our age, our brains can continue to grow and renew. In fact, according to renowned brain researcher Dr. Marian Diamond, senior citizens have even more highly developed neuronal networks than younger people, meaning they're even more responsive to intellectual

Chatting on Your Cell Phone?
Use an earpiece to keep the body of the phone away from your brain and minimize radiation exposure. (Studies aren't conclusive, but why not protect yourself just in case?)

Can Mental Activity Stave Off Alzheimer's?

Older adults who stay mentally active may be at lower risk for developing Alzheimer's disease, says recent (albeit limited) research. That includes reading, playing cards and other games, working crossword puzzles, going to museums—even watching television or listening to the radio. Although this "use it or lose it" approach hasn't been proved, no harm can come from putting your brain to work on a regular basis!*

*Wilson, R. S., et al., "Participation in Cognitively Stimulating Activities and Risk of Incident Alzheimer's Disease," *Journal of the American Medical Association* 287 (2002): 742–748.

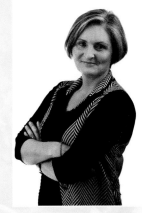

Exercise your brain regularly with books of brain teasers or other mental exercises. Here are some great choices:

- *Mensa Mind Teasers*, by Philip J. Carter and Kenneth A Russell (Sterling Publishing, 2007)
- *Will Shortz Presents Sudoku to Soothe Your Soul*, by Will Shortz (St. Martin's Press, 2008)
- *Get Your Brain in the Fast Lane*, by Michel Noir and Bernard Croisile (McGraw-Hill, 2006)

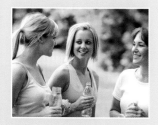

enrichment. At birth, our neurons are just little spheres, sending out tiny preliminary branches of dendrites. But as we grow, our neurons continue to reach out and gather information, communicating and creating a network of interconnectivity.

If we exercise our brains and increase these connections through continual stimulation, we can protect ourselves from memory loss and maintain our cognitive ability. After all, studies show that better-educated people have less risk of Alzheimer's, and that engaging in manual activities that require thought and action can increase and speed up cognition. So go play Bingo, engage in do-it-yourself projects, paint, participate in sports, or grow a garden! Just remember to vary your intellectual activities on a regular basis to keep stretching your brain.

Cognitive Training for Your Brain

One important study tracked 5,000 people between the ages of 20 and 90. When participants began experiencing mental decline, they were given a series of one-hour trainings designed to improve inductive reasoning and spatial orientation. The results? Over half improved significantly—showing that mental enrichment can increase intelligence at any age. In other words, if you haven't been using your brain, fire up the mental treadmill and watch your thinking power bounce back! Here are some mental practices you can follow to boost your brain's learning capacity:

- Practice the art of focusing. Think about what you're doing ("I'm putting my keys on the table"). Or try finding something you want to learn how to do and build some new circuitry by actually doing it!
- Mentally repeat information you've just learned to ensure it transfers to your long-term memory. Attaching emotion to an event can help you remember it as well.
- Think about what you're trying to learn. ("So why exactly is high-glycemic food bad for me?")
- Mentally summarize what you've just learned.
- Organize information into categories. Try classifying your grocery list, for example.
- Use acronyms or create associations between things to tie information together and ground it in your memory.

Pump It Up: Physical Exercise for Brain Health

Statistics actually support the saying "What's good for the heart is good for the head." Adults who exercise at least three times a week have a 30–40 percent lower risk of developing dementia later in life than those who don't exercise. So just why is exercise so important for the brain? We can break it down into three factors:

- It provides a healthy brain environment.
- It stimulates nerve growth factor (NGF).
- It reduces stress.

Let's take a look at these great benefits, one by one.

A Healthy Brain Environment

Exercise increases blood flow to the brain, delivering nutrients and oxygen and flushing out waste and necrotic debris such as beta-amyloid—toxic protein fragments that can gunk up transmissions in the hippocampus, your memory command center. In fact, exercise even helps prevent beta-amyloid from being produced in the first place.

What else can exercise do? It increases neurotransmitters such as norepinephrine and dopamine, makes beneficial CoQ_{10} more easily available, boosts neuropeptides such as endorphins, and decreases damaging cortisol. It stabilizes blood sugar and can relieve depression just as effectively as medication can. And it plays a key role in lowering blood pressure—which improves cognition, slows Alzheimer's, and is an important determinant of long-term brain health.

And the great thing is, you don't even need to be an elite triathlete to enjoy this wealth of benefits. It turns out that plain old walking is especially good for the brain—it increases blood circulation, but it's not so strenuous as to cause your legs to take up the extra oxygen and glucose like other types of exercise can. And according to a recent study, walking is even more effective than weight training in preserving and enhancing brain health.

In fact, studies show again and again that this type of moderate exercise produces dramatic results. Here are findings from some of those studies:

- Sedentary individuals were twice as likely to get Alzheimer's as those who exercised three times a week.

- People 85 and older who remained active were spared significant heart disease and enjoyed 80 percent better memory functions than their inactive peers.

- Seniors who walked regularly showed significant improvement over sedentary older people, improving their learning ability, concentration, and abstract reasoning.

- Woman walkers in their seventies experienced much less cognitive decline than their sedentary peers, and each additional mile they walked further decreased the decline by 13 percent.

- Exercisers exhibited much less decline in frontal and prefrontal regions of the brain, preserving executive function such as planning, organization, and mental multitasking.

High Blood Pressure and Brain Risk
Having diastolic blood pressure of 90 or above for twenty years raises your risk of dementia to five times that of someone whose diastolic blood pressure is under 90.

Exercise to Ward Off Stroke!
According to recent research, older people who walked as little as twenty minutes a day reduced their risk of stroke by 57 percent.

- Moderate exercise has been shown to improve brain cell survival in neuro-degenerative disease.

- Running boosts brain cells in the hippocampus, the area of the brain responsible for memory.

As you can see from these studies, it's never too late to start. In fact, exercising to boost your brain is more important than ever as we age. Older people who have heart disease and high blood pressure suffer cognitive decline because the blood flow to their brain is decreased. After all, the brain uses about 25 percent of our blood supply—and exercise plays a critical role in increasing the strength of the entire circulatory system.

Nerve Growth Factor (NGF)

Nerve growth factor (NGF) and brain-derived neurotrophic factor (BDNF)—two powerful substances produced in the brain—are stimulated by exercise and suppressed by stress and high levels of saturated fats and refined sugars.

So why are these substances so important? NGF and BDNF repair and rescue damaged neurons, increase production of neurotransmitters, and protect the neurons from oxygen stress radicals. They can help improve intelligence, and are guardians that bathe, protect, and heal our precious neurons.

And all we have to do to help them out is to go take a brisk walk! In fact, walking is just what the doctor ordered to clear your head.

Stress Reduction

Most of us rarely experience true relaxation (outside of vacation, that is). Yet this state—being relaxed, creative, intuitive, vibrant, intelligent—should be our brain's normal default state. It's how we're supposed to be.

When we're stressed, our brain can't function optimally, and when stress becomes chronic, it can decrease brain health and accelerate cellular aging. In fact, reducing the amount of stress in our life is so critical to brain health that I've devoted the whole next section of this chapter to mental techniques that can help you relax and become more stress-free so you can take control of your life and choose the outcome that supports your long-term goal—a healthy brain.

First, let's look deeper into what's sometimes called the *stress response*. The human stress response served our ancestors well 10,000 years ago. For them, stress was almost always induced by physical danger, and those dangers demanded a physical response. So when they came face-to-face with a preda-

Dr. A Says . . .

Studies show again and again that even moderate exercise like walking can improve brain health dramatically. And best of all, it's never too late to start.

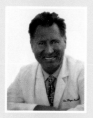

Boost Your Brain. . . with Curry?

What do exercise, falling in love, reducing calories, and eating Indian food have in common? They all boost your level of BDNF (brain-derived neurotrophic factor), a powerful protector of cognitive intelligence. Curcumin, a spice from the turmeric plant that's been shown to increase BDNF, is an important ingredient in curry and many spicy types of mustards. So dig in—for a better brain!

tor, and their brains shot out norepinephrine, epinephrine, and cortisol, they used those chemicals to get the heck out of Dodge.

But today, that stress response can turn on us. In the course of our modern, chaotic lives, our stress response may be activated several times a day—but unlike in ancient times, it's almost always in response to mental threats that don't elicit a physical response like running or fighting. Instead, we internalize the stress, bathing our brain and heart with damaging substances that create systemic inflammation.

And here's something interesting—because the initial stress response gives us a jolt of energy and self-confidence, we can actually become addicted to it. The result? Chronic stress and a decline in brain function. Over time, ongoing stress reduces the neurotransmitters in the frontal lobe of our neocortex, where most of our abstract thinking occurs, and shunts norepinephrine away from the limbic system, which controls emotions. That can lead to anxiety, poor work performance, depression, and feelings of helplessness and lack of meaning.

Now how can we prevent those excess stress chemicals from just sitting there inside us causing all that damage? Exercise, of course! Exercise is a wonderfully effective way to dispose of those stress chemicals in just the way your body was designed to. All kinds of exercises are effective for this, but activities that mimic aggression such as kicks, lifts, or thrusts are especially therapeutic, as is physical labor like digging or whacking weeds. Not only will you burn off the stress you're feeling at the moment, you'll also create resistance to future stress and help your brain grow.

Stress Reduction: The Relaxation Response

Now that you've seen how exercise can help reverse the ill effects of stress, let's add to your arsenal with some specific techniques to help you respond to stress whenever it occurs and put your brain back into its normal, default state—relaxation.

To do that, I'm going to teach you to develop a Habit of Health that's just the opposite of the stress response, called the *relaxation response*. Originally developed by Dr. Herbert Benson at Harvard, the relaxation response is based on meditation. But it takes from that spiritual practice just the parts that have to do with mental relaxation, enabling anyone to use this wonderful mechanism to reduce stress and improve brain health.

What we're going to do in essence is teach your neocortex—the part of your brain that's responsible for producing higher thought—to tell the emotional areas of your brain to relax. This stimulates the release of brain chemicals that change the body's state from one of stress to one of relaxation. It puts the brakes on our normal ways of thinking, slowing us down so that we actually begin to experience short pauses in which we have no thoughts at all. Our body's autonomic functions such as heart rate and breathing naturally begin to slow down, and we feel calm. Stress chemicals recede, and our brain gets a needed rest.

It's a remarkable process, and there are a number of books available that can teach you the proper techniques in depth. But for now, I'd like to show you

A Habit of Health: Keeping your brain in shape with daily exercise

Counter the *stress response* with the *relaxation response,* a meditation-based technique to calm body and brain.

Want to learn more? For
a great introduction to
meditative techniques,
you might enjoy reading
Notes to Myself, by
Hugh Prather.

A Habit of Health:
Practicing the relaxation
response

some very basic methods that anyone can use to reach this relaxed and healthy
stress-free state.

A Simple Relaxation Meditation

The goal here is to clear your mind of all thoughts—to turn off the mental
merry-go-round that's feeding your brain and body with tension and creating
a negative mental state.

Step 1: Set aside ten to twenty minutes. Good choices might be in the morning
before breakfast or just before your evening meal.

Step 2: Find a cozy spot—a quiet, serene place where you can be alone with
your thoughts without interruption. Make sure to turn off any electronic
communication devices. Silence is the overriding principle.

Step 3: Sit up straight on the floor, in a comfortable, relaxed position with your
legs crossed. (Alternatively, you may sit in a chair with your feet flat if sitting
on the floor is difficult or uncomfortable for you.) Place your hands together
in your lap, with your right hand resting in your left, palms up. Begin taking
slow breaths using the abdominal breathing technique described in chapter 19
(see page 241).

Step 4: Close your eyes and let any tension release. Imagine that stress is seeping
out of every pore in your skin. Starting with your feet, relax your muscles all
the way to the top of your head.

Step 5: Now let's turn off the internal dialog in your brain and stop the thought
process. Slowly repeat a word or phrase that you find calming, such as love,
quiet, peace, or a spiritual word that creates a serene state. Don't let other
thoughts such as memories or events enter your brain. Just keep repeating
that one word or phrase (your *mantra*) silently. This will help keep distracting
thoughts from seeping into your gray matter.

　　If thoughts come to you—which will happen until you perfect the technique and it becomes a Habit of Health—just repeat the word *relax,* take a deep
breath, and let the thought go as you exhale. Then return to your mantra.

Step 6: Once you've continued your internal chant for the length of time you've
selected (long enough to reach a state of relaxation and calm), sit quietly for a
minute or two. As you come back to your normal state, merge with the calmness
of the meditative state and take one last deep inhalation. Hold your breath for
about fifteen seconds, exhale, and relax.

You've just created a new state of composure and control.

Progressive Relaxation for Body and Mind

Here's a great way to reset your body-mind connection. This is my favorite
mind-body relaxation technique because it makes you more aware of the
tension level in each part of your body and teaches you to shift your brain's

directive from tension to relaxation using very precise control. As you relax your muscles, you'll enable background tension to dissipate as well.

Step 1: Find a quiet, comfortable place to lie down.

Step 2: Close your eyes and let all the tension melt from your body. Begin focusing on the toes of your left foot. Sense the level of tension, and then slowly relax every fiber in those toes, allowing the tension to flow out of you until it's completely gone. Now shift your attention from your toes to your foot, and repeat. Continue in the following progression:

left toes > left foot > left calf > left thigh > left hip
right toes > right foot > right calf > right thigh > right hip
buttocks > belly > lower back > chest
left fingers > left hand > left forearm > left upper arm > left shoulder
right fingers > right hand > right forearm > right upper arm > right shoulder
upper back > neck > face > scalp

Finally, let the last bit of tension escape from the top of your head.

Step 3: Spend a few minutes absorbing this new state of relaxation. As you go about your day, notice if tension begins to creep into certain areas. If it does, stop what you're doing as soon as possible and relax those areas using an abbreviated version of the technique above. This will help prevent areas of tension from becoming stress reinforcers and stave off musculoskeletal dysfunction.

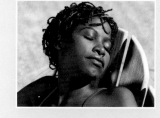

Get Help!

Remember, you can't hope to enjoy optimal health and extend life without addressing this critical area! If you're experiencing health-robbing stress, it's worth your time to seek someone who can help you reduce and eliminate

---

More Stress Reducers

Try these techniques to create relaxation and lower internal stress.

- *Deep breathing.* Whenever you have a few moments and need to relax, revisit the deep breathing techniques we covered in chapter 19. Remember, these are especially useful during the challenge portion of Stop-Challenge-Choose, the mental exercise you learned in chapter 19 to help you regain control and inhibit stress.
- *Prayer.* This healing stress reducer is especially beneficial for those who are experiencing severe situational stress as a result of illness or the loss of a family member or friend.
- *Yoga.* For a complete mind-body practice, explore these ancient exercises that combine movement, breathing, posture, mantra, meditation, and even special healing finger positions.

A study of 1,350
patients with severe
cardiac disease found
that those with no
support system were
three times more likely
to die as a result of
their illness.

chronic stress from your life. Take a yoga class, reread chapter 21 on well-being, learn to say *no*, use your support network, get a pet, or find a soul mate and fall in love! And if you find you can't harness stress on your own, please seek professional help.

You can't live long and thrive if your mind isn't in its natural state—relaxed.

Brain Food: Nutritional Enhancement

We now turn to our third essential component of brain health and longevity—food for your brain. Certain foods and supplements are particularly important for brain health and longevity, while others create conditions that leave your brain open to attack.

The brain is a fatty organ. In fact, your neurons are about 60 percent fat. This high fat content makes your brain especially vulnerable to attack by destructive oxygen radicals. When you eat saturated fats in particular, you bathe your brain in oxygen radicals from saturated and polyunsaturated oils. If you were to pour these oils into an open container, they would oxidize quickly, becoming cloudy and rancid as they filled with damaging oxygen radicals. That same scenario takes place in your body as oxygen-rich blood mixes with unhealthy fats and rushes to your brain.

In addition, excess dietary fat can impair cerebral circulation and clog your arteries with LDLs (bad cholesterol), decreasing the elasticity of your brain's blood vessels. That's why it's so important to avoid saturated and polyunsaturated fats such as margarine, as well as all sources of trans-fat.

To protect your brain, confine your fat and oil intake to these healthy choices:

- Extra virgin olive oil
- Flaxseed oil
- Canola oil
- Fatty fish and fish oils, including eicosapentaenoic acid (EPA) and docasahexanoic acid (DHA)

And to further decrease oxygen radical formation, reduce the total number of calories you eat and choose only the lowest-glycemic carbohydrates. In addition, be sure to include in your daily intake the full antioxidant supplement battery you learned about in the optimization program in chapter 20, including vitamins E and C, beta-carotene, zinc, selenium, and CoQ_{10}. These will help your body create an environment rich in radical scavengers to protect your brain.

And finally, don't forget herbs and spices! The following choices are especially useful in helping the brain replenish its neurotransmitters and remove dangerous beta-amyloid:

- Turmeric (curcumin)
- Basil
- Lemon balm

> ### *Foods for Better Blood Flow*
>
> Chocolate—in the form of pure cocoa or 70 percent dark chocolate—contains flavonoids that help keep your cerebral blood vessels open, something that's particularly important when we're over fifty-five. Other flavonoid-rich foods include wine (especially red wine), grape juice, and black tea. Just be sure to avoid foods that are high glycemic!

- Black pepper
- Sage
- Mint
- Salvia
- Lemon rosemary

Supplements for Your Brain

The supplements you added as part of your optimization program are a great start, but there are a few more that are particularly important for brain health. For a serious boost to brain longevity, try the following:

- Vitamin E (400 IU mixed tocopherols with a gram [1,000 mg] of vitamin C)
- Vitamin B_6 (40 mg), vitamin B_{12} (800 mcg), folic acid (100 mg), and niacin (100 mg) in the form of a mega B complex
- Acetyl-L-carnitine (100 mg)
- Alpha lipoic acid (200 mg)
- Phosphatidylserine (100–300 mg)
- Coenzyme Q_{10} (100 mg)
- Zinc (20 mg)
- Selenium (200 mcg)
- Magnesium (400 mg)
- Vitamin A (2,500–5,000 IU)

And, although conclusive research is still pending, you might want to consider these:

- Ginkgo biloba (90 mg)
- Lecithin (1,500 mg)
- Green juice products and green tea (1–2 servings per day)

With the addition of these brain-boosting nutritional supplements, a regular course of brain and body exercises, and some healthy stress-reducing techniques, you now have a whole new additional set of Habits of Health for your brain! Use them to protect this most important organ from harm and ensure that you stay in the best possible shape to enjoy the longer life that's now within your grasp.

Dr. A Says . . .

As always, check with your physician before beginning any supplement protocol. And while you're at it, ask him about taking 162 mg of baby aspirin as part of your brain and cardiovascular longevity program.

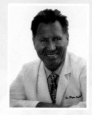

Chapter 26
Reaching a State of Ultrahealth

Once you settle into your Ultrahealth program, you'll want to track your progress closely, especially for the first year. I suggest quarterly visits to your physician to make sure your body is responding properly. I expect your doctor will be very interested in your progress, because you represent a new type of patient, with outstanding health parameters like these:

- You'll be coming off most or all of your medication.
- Your lab results will be to the far left (low normal) of the reporting range.
- Your lipid profile may fall into the 50–70 range for LDLs (bad cholesterol).
- Your fasting blood sugar may drop into the low 70s.

Let's focus on three critical parameters that together really serve to define your Ultrahealth state:

- Your hs-CRP
- Your body mass index (BMI)
- Your percentage of body fat (body composition)

Your Major Ultrahealth Goals. Achieving a state of Ultrahealth puts you in an elite group of individuals whose most critical parameters of health—hs-CRP, BMI, and body fat percentage—put them on target for the very best health and longevity.

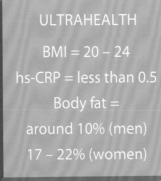

ULTRAHEALTH

BMI = 20 – 24
hs-CRP = less than 0.5
Body fat =
around 10% (men)
17 – 22% (women)

Your hs-CRP

Initial goal: less than 1.0 mg/L
Ultrahealth goal: less than 0.5 mg/L

The hs-CRP test (high-sensitivity C-reactive protein) is probably the best single indicator of how well your body is performing in terms of cellular aging. A low level lets you know that your body is negotiating successfully through our complex world and that you're in the best possible condition for long-term health and longevity.

If your goal is to reach optimal health, an hs-CRP level of less than 1.0 is a great start. But with Ultrahealth enhancements, you have a system that can help you reach an even healthier state. When your CRP reaches less than 0.5, you'll know that your body is positioned to thrive for a very long time indeed.

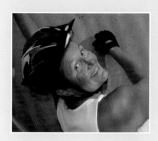

Does Your Inflammation Level Put You at Risk?

The American Heart Association and Centers for Disease Control have defined the following categories for disease risk based on CRP level:

Low risk: less than 1.0 mg/L

Average risk: 1.0 to 3.0 mg/L

High risk: above 3.0 mg/L

Your Body Mass Index

Initial goal: under 25
Ultrahealth goal: 20–24

At the beginning of your journey, we checked your body mass index (BMI) to assess your risk for cardiovascular disease, diabetes, and a variety of cancers, and we worked to get your BMI into a healthy range of under 25. But now we're returning to this old friend from a completely different orientation—to move you into and keep you in the zone of Ultrahealth. So just what does that mean?

The World Health Organization and the National Institutes of Health have proposed a normal BMI range of between 18.5 and 24.9. Values above or below this range increase the risk of premature death—above, because being overweight or obese leads to a whole host of serious diseases; and below, because a very low BMI probably reflects weight loss that's a result of diseases already present.

Many of the studies I've shared with you throughout the book support an association between high BMI and risk for diseases such as diabetes (see chart, below). Conversely, there's a proven connection between a BMI at the low-normal end of the range and optimum metabolic and cardiovascular health. And, research studies aside, I can tell you personally that I've had the opportunity to evaluate Calorie Restriction Society members who enjoy incredible cardiovascular and metabolic parameters and are thriving, happy human beings!

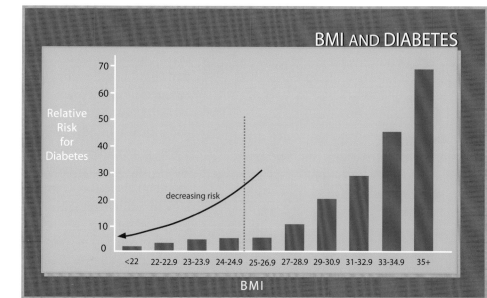

BMI AND DIABETES

Relative Risk for Diabetes

decreasing risk

<22 22-22.9 23-23.9 24-24.9 25-26.9 27-28.9 29-30.9 31-32.9 33-34.9 35+

BMI

BMI (Body Mass Index) and Diabetes.

As you can see from the chart, as your BMI goes down, so does your risk for developing type 2 diabetes. That's one of the reasons that a BMI of around 20 is ideal for ultimate health and disease resistance.*

American Journal of Epidemiology 132 (1990): 501–513.

While there may be some advantages to a BMI slightly lower than 20, until we have more information to support those benefits, I believe it's important to give the body a buffer and a bit of reserve. (In fact, I actually think you're better off focusing on CRP reduction as a goal.) That's why we've set your Ultrahealth BMI goal in the range of 20 to 24, a range that provides leeway for genetic and lifestyle differences and that reinforces an important point—that weight reduction is not the focus, but rather the result, of obtaining Ultrahealth.

Just remember to get a check-up and have blood work done by your physician as you approach the lower end of this range (around 20). We're exploring new ground here, and you and your lab results will help us find out more as we move to the next level and redefine health for the twenty-first century!

Your Percentage of Body Fat

Initial goal: 15–18% for men and 22–25% for women
Ultrahealth goal: around 10% for men and 17–22% for women

The amount of body fat we have varies according to genetics, culture, and environment, but our general goal is around 10 percent for men and between 17 and 22 percent for women.

Why such a difference between the sexes? Because in addition to *storage fat*, the fat we gain or lose as our weight changes—which normally makes up about 12 to 15 percent of a woman's total body weight—women carry gender-specific *essential fat* in their breasts, pelvis, hips, and thighs. This essential fat is biologically necessary for child bearing and other hormone-related functions, and should account for at least 10 to 12 percent of a woman's total weight. Together, these two types of fat make up the total percentage for women. But as always, for the best analysis of your individual needs, see your doctor.

Body Fat Percentage by Body Type, from the American Council on Exercise.
As we become lean and fit, our percentage of body fat decreases. For Ultrahealth, you should aim for a percentage in the "lean" category.

BODY FAT PERCENTAGE

BODY TYPE	Female (% Body Fat)	Male (% Body Fat)
Athletic	17	10
Lean	17 – 22	10 – 15
Normal	22 – 25	15 – 18
Overweight	25 – 29	18 – 20
Overfat	29 – 35	20 – 25
Obese	35+	25+

What about Dietary (Calorie) Restriction?

Throughout this book, we've discussed the importance of gaining command over your calorie intake, and have used that control as the vehicle for taking you on this journey.

First, we used it to help you reach a healthy weight. Then, as your body became able to move more freely, we found a balance between energy in and energy out. And then we set our sights on helping you reach optimal health. At each of these levels, we've also added Habits of Health, building a foundation of behaviors that will last you a lifetime.

Now, through the Habits of Longevity, we've taken your newfound mastery of energy intake, as well as those important supporting habits, and given you access to a state of health that few adults have ever experienced, or ever will. The final verdict on dietary (calorie) restriction as a longevity enhancer isn't in, nor do we yet know the absolute optimal intake needed to slow the aging process. But what we do know is this—that evidence suggests that dietary restriction, when accompanied by a balanced, nutrient-dense diet, should provide the same benefits of disease reduction and metabolic adaptation in humans as it does in animal studies.

And even if it turns out that dietary restriction doesn't extend mankind's maximum life span, its ability to help us spend more time in a healthier state is enough to be excited about. After all, who knows what possibilities are about to unfold? By living and thriving in Ultrahealth, you'll be in great position to take advantage of all the new advancements that science will undoubtedly reveal.

Let's get ready by taking a look at some of the techniques, both present and up-and-coming, that may well turn out to hold some of those secrets.

Wine: The Fountain of Youth?

Nothing more excellent nor more valuable than wine
was ever granted mankind by God.

–Plato

In 1991, CBS's *60 Minutes* broadcast its now famous "French Paradox" story, which reported that the French, despite a diet high in saturated fats, enjoy a lower death rate from heart disease than citizens of other Western nations. That single report sent baby boomers into a frenzy, envisioning trips to Napa Valley to fill their wine cellars with this new fountain of youth. Finally, a fun way to live longer without all that work!

Three thousand scientific articles and more than four hundred research projects later, we still don't definitively understand the importance of wine and alcohol to health or their role in life extension. Look online and you'll find over 180,000 Web sites with information on wine-related health studies. The general consensus is that wine taken in moderation does indeed benefit health. But just what is moderation, and what are the benefits?

Moderate drinking is defined as one drink a day for women and for men over 65, and two drinks a day for men under 65. This level of consumption has consistently been associated with lower levels of inflammation and lower risk for type 2 diabetes and heart disease.

According to a recent study, one drink a day can help the heart by relaxing the blood vessels, but more than that can actually increase heart rate. And all types of alcohol, including wine, have a blood-thinning effect that helps the circulatory system by making the blood platelets less sticky. But among the many varieties of alcoholic beverages, red wine stands out for its many additional health benefits, including its over 200 health-enhancing antioxidant

Heart disease in France is 60 percent lower than in the U.S. Could it be the red wine?

Health Benefits from Wine and Other Types of Alcohol

The antioxidant compounds in wine and other types of alcohol appear to have some amazing effects on the body—but remember, these positive effects come from **moderate** drinking and are outweighed by negative effects when too much alcohol is consumed.

Health benefits of polyphenols

- Raise HDL (good cholesterol)
- Lower LDL (bad cholesterol)
- Anticoagulate (thin the blood)
- Vasodilator (open the blood vessels)
- Reduce oxidative stress
- Decrease blood pressure
- Reduce risk of ischemic stroke in men (1–2 glasses red wine a day, 3–4 times a week)
- Reduce lipoproteins (fats) after eating, a possible explanation of the French Paradox

Health benefits of resveratrol (found in concentration in red wine)

- Anticarcinogen
- Inhibit the initiation and progression of cancer in a wide variety of tumor cells
- Anti-inflammatory
- Neuroprotective
- Antimicrobial
- Vasodilator (open the blood vessels)
- Stimulate life-extending enzymes

---

compounds called *polyphenols*. (White wine has similar antioxidants, but in concentrations so low that it would take twelve glasses of white wine to equal the benefits of one glass of red.)

Red wine is thought to have unique life-extension potential because of a high concentration of one of these polyphenols, resveratrol—which appears to be a particularly potent polyphenol, with an amazing range of health-enhancing antioxidant, anti-inflammatory, and antimicrobial effects. It's been shown to suppress tumor cells; help repair DNA; contribute to metabolic balance; improve diseases such as cardiovascular disease, cancer, and diabetes; and even fight H. pylori, the bacteria implicated in stomach ulcers. It's also been shown to stimulate a gene in mice that increases their sensitivity to insulin and prevents diabetes.

In addition to these general health benefits, red wine has been receiving a lot of attention lately for its ability to extend the life span in worms, fruit flies, and short-lived fish. It appears that resveratrol activates sirtuins, substances that attack cancer cells while leaving healthy cells intact—the same substances, in fact, that are activated by calorie restriction.

Wine may even play a role in the prevention of Alzheimer's disease. In a recent study, researchers at the University of Bordeaux tracked nearly 4,000 local residents over age 65. They found that light drinkers—those who drank up to two glasses of wine a day—were 45 percent less likely to develop Alzheimer's than nondrinkers. A Dutch study showed similar results in protection against dementia. So light drinking may indeed be protective well beyond its anti-stroke effect!

In Vino Veritas? Some Wine FAQs

Which types of wine have the most benefits?

Resveratrol, one of the most potent health enhancers in wine, is found in varieties of red wine such as pinot noir, cabernet, and syrah. Because resveratrol is made by the grape as a natural defense against cool and damp climates, ultraviolet light (common at higher altitudes), and fungal infections, grapes grown in areas with those conditions should have the greatest concentration of resveratrol.

Beneficial polyphenols are concentrated in the skins and seeds of grapes, making red wine, which is fermented with the skins, higher in beneficial substances than white wine.

Should I start drinking red wine?

If you're not currently drinking alcohol, I don't think the evidence is strong enough at this point to warrant starting. However, if you already drink alcohol, changing to red wine probably makes sense. Just be sure to limit your daily consumption to one drink if you're a woman or man over 65, and two drinks if you're a man under 65.

To help you stay within that guideline, take a look at the illustration at right, which compares four wine glasses of varying size. It may surprise you to learn that each of those glasses contains five ounces of wine—the recommended serving. A bottle of wine holds four of these five-ounce glasses plus one four-ounce glass, or about five total servings.

If you prefer not to drink, you do have the option of taking resveratrol supplements. The dosage I suggest is 100 mg per day. And of course, some people shouldn't drink alcohol at all (see box, page 324, Contraindications for Alcohol Consumption). Remember, alcohol is an extremely dangerous substance when abused, and overconsumption can diminish your health and actually increase your rate of cellular aging.

Will drinking wine or taking resveratrol supplements help me live longer?

Maybe. But until we learn the full effect, I recommend that you include wine in your Ultrahealth program only if you're already consuming alcohol. And

Various Five-Ounce Servings of Red Wine. Be careful with serving size! Remember, drinking a *moderate* amount of wine is key—just one five-ounce glass per day for women and men over 65, and two five-ounce glasses per day for men under 65. As you can see from the various five-ounce servings shown here, a large glass can hold quite a bit more than that!

Ready to Open That Bottle?
Don't Forget to Count Calories!

The alcohol content of wine varies widely, but is usually between 10 and 14 percent. Obviously, the higher the alcohol content, the higher the calories. A bottle of wine contains 750 milliliters of liquid, or 25.42 ounces—about five 5-ounce or six 4-ounce servings. So at twenty calories per ounce, a full bottle has approximately 525 calories.

> ### Contraindications for Alcohol Consumption:
> ### Who Shouldn't Drink Alcohol
>
> If you do choose to drink alcoholic beverages, don't exceed one drink per day for women and men over 65 and two drinks per day for men under 65. And if you fall into one of the following categories, please don't drink alcohol at all:
>
> - Children and adolescents
> - People of any age who can't restrict their drinking to moderate levels
> - Women who may become pregnant or who are pregnant
> - People who plan to drive, operate machinery, or take part in other activities that require attention, skill, or coordination
> - People taking prescription or over-the-counter medications that can interact with alcohol
> - People with specific medical conditions
> - People recovering from alcoholism

remember, a five-ounce glass of red wine has about 106 calories and a glass of white about 100 calories that must be taken into account!

What's on the Horizon?

As a young boy, I loved reading Jules Verne's books about submarines, airplanes, and space travel, as well as a host of science fiction stories about inventions that hadn't even been created. His books, including *Journey to the Center of the Earth, Around the World in Eighty Days,* and my favorite, *Twenty Thousand Leagues Under the Sea,* have been translated more often than nearly any other author's (only Disney productions and Agatha Christie's works can boast more). Clearly, we're all fascinated by the ability of science to create endless possibilities.

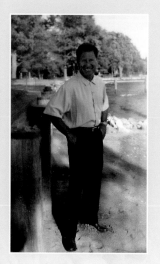

Author and futurist Ray Kurzweil reminds me a lot of Jules Verne. He believes that the cavalry that's going to help us live forever is just around the corner. He has vision, creativity, and most important, he's living a healthy lifestyle. Here's an extract from an interview he gave CNN.*

> Futurist and author Ray Kurzweil pops a couple hundred supplements a day, eats an extremely healthy diet and exercises. Kurzweil says he plans to live long enough to live forever.
>
> Kurzweil's strategy for immortality is based on the premise that science moves forward exponentially, with breakthroughs building on each other and coming at a faster and faster rate. As a result, he thinks life expectancy will start extending to the point where he can live indefinitely.
>
> Kurzweil is dead serious about this.

*David S. Martin, "The Future of Longevity," interview with Ray Kurzweil, CNN, May 9, 2007, http://www.cnn.com/2007/HEALTH/03/23/chasinglife.fountainyouth/index.html.

"It's going to be a very different situation ten or fifteen years from now," says Kurzweil, author of *The Singularity Is Near: When Humans Transcend Biology.*

"We have very sharply designed interventions that can stop disease. So for baby boomers, we'd like to be in good shape ten or fifteen years from now when we have the sort of full flowering of the biotechnology revolution."

Science is indeed making progress decoding the factors necessary to extend life. We're beginning to learn how telomeres unravel, a discovery that could teach us how to increase the production of telomerase and perhaps prevent this built-in aging process. We're learning more about several potent inducers of cell survival, such as the class of enzymes called sirtuins, which we discussed earlier, and which have the ability to specifically change NAD-dependent histone deacetylases, protecting our DNA and helping our mitochondria become more resilient to aging. Using complex computers, we're identifying genes that play a role in longevity. In just the past few years, Dr. Nir Barzilia, of Albert Einstein College of Medicine, has discovered, by studying the genes of centenarians, three longevity genes that shield against heart disease.

Eventually we'll unlock the secrets of aging, just as sure as we've created submarines that can visit the Titanic 10,000 feet below sea level, learned to fly faster than the speed of sound, and put a man on the moon.

For certain, Ray Kurzweil's advice is accurate in at least one regard. In order for any of these wonderful scientific advancements to help us live longer, we must do our part to fulfill that destiny—by maintaining a healthy lifestyle and optimal health, for today and for that boundless future.

• •

Dr. A's Habits of Health provide that for you now, and they'll provide it for you then!

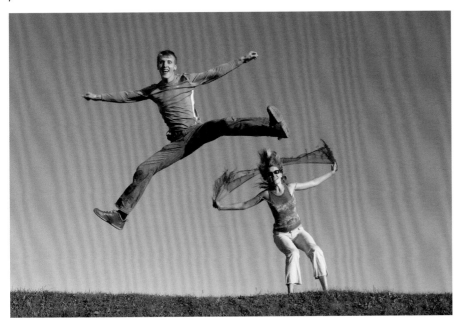

Appendix A

Physician Information

Your patient has made the fundamental choice to create health in his or her life by taking part in a comprehensive health-modification program, the first step of which is reaching a healthy weight.

I've asked them to share this information with you to ensure that they have the proper medical supervision as they undergo this transformation to optimal health. The following is a brief description of the program and some suggested medical support.

- **Phase I: Weight Loss**
  - ✓ Calorie reduction
  - ✓ Dietary focus on low-glycemic carbohydrates, healthy fats, and proteins
  - ✓ q. 3-hour portion control using medically formulated, low-calorie portion-controlled meal replacements (PCMRs)
  - ✓ Instruction in healthy eating system
  - ✓ Increased daily movement

- **Phase II: Lifestyle Change**
  - ✓ Healthy eating for life
  - ✓ Increased exercise through daily walking plan and resistance training
  - ✓ Improved sleeping patterns
  - ✓ Support through personal coach, online tracking, and/or bionetwork health community
  - ✓ Ongoing instruction through Habits of Health book, workbook, and DVD
  - ✓ Behavioral changes through focus on motivation and choices to support health

- **Phase III: Creating a Microenvironment of Health**
  - ✓ Removal of inflammatory stimulators (i.e., water, air, and home toxins)
  - ✓ Stress reduction
  - ✓ Enhancement of healthy nutrients

Your patient will be eating a reduced amount of energy-dense, low-glycemic food and will lose on average 2–5 pounds per week for the first 2 weeks and 1–2 pounds per week thereafter. As a result, their blood sugar, cholesterol, triglycerides, blood pressure, and hs-CRP will decrease significantly. Diabetics should lower their hypoglycemic medications and increase blood sugar monitoring as they begin this new eating pattern to avoid hypoglycemia.

Suggested Diagnostics

In addition to routine blood chemistry, suggested labs include lipid profile for a baseline, hs-CRP, and EKG. A cardiovascular assessment is suggested in high-risk individuals especially if they have considerable weight to lose or have been inactive.

Significant Disease Caution

The presence of significant medical conditions and certain medications may contraindicate the use of this program. Do not use the Medifast Program if you are pregnant. If you have a serious acute or chronic illness (i.e., heart attack, cancer, liver disease, kidney disease, anorexia, bulimia, etc.), do not use Medifast until your health care provider says you have recovered or that your condition is stabilized.

For more information on our program, go to www.habitsofhealth.net or contact a health coach.

Appendix B

Evening Meal Recipes

Day 1   BROILED COD (SCROD) with LEMON PEPPER

Makes two portions.

12 ounces cod (or similar white fish)
½ lemon
1 tsp. black pepper

1. Turn broiler to high. Cover broiler pan with foil and spray with nonstick cooking spray.
2. Cut scrod into two pieces.
3. Squeeze lemon juice over fish.
4. Sprinkle with fresh-ground black pepper.
5. Place fish on broiler pan and place under broiler for 5–6 minutes or until fish is white and flaky throughout. (Do not overcook or fish will become dry.)

Day 2   GRILLED HERBED CHICKEN BREAST

Makes two portions.

10 ounces boneless/skinless chicken breast
Mixture of black pepper, garlic powder, basil, and oregano (½ tsp. each)

1. Preheat grill or sauté pan.
2. Divide chicken into two pieces and sprinkle top and bottom with herbs.
3. Place chicken top-side down on heated grill/pan. Cook for 3–4 minutes and turn. Cook for an additional 3–4 minutes or until cooked through. (Internal temperature should be 165 degrees.)
4. Remove from grill/pan and serve.

Day 3   ROASTED PORK TENDERLOIN

Makes two portions.

10–12 ounces pork tenderloin
½ tsp. pepper
½ tsp. garlic powder
1 tsp. tarragon
pinch salt

1. Preheat oven to 350 degrees.
2. Season pork with the herbs.
3. Place pork in roasting pan in preheated oven.
4. Roast for 10–12 minutes or until internal temperature reaches 155 degrees.
5. Remove from oven and let rest for 5 minutes. Slice on a bias and serve.

Day 4   MONTREAL GRILLED BEEF

Makes two portions.

10–12 ounces lean beef (e.g., sirloin, flank steak)
1½ tbsp. Montreal seasoning mix

1. Preheat grill.
2. Rub meat top and bottom with Montreal seasoning mix and let sit for ten minutes at room temperature.
3. Place beef on grill and cook for 4–6 minutes. Turn over and cook for 3–4 minutes more or until desired doneness.
4. Remove from grill and let rest for 5 minutes. Slice and serve.

Day 5   HERBED POACHED SALMON

Makes two portions.

12 ounces fresh salmon
1 quart poaching liquid (1 quart water, ½ cup lemon juice, 1 tsp. black pepper)
1 bunch fresh dill, chopped
½ tsp. ginger powder

1. Place the poaching liquid with the dill and ginger in a pan large enough to hold the salmon. There should be enough liquid to cover the salmon.
2. Heat poaching liquid until tiny bubbles start to form (around 180 degrees).
3. Place salmon in pan and poach for 6–8 minutes or until salmon is cooked through. Salmon should be firm and slightly flaky.
4. Remove salmon from pan and drain excess liquid from fish. Place on a heated plate and serve.

Day 6   SAUTEED CHICKEN with LEMON and CAPERS

Makes two portions.

Two 6-ounce boneless/skinless chicken breasts
Juice from ½ lemon
2 tbsp. capers
½ tsp. black pepper
2 pinches salt

1. Preheat sauté pan.
2. Season chicken with salt and pepper.
3. Spray pan with nonstick cooking spray.
4. Place chicken top-side down and cook for 3 minutes. Turn over and cook for 2 minutes more.
5. Add lemon juice and capers. Cook for 2–3 minutes or until cooked through.
6. Place chicken on plate and pour pan drippings over each portion.

Day 7 GRILLED CHINESE FIVE-SPICE BEEF

Makes two portions.

10 ounces sirloin or London broil

3 tbsp. Chinese five-spice powder

1. Rub beef top and bottom with seasoning and let sit for 5–8 minutes.
2. Heat grill or sauté pan until hot. (If using sauté pan, spray with nonstick cooking spray.)
3. Place beef on grill and cook for 3 minutes. Turn over and cook an additional 3–5 minutes or until desired doneness.
4. Remove beef from heat and let rest for 5 minutes.
5. Slice thin and divide into two portions.

Day 8 MARINATED TURKEY CUTLET

Makes two portions.

12 ounces uncooked turkey breast

¼ cup white wine

3 tbsp. lemon juice

1 tbsp. minced garlic

1 tsp. chopped fresh rosemary

1 tsp. chopped fresh sage

½ tsp. salt

½ tsp. pepper

1. Combine all ingredients except for turkey and mix well.
2. Cut turkey breast into two pieces
3. Place turkey in pan and pour marinade over top. Cover with plastic wrap and refrigerate overnight.
4. Preheat grill.
5. Place turkey breast on grill and cook for 5–6 minutes. Turn over and cook for 4–5 minutes more or until cooked through. (Internal temperature should be 160 degrees.)
6. Remove from grill and let rest for 5 minutes. Plate and serve.

Day 9 SIRLOIN and VEGETABLE KABOBS

Makes two portions.

14 ounces top sirloin steak, cut into 1½ inch cubes

½ green pepper, cubed

½ red pepper, cubed

8 button mushrooms

8 cherry tomatoes

Marinade (combine 1 tsp. dry mustard, ½ tsp. pepper, ¼ cup balsamic vinegar, 1 tsp. garlic powder, 1 tsp. lemon juice, ½ tbsp. chopped parsley, ¼ cup water)

1. Place meat in pan and cover with marinade mix. Refrigerate overnight.
2. Soak wooden skewers in water for 30 minutes.
3. Remove meat from marinade. Place sirloin, green pepper, mushroom, cherry tomato, and red pepper on skewers, alternating items.
4. Preheat grill.

5. Place skewers on grill and cook for 3–4 minutes. Turn and continue cooking until meat reaches desired doneness.
6. Remove from grill and serve.

Day 10 GRILLED SEA BASS with TOMATO SALSA

Makes two portions.

14 ounces sea bass
1 tsp. olive oil

For salsa:
4 ounces diced cucumber
4 ounces diced tomato
¼ cup chopped green onion
⅛ cup lime juice
1 tsp. minced garlic
½ tsp. cumin powder
¼ cup chopped cilantro

1. Combine salsa ingredients and let sit for at least two hours.
2. Preheat grill.
3. Cut sea bass into two pieces.
4. Brush fish with oil and place on grill.
5. Cook for 2 minutes. Turn over and cook for 2–3 minutes more or until cooked through.
6. Remove from grill and serve with 3 tbsp. salsa per portion.

Day 11 SAUTEED CHICKEN with BASIL and LEMON

Makes two portions.

12 ounces boneless/skinless chicken breast
1 tsp. black pepper
pinch of salt
3 tbsp. lemon juice
8 sliced basil leaves or 2 tsp. dry basil

1. Divide chicken into two pieces.
2. Sprinkle salt and pepper over each portion of chicken.
3. Heat sauté pan.
4. Place chicken in pan and cook for 3–4 minutes. Turn over and cook an additional 3–4 minutes.
5. Add lemon juice and basil to chicken and cook for 2 minutes more or until chicken is cooked through.
6. Remove chicken from pan, place on a plate, and pour pan drippings over chicken.

Day 12 SEARED SEA SCALLOPS

Makes two portions.

12 ounces sea scallops
Fresh ground black pepper to taste
Lemon or lime juice

(continued next page)

(Seared Sea Scallops continued)

1. Preheat grill.
2. Grind black pepper over scallops.
3. Place scallops onto hot grill and cook for 2–3 minutes. Turn over and cook for 1–2 minutes more. (Do not overcook or scallops will become tough.) Scallops will be opaque when cooked.
4. Remove from grill and place on plate. Squeeze lemon or lime juice over scallops.

Day 13 SAUTEED GINGER BEEF

Makes two portions.

12 ounces beef sirloin or top round
¾ cup water
½ cup rice vinegar
2 tbsp. minced fresh ginger
1 tbsp. minced garlic
¼ cup sliced green onion
1 tsp. olive oil

1. Cut beef into quarter-inch strips.
2. Combine water, vinegar, ginger, and garlic.
3. Cover beef with marinade and let sit for 10 minutes.
4. Heat sauté pan and add oil.
5. When pan is hot, remove beef from marinade and drain excess liquid.
6. Place beef in pan and cook for 3–4 minutes. (Do not overcook or beef will become tough.)
7. Remove beef from pan and set aside. Add marinade to pan and cook until liquid is reduced by half.
8. Pour liquid over beef as desired and sprinkle with green onions.

Day 14 BALSAMIC GLAZED CHICKEN with ROSEMARY

Makes two portions.

Two 6-ounce boneless/skinless chicken breasts
2 tbsp. diced onion
1 tbsp. minced garlic
½ cup balsamic vinegar
½ cup water
1 tsp. olive oil
1 sprig fresh rosemary, chopped fine
¼ tsp. black pepper

1. Combine onion, garlic, vinegar, pepper, water, oil, and rosemary in a bowl.
2. Add chicken and marinate for 2–3 hours or overnight.
3. Remove chicken from marinade and pat dry.
4. Heat grill or set broiler to high and cook chicken for 4–5 minutes. Turn and cook for 3–4 minutes more or until cooked through.
5. Remove from heat and serve.

Appendix C

Buying a Pedometer

Pedometers are a great way to find out how many steps you take in a day—whether through NEAT activities such as your daily chores or as part of your formal EAT Walking Program. They've even been found to improve health by motivating users to increase the amount of physical activity they get, according to a study in the *Journal of the American Medical Association.** But with so many models out there to choose from, it can be hard to know what's best. Here are some tips to make choosing a pedometer that suits your needs a little easier.

Features. Basic, inexpensive pedometers simply count steps. More advanced models also give calorie counts and measure distance by multiplying the number of steps by stride length—but these features have been found to be fairly problematic to use and are often inaccurate. A more accurate, but more expensive, option is a GPS-based pedometer. Other common options include alarms, backlights (useful if you walk early in the morning or late in the evening), memory functions, pulse meters, even radios! But before you spend the extra money, think about which of those additional features you're likely to use.

Accuracy. Reports show that the accuracy of many pedometers varies, particularly at low speed. Several Web sites, including www.medicinenet.com, www.ConsumerSearch.com, and www.pedometers.com, offer suggestions and reports on accuracy of various models, or check out the user reviews on sites like www.amazon.com. Once you do choose a model, be sure you position it correctly, according to manufacturer's instructions. Most pedometers are worn at the waist, and should be placed as close to the hipbone as possible.

Style. Like many cell phones, pedometers come in open-face and flip-down styles. You may find that one type is more comfortable to wear, or gives you better access to the buttons and screen. If you buy an open-face model, try to find one with a protective cover so the buttons don't get accidentally bumped. Whichever type you choose, make sure the screen is easy to read. Ideally, you want to be able to read the information without taking off the pedometer.

And of course, don't forget to record your daily steps in your NEAT and EAT logs to make sure you're meeting or even exceeding your goals!

*Bravata, D. M., et al., "Using Pedometers to Increase Physical Activity and Improve Health," *Journal of the American Medical Association* 298 (November 21, 2007): 2296–2304.

Note: The charts in appendix D can be downloaded from the Web site at www.habitsofhealth.net.

Appendix D

NEAT Scoring Sheet

Category	NEAT Points	Energy Expenditure
Stance (Posture)		
Core position focus	1 point per minute	1 kcal/min
Balance ball	10 points per hour	10 kcal/hour
Sitting to moving	1 point	1 kcal
Standing		
Standing upright	1 point per minute	1 kcal/min

Strolling (Walking)

1. Record your total steps per day (TSD).
2. Divide your TSD by your Energetic Step Value ESV (see chart) to find your NEAT points.

Energetic Step Value (ESV) (steps required to burn 1 kcal). Locate your BMI in the left-hand column of the chart to find out how many steps you must take to burn one calorie. This number is your Energetic Step Value (ESV), which you'll use to calculate the total number of NEAT points you earn from walking.

ENERGETIC STEP VALUE (ESV)
(steps required to burn 1 kcal)

Body Mass Index BMI	ESV (Female)	ESV (Male)
18 – 24.9 Healthy	36 steps per kcal	28 steps per kcal
25 – 29.9 Overweight	30 steps per kcal	24 steps per kcal
30 – 34.9 Class I Obesity	24 steps per kcal	20 steps per kcal
35 – 39.9 Class II Obesity	18 steps per kcal	16 steps per kcal
Over 40 Class III Obesity	12 steps per kcal	11 steps per kcal

Stairs

1. Record the flights of stairs you climb (up and down) per day.
2. Multiply that number by your NEAT points per flight (see chart) to find your total NEAT points.

NEAT POINTS PER FLIGHT OF STAIRS

Body Mass Index BMI	NEAT Points per flight (up and down)
<25	3
25 – 30	4
30 – 35	5
35 – 40	6
>40	7

NEAT Points per Flight of Stairs. Locate your BMI in the left-hand column to find out how many NEAT points you earn for each flight of stairs you climb.

Samba

Listening to music (up-tempo)	1 point per minute	1 kcal/min
Slow to moderate dancing	3 points per minute	3 kcal/min
Fast to intense dancing	5 points per minute	5 kcal/min

Switch

Minor manual task	1 point per task	1 kcal
Manual chore	3 points per minute	3 kcal/min

Daily NEAT Activity Log

	Stance	Standing	Strolling	Stairs	Samba	Switch
7:00 – 8:00 am						
8:00 – 9:00 am						
9:00 – 10:00 am						
10:00 – 11:00 am						
11:00 – 12:00 am						
12:00 – 1:00 pm						
1:00 – 2:00 pm						
2:00 – 3:00 pm						
3:00 – 4:00 pm						
4:00 – 5:00 pm						
5:00 – 6:00 pm						
6:00 – 7:00 pm						
7:00 – 8:00 pm						
8:00 – 9:00 pm						
9:00 – 10:00 pm						
Total						
	Core position (minutes) ———— Balance ball (hours) ———— Sitting to moving ————	Minutes ————	Total steps per day (TSD) ———— Energetic Step Value ————	Flights per day ———— NEAT points per flight ————	Music (minutes) ———— Slow dance (minutes) ———— Fast dance (minutes) ————	Tasks ———— Chores (minutes) ————
NEAT Points						
NEAT Point Guide	Core position focus 1 point per minute Balance ball 10 points per hour Sitting to moving 1 point	Standing 1 point per minute	TSD ÷ ESV = total NEAT points	Flights (up and down) x points per flight = total NEAT points	Upbeat music 1 point per minute Slow dance 3 points per minute Fast dance 5 points per minute	Manual task 1 point Manual chore 3 points per minute

Weekly NEAT Activity Log

NEAT Points	Monday	Tuesday	Wednesday	Thursday	Friday	Saturday	Sunday	Total NEAT Points
Stance								
Standing								
Strolling								
Stairs								
Samba								
Switch								

NEAT Goal Setter

Your goals for this initial stage of your lifetime movement plan are as follows:

- 120 NEAT points per day for the first thirty days.
- 200 NEAT points per day for the second thirty days.

Depending on your current lifestyle and activity level, I suggest you focus on adding one additional activity per day for the first week, then one additional activity in each category starting the second week, until you've reached 200 NEAT points per day.

	ADD 1 NEW NEAT "S" ACTIVITY PER DAY
DAY 1	
DAY 2	
DAY 3	
DAY 4	
DAY 5	
DAY 6	
DAY 7	

Starting in the second week, add one additional NEAT "S" activity per week in each category.

	S	+ S	+ S	+ S	+ S	+ S
WEEK 2 Add 1 activity per category						
WEEK 3 Add 1 activity per category						
WEEK 4 Add 1 activity per category						

Appendix E
Exercises

The following exercises have been reviewed and approved by Greg Freitag, MS, CSCS, exercise physiologist at Johns Hopkins Weight Management Center.

DAILY STRETCHES
Abdominals

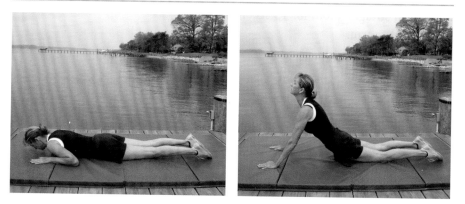

Lie face down on your mat. Point your toes and bend your arms, palms face down on the mat. Exhale as you extend your arms and raise your body, keeping your head in line with your spine. Hold for 15 seconds.

Chest

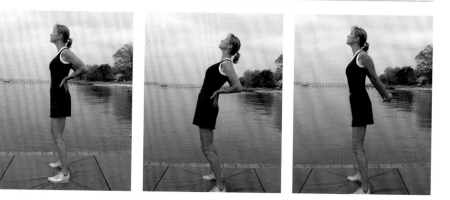

Stand with your feet shoulder-width apart. Place your hands in the small of your back and arch your back until you feel the stretch. As a variation, clasp your hands behind your back and pull outward. Hold for 15 seconds.

(partial text visible from previous page)

CORE
Level On...

Choice A:
Lie on your
palms unde
your knees
Take a deep
contract you
shoulders a
just 2–5 inc
and lower b
with your sp
than bendii
for 4 secon

Choice B:
Stand up
knees sligh
if you're h
and rotate
side, back t
and delibe
repetitions.

Choice C
Stand with
bent. Keep
hand on y
the right fo
on the oth
increase th

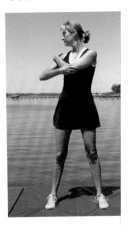

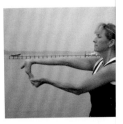

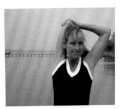

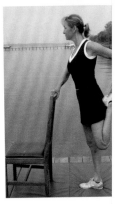

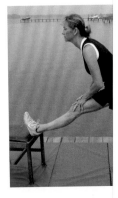

Level Two

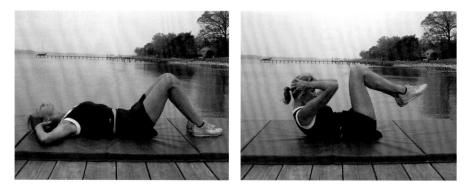

Choice A: Total Crunch

Lie on your back on a mat or on a cushioned rug, palms under your head, fingers unlocked. Bend your knees and place your feet flat on the floor. Take a deep breath and slowly let it out as you contract your abdominal muscles. Slowly bring your knees up toward your head and crunch your upper torso to your knees. Lift for 8 seconds, hold for 4 seconds, lower for 8 seconds. Do five repetitions.

Choice B: Twist Crunch

Lie on your back with your hands behind your head, knees bent at a 90 degree angle. Slowly rotate one elbow toward the opposite knee, curling your upper body (8 seconds). Hold (4 seconds) and slowly return to start. Do five repetitions on each side.

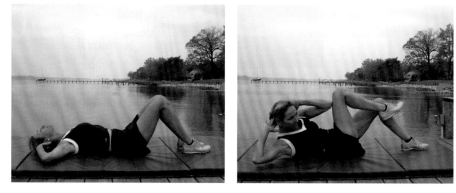

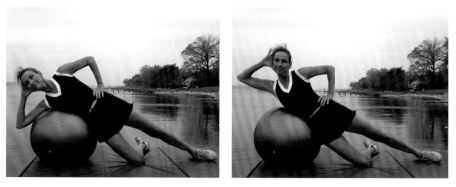

Choice C: Side Crunch on Ball

Lie sideways on an exercise ball, waist and hips touching the ball. Bend your lower leg, keeping your upper leg extended, and bend your lower arm and place your hand on your temple. If you need to, rest your upper hand on the ball for balance. Lift your torso slowly, using your oblique muscles and squeezing your rib cage (8 seconds). Hold (4 seconds) and return to start (8 seconds), using controlled movements. Do five repetitions on each side.

CHEST
Level One

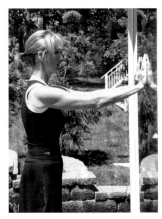
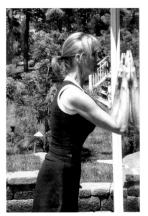

Choice A: Wall Push-Off

Stand at arm's length from a wall, palms shoulder-width apart on the wall. Slowly bend your elbows, bringing your body toward the wall until your face is close to the wall (8 seconds). Hold (4 seconds) and slowly return to start (8 seconds). Keep your abdominal muscles tight and don't move your feet. Do five repetitions.

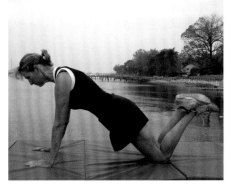
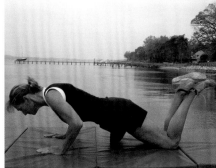

Choice B: Push-Up on Knees

Get on all fours on your mat, knees hip-width apart and hands slightly wider than your shoulders. Point your fingers forward. Slowly lower your upper body, keeping your abdominals tight and your body in a straight line (8 seconds). Your elbows should bend back, not out. Hold (4 seconds) and lift yourself back up (8 seconds). Do five repetitions.

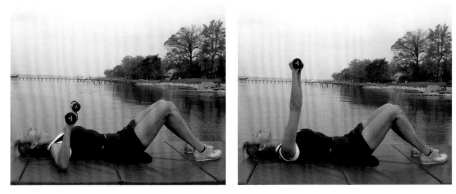

Choice C: Flat Press on Mat

Lie on your mat, face up, holding a dumbbell or soup can in each hand. Extend your arms upward, pressing the ends of the weights together, then slowly bend your elbows to lower the weights (8 seconds). Stop just before your arms touch the floor and hold (4 seconds). Slowly return to start (8 seconds). Do five repetitions. To increase the challenge, try performing this exercise while lying on an exercise ball.

Level Two

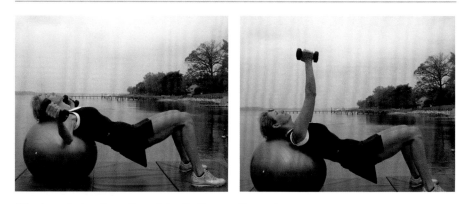

Choice A: Incline Dumbbell Fly on Exercise Ball

Begin this exercise using light weights, then add more weight progressively as you're able. Holding a pair of dumbbells or soup cans, lie on an exercise ball with your head and neck supported by the ball. Your lower back and hips should be off the ball, with your bottom a few inches from the ground. Extend the dumbbells over your chest, palms facing each other, elbows slightly bent. Slowly lower the weights down and outward (8 seconds), hold (4 seconds), and slowly raise them back over your chest to the starting position (8 seconds). Do five repetitions.

Choice B: Incline Push-Up

Lean against a chair or stairway and walk your feet back far enough so that your body is in an incline position. Keep your head in alignment with your straight back and tighten your abdominals. Lower yourself toward the chair or step (8 seconds), hold (4 seconds), and slowly return (8 seconds). Do five repetitions.

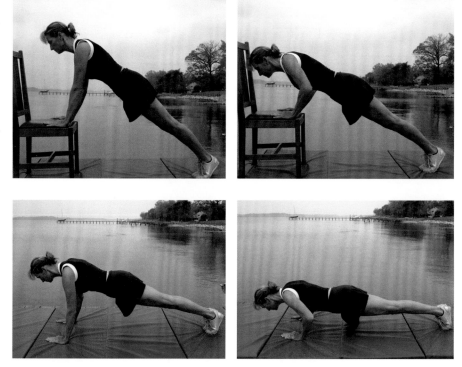

Choice C: Plank Push-Up

Stand at the end of your mat. Lean over and walk your hands out until your body is in a plank position. Keeping your body straight and your abdominals tight, slowly begin to lower your body by bending at your elbows. Make sure your elbows are bending back and not out. Lower for 8 seconds, hold for 4 seconds and push up for 8 seconds. Do five repetitions.

BACK (LATISSIMUS DORSI)
Level One

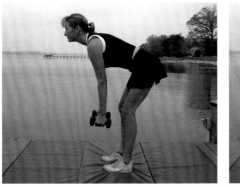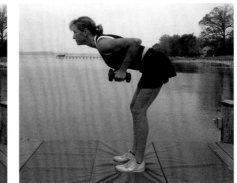

Choice A: Bent-Over Row

Holding a pair of light dumbbells or soup cans, bend forward at the waist. Your feet should be hip-width apart and your knees slightly bent. Extend your arms toward your feet, palms facing in. Make sure you're looking forward, with a slight arch in your back. Slowly bend your elbows, pulling the weights up (8 seconds), hold (4 seconds), and return (8 seconds). Do five repetitions.

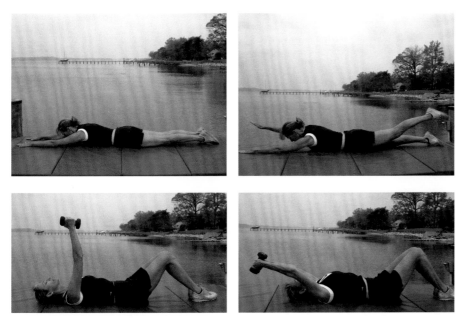

Choice B: Swimming

Lie face down on a mat, arms extended above your head. Look forward, keeping your face off the mat. Alternate lifting your opposite arm and leg (4 seconds), hold (4 seconds), and slowly return (4 seconds). Do five repetitions.

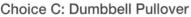

Choice C: Dumbbell Pullover

You can begin this exercise without weights if you prefer and gradually add them as you're able. Holding a pair of dumbbells or soup cans, lie on your mat with your knees bent. Make sure your lower back is flat against the mat and your abdominals are tight. Keeping your arms slightly bent, raise them above your head and then slowly lower them to the floor behind your head (8 seconds). Hold (4 seconds), then slowly lift your arms back to start (8 seconds), keeping your back muscles contracted and your abdominals tight. Add more weight as you're able. Do five repetitions.

Level Two

Choice A: Hyperextension on Exercise Ball

Lie face down with an exercise ball under your hips and lower abdomen, palms on the floor about shoulder-width apart. Your feet should be about three inches from the ground. Keeping your feet together and your legs straight, slowly raise your heels toward the ceiling (8 seconds), hold (4 seconds), and lower them back down (8 seconds). Do five repetitions.

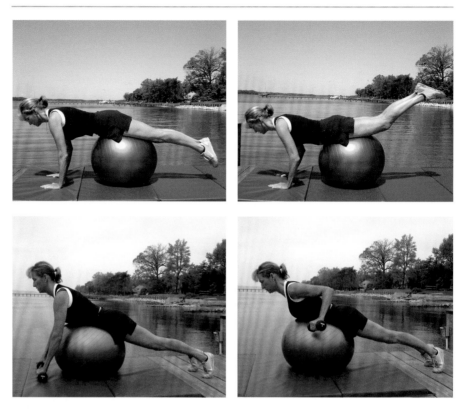

Choice B: Dumbbell Row with Exercise Ball

Holding dumbbells or soup cans, lie on an exercise ball so that the middle of your abdomen is touching the ball. Raise your head and chest, creating a slight arch in your back. Your legs should be straight behind you, with your arms hanging down, palms facing the ball. Using your back muscles, slowly pull the dumbbells up and back toward your hips using a rowing motion (8 seconds). Hold, squeezing your shoulder blades together (4 seconds), then slowly return to the starting position (8 seconds). Do five repetitions.

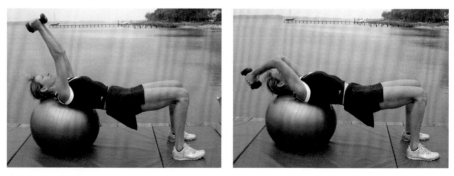

Choice C: Exercise Ball Pullover

Holding either one dumbbell or soup can or a small medicine ball, lie on an exercise ball with your head and neck supported. Your knees should be bent, hips raised, and abdominals tight. Maintain this position throughout the exercise. Slowly lower the weight behind your head (8 seconds), hold (4 seconds), and slowly raise the weight (8 seconds), contracting your back muscles and tightening your abdominals. Do five repetitions.

SHOULDERS
Level One

Choice A:
Seated Shoulder Press

Sit on a chair with your legs about shoulder-width apart. Keep your back straight, your abdominals tight, and your chin raised. Start with light weights (2 pounds) or soup cans and add weight as you feel

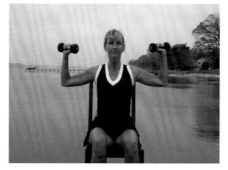

able. Holding a can or dumbbell in each hand, bend your elbows and lift your arms until your hands are at ear level, palms facing forward. Slowly extend your hands above your head (8 seconds), hold (4 seconds), and lower your hands back to your ears (8 seconds). Do five repetitions. This exercise can be done in a standing position if you prefer.

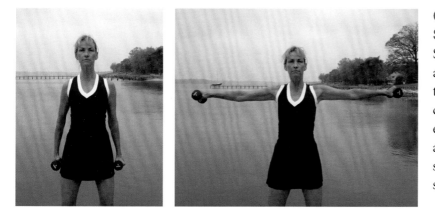

Choice B:
Standing Dumbbell Raise

Stand with your feet shoulder-width apart, back straight and abdominals tight. Holding dumbbells or soup cans, place your arms by your sides, elbows slightly bent. Slowly raise your arms up and out (8 seconds), hold (4 seconds), and lower back to start (8 seconds). Do five repetitions.

Choice C: Seated Reverse Lateral

Holding a pair of dumbbells or soup cans, sit on an exercise ball or chair, back straight and abdominals tight. Extend your arms over your head, elbows slightly bent, palms facing each other. Slowly lower the weights to shoulder height (8 seconds), hold (4 seconds), and raise them back up (4 seconds). Do five repetitions.

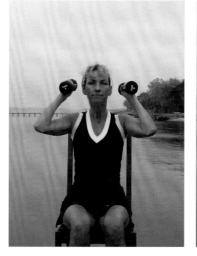

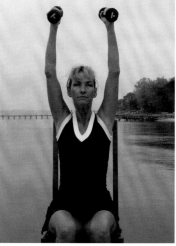

Level Two

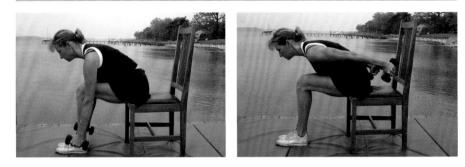

Choice A: Seated Rear Deltoid Raise

Sit on the edge of a chair or bench, feet flat on the floor. Holding a pair of dumbbells or soup cans, lean forward until your chest is almost touching your knees. With your arms next to your legs, palms facing each other and elbows slightly bent, slowly raise the weights up and outward until your arms are almost parallel to the floor (8 seconds). Contract the muscles in the back of your shoulders and hold (4 seconds), then slowly return (8 seconds). Do five repetitions.

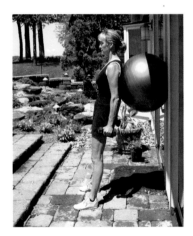

Choice B: Front Deltoid Raise with Exercise Ball

Holding a pair of dumbbells or soup cans, stand with an exercise ball between you and the wall, with the ball touching your shoulder blades. Place your feet slightly forward, so they're a bit farther from the wall than the rest of your body. With your elbows slightly bent, raise the weights to eye level (8 seconds), hold (4 seconds), and slowly lower (8 seconds). Do five repetitions.

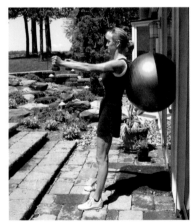

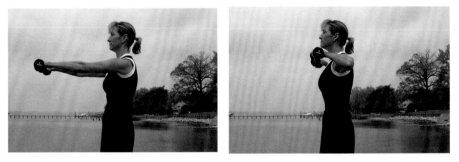

Choice C: Upright Row

Holding a pair of dumbbells or soup cans, stand with your feet together, knees slightly bent. Extend your arms in front of you, palms facing down and elbows slightly bent. Keeping your back straight and your abdominals tight, slowly lift the weights toward your chin (8 seconds), hold (4 seconds), and lower (8 seconds). Do five repetitions.

ARMS
Level One

Choice A: Standing Dumbbell Curl

Stand with your feet shoulder-width apart, knees slightly bent. Holding dumbbells or soup cans, place your arms at your sides, palms facing out. Keep your abdominals tight and your back straight, and extend your arms. Slowly bend your elbows and curl your arms up (8 seconds), hold (4 seconds), and lower (8 seconds). Do five repetitions.

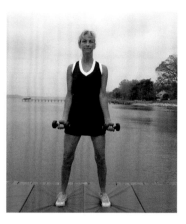
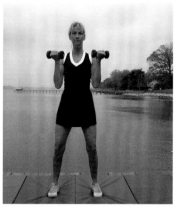

Choice B: Standing Dumbbell Kickback

Hold a pair of dumbbells or soup cans at your side, palms facing in. Keeping your back straight, bend at the waist and look forward, creating a slight arch in your back. Bend your knees slightly. Raise your elbows as high as possible, keeping them close to your body. This is the start position. Slowly extend your hands back without moving your upper arms (8 seconds), hold (4 seconds), then return to start and squeeze (8 seconds). Do five repetitions.

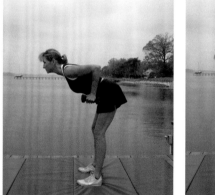
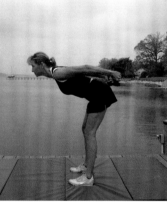

Choice C: Overhead Triceps Extension on Exercise Ball

Holding one dumbbell or soup can, sit on an exercise ball or bench with your back straight, feet shoulder-width apart. Extend your arms over your head, with your elbows slightly bent and your biceps tight against your head. Bending your elbows slowly, lower the weight toward your back (8 seconds), hold (4 seconds), and lift the weight back to start (8 seconds). Do five repetitions.

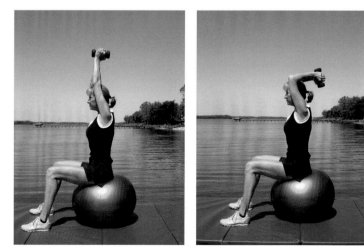

Level Two

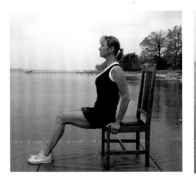
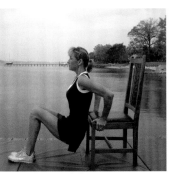

Choice A: Chair Dip

Sit on the edge of a chair with your legs out in front of you, and grip the sides of the chair with your hands. Bending your knees and elbows, slowly lower yourself in front of the chair (8 seconds), hold (4 seconds), and slowly lift yourself back up to start (8 seconds). Do five repetitions. To increase the challenge, place your feet on an exercise ball in front of you.

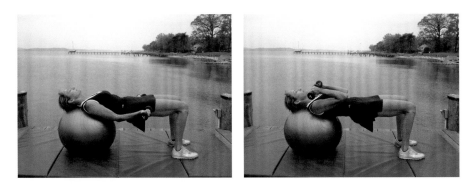

Choice B: Incline Curl on Ball

Sit on an exercise ball, holding a pair of dumbbells or soup cans. Roll forward until your head, neck, and upper back are supported by the ball. Your knees should be bent and your feet flat on the floor. Place your arms by your sides, palms facing up. Bending your elbows, slowly curl your arms up (8 seconds), hold (4 seconds), and return to start (8 seconds). Do five repetitions.

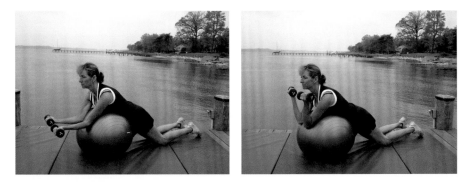

Choice C: Preacher Curl on Exercise Ball

Holding dumbbells or soup cans, lean over an exercise ball with your knees on the floor. Place your elbows and upper arms on the ball and extend your arms in front of you, palms facing up. Slowly curl your arms (8 seconds), hold (4 seconds), and return (8 seconds). Do five repetitions.

Lower Body

CORE
Level One

Choice A: Leg Drop

Lie on your back with your legs bent and your feet off the ground at a 45 degree angle. Cross your arms over your chest or place them under your buttocks if you need more support for your back. Slowly lower both legs to the floor (8 seconds), tap the floor with your toes and hold (4 seconds), and slowly return to start (8 seconds). Do five repetitions. If you find this exercise too difficult, try lifting one leg at a time, alternating legs.

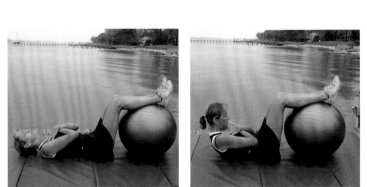

Choice B: Elevated Leg Crunch

Lie on your back with your feet at a 90 degree angle. Cross your arms over your chest, tighten your abdominal muscles, and raise your head and shoulders slowly off the floor (8 seconds). Hold (4 seconds) and slowly lower your head and shoulders back to start (8 seconds). Do five repetitions.

Choice C: Segmental Roll

Lie on your back with your knees bent and your back in a neutral position. Tighten your abdominals. Keeping your shoulders on the ground, let your knees fall slowly to the left, going only as far as is comfortable (8 seconds). Hold (4 seconds) before slowly returning to start (8 seconds).

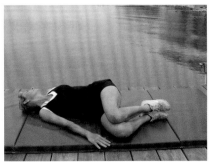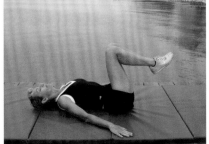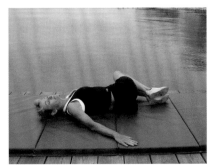

Level Two

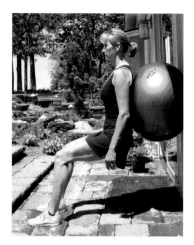

Choice A: The Invisible Chair

With your back supported by an exercise ball against a wall, sit as if you were sitting in an imaginary chair. (If you feel that you could fall from this position, you may place a stool below you to catch you.) Your heels should be directly below your knees, making a 90 degree angle, with your shoulders and back against the ball. Place your palms on your knees or by your side. Hold the position for as long as you can.

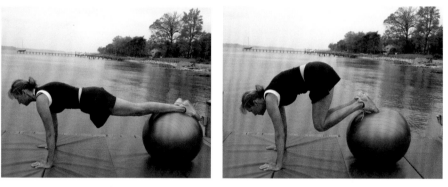

Choice B: Jackknife on Ball

Lie on an exercise ball and walk yourself out until your legs are extended and only your shins and feet are on the ball. Your hands should be shoulder-width apart. Slowly roll the ball toward you by bending your knees and tightening your abdominals (8 seconds). Hold (4 seconds) and slowly return (8 seconds). Do five repetitions.

Choice C: Side Plank

Lie on your left side and lift your body up, supported by your left arm. Your left shoulder should be directly above your left elbow. Keep your entire body in alignment. Raise your upper arm to the sky and hold for as long as you can. Repeat on the other side.

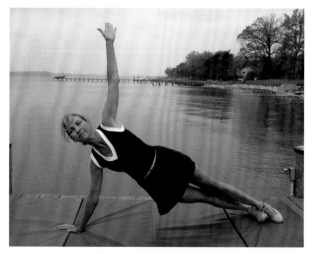

THIGHS
Level One

Choice A: Beginner Squat

Using either one or two chairs (one on each side) for support, stand with your feet shoulder-width apart. Keeping your back straight, abdominals tight, and chest lifted, slowly lower yourself into a squat (8 seconds), hold (4 seconds), and return to standing (8 seconds). Do five repetitions.

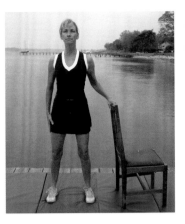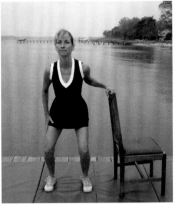

Choice B: Plié Squat

Hold one dumbbell with both hands. Take a wide stance, with your feet apart and toes turned out. Slowly lower yourself into a plié position by bending your knees outward (8 seconds), hold (4 seconds), and return to start (8 seconds). Do five repetitions.

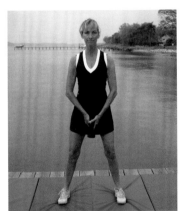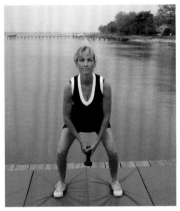

Choice C: Side Leg Lifts

Stand holding onto a chair or, alternatively, lie on the floor for more challenge. Keeping your body still, raise your outer leg up and out (8 seconds), hold (4 seconds), and return to start (8 seconds). Do five repetitions on each side. To increase the challenge, add ankle weights.

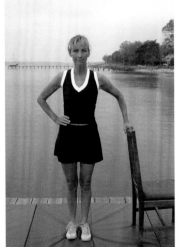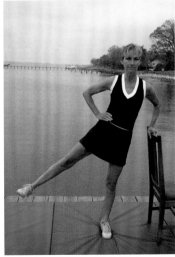

Level Two

Choice A: Chair Squat

Stand in front of a chair with your back straight, abdominals tight, and head up. Stretch your arms out in front of you or cross them over your chest. Slowly lower your body as if you were going to sit in the chair (8 seconds). Hold just above the chair (4 seconds) and slowly return to standing (8 seconds). Do five repetitions.

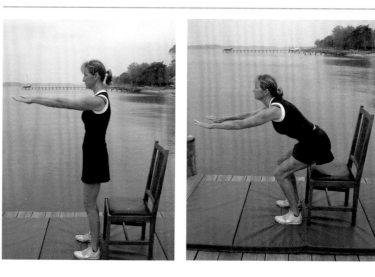

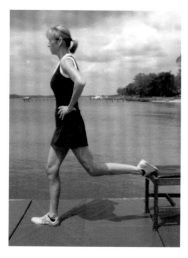

Choice B: One-Leg Squat

Stand about three feet in front of a chair and place one foot on the seat of the chair. With your back straight, abdominals tight, and chest up, slowly bend your front knee and lower yourself into a lunge position (8 seconds). Hold (4 seconds) and slowly straighten back up (8 seconds). Do five repetitions on each leg.

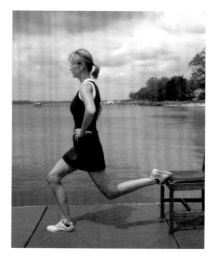

Choice C: Alternate Weighted Leg Extensions

Using ankle weights, sit straight up in a chair, holding the sides for support. Slowly extend one leg (8 seconds), hold (4 seconds), and lower it back down (8 seconds). Do five repetitions on each leg.

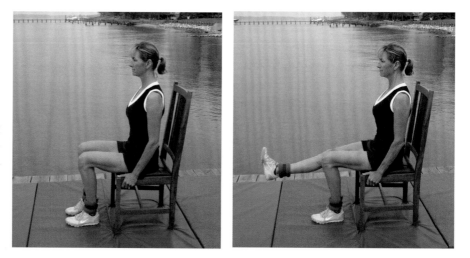

GLUTEALS
Level One

Choice A: Dumbbell Squat

Hold a pair of dumbbells or soup cans at your sides and stand with your feet shoulder-width apart. Keep your back straight, abdominals tight, head lifted, and face forward. Slowly bend at the knees as if you're going to sit down (8 seconds), hold (4 seconds), and slowly straighten your legs back to standing position (8 seconds). Do five repetitions.

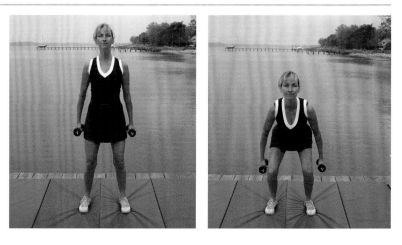

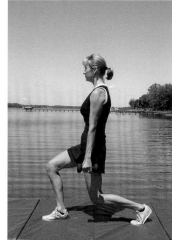

Choice B: Dumbbell Lunge

Stand straight, holding a dumbbell or soup can in each hand or a medicine ball in front of you at chest level, and look straight ahead. Place your legs shoulder-width apart. Step forward with one foot and slowly bend at the knee until your thigh is parallel to the floor (8 seconds). Hold (4 seconds) and slowly straighten the knee (8 seconds). Do five repetitions on each leg.

Choice C: Step-Up

Stand in front of a step. Keeping your back straight, abdominals tight, and head up, lift one foot onto the step. Slowly bring the other leg up and bend that knee toward your chest (8 seconds). Hold (4 seconds) and slowly lower the leg to start position (8 seconds). Do five repetitions on each leg.

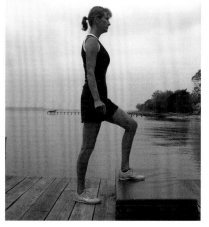

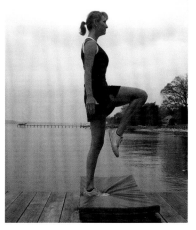

Level Two

Choice A:
Dumbbell Step-Up

Use the same motion as in the previous exercise (Step-Up), adding weights, soup cans, or a medicine ball.

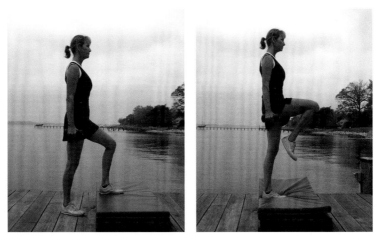

Choice B:
Gluteal Hot Buns

Lie on your back with your knees bent and your feet flat on the floor, arms at your sides. Slowly raise your hips to the ceiling, contracting your gluteals (8 seconds). Hold (4 seconds) and lower (8 seconds). Do five repetitions. If you prefer, you can do this exercise with your legs bent over an exercise ball.

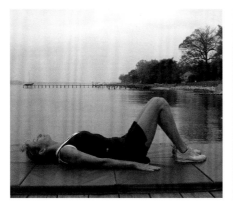
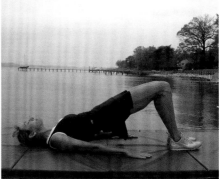

Choice C:
Donkey Kickback

Get on all fours. Keeping your back straight and head raised throughout, flex one foot and slowly raise it to the ceiling (8 seconds). Hold (4 seconds) and slowly lower your foot (8 seconds). Do five repetitions on each side, alternating legs. To increase the challenge, use ankle weights.

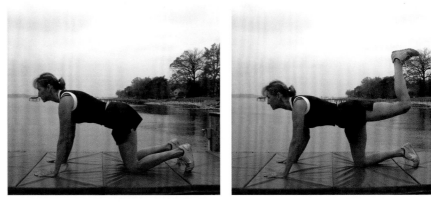

HAMSTRINGS
Level One

Choice A: Dead Lift with Dumbbells

Holding dumbbells or soup cans, stand with your feet about hip-distance apart, hands in front of your thighs. Keeping your back straight, abdominals tight, and shoulders back, bend slowly from the hips and lower the weights toward the floor as far as is comfortable (8 seconds). Keep your gaze forward. Hold (4 seconds) and then raise yourself back up to start position by slowly pushing into your heels (8 seconds). Don't let your shoulders round forward as you lift. Do five repetitions.

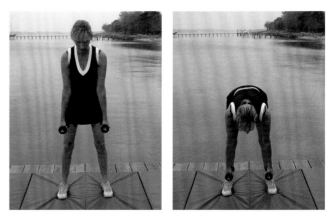

Choice B: Pillow Squeeze

Sit straight up in a chair with a pillow between your thighs and tighten your abdominals. Place your hands near your hips and grip the seat of the chair. Take a deep breath in and as you exhale squeeze the pillow with your thighs (8 seconds). Hold (4 seconds) and release slowly (8 seconds). Do five repetitions.

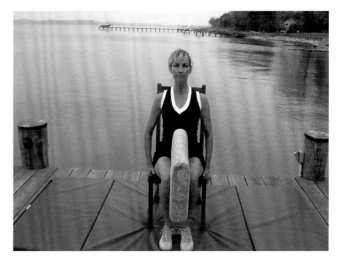

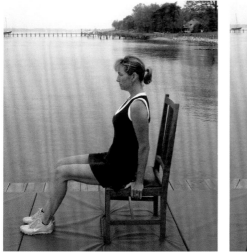

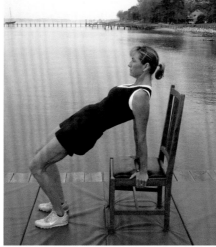

Choice C: Butt Bridge

Sit on the edge of a sturdy chair. Rest your hands on the chair near your hips and place your feet on the floor. Exhale as you lift your hips toward the ceiling, using your hands and feet to support your body (8 seconds). Hold (4 seconds) and slowly lower yourself back down (8 seconds). Do five repetitions.

Level Two

Choice A:
Hamstring Rolls on Ball

Lie on your mat with your heels and calves on an exercise ball and your legs extended. Lift your hips so that your body is in a straight line. Press your heels into the ball and slowly roll the ball toward you, keeping your feet on the ball (8 seconds). Hold in the flexed position (4 seconds) and then slowly roll the ball away from you until your legs are once more extended (8 seconds). Do five repetitions.

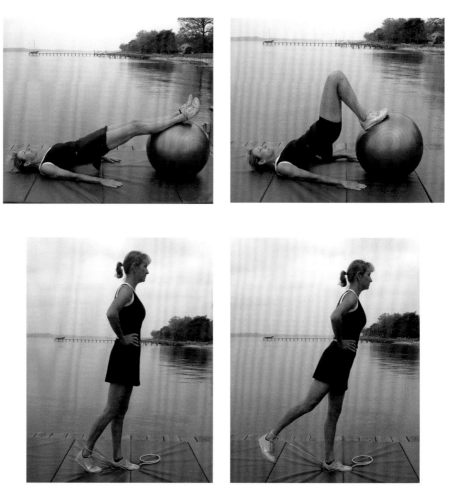

Choice B: Elastic Band Kickbacks

Place the loop of an exercise band on one ankle and step on the other end to create tension. Keeping your leg straight, slowly kick your banded foot backward about one foot (8 seconds). Hold (4 seconds) and slowly return to start (8 seconds). Do five repetitions on each leg.

Choice C: Hamstring Curl

Using ankle weights, lie on your stomach with your legs extended. Slowly curl your feet upward until your heels touch your buttocks (8 seconds). Hold (4 seconds) and slowly lower your feet back to the floor (8 seconds). Do five repetitions.

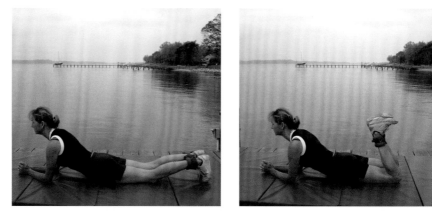

CALVES
Level One

Choice A: Step Heel Raise

Stand on a step using just the balls of your feet. Holding onto the banister and keeping your legs straight, slowly lift yourself up on your toes (8 seconds), hold (4 seconds), and slowly lower your heels until they're slightly lower than the step (8 seconds). Do five repetitions. To increase the challenge, add ankle weights or hold dumbbells or soup cans.

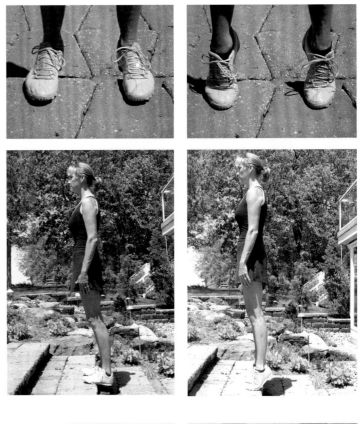

Choice B: Duck-Foot Calf Raise

Use the same motion as in Choice A, but have your heels touching and your toes pointed outward.

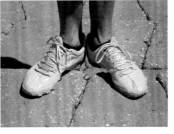
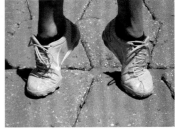

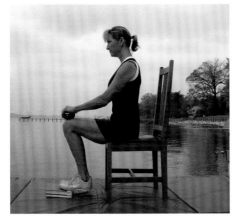
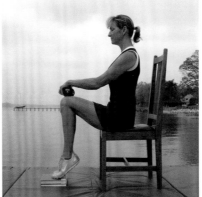

Choice C:
Seated Calf Raise

Sit straight up in a chair with the balls of your feet shoulder-width apart on a book or block. Place a weight (dumbbells, soup cans, or medicine ball) across your lap. Slowly lift your toes as high as you can (8 seconds), hold (4 seconds), and return to start (8 seconds). Do five repetitions.

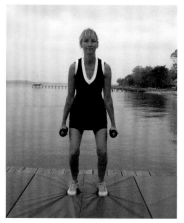

Level Two

Choice A: Jump-Ups

Hold a medicine ball, dumbbells, or soup cans and place your feet shoulder-width apart. Slowly bend at the waist, then explode with energy and jump up, landing on the balls of your feet. Hold for 4 seconds. Do five repetitions.

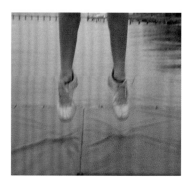

Choice B: Rocking Dumbbell Calf Raise

Stand with your feet shoulder-width apart. Hold dumbbells or soup cans at shoulder level or hold a medicine ball in front of your chest. Slowly rock back on your heels so that your toes come off the ground about 2 inches, then rock forward and hold (4 seconds) and return to your heels. Do five repetitions.

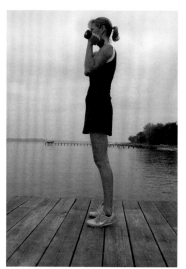

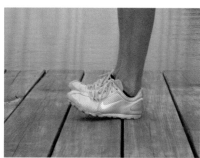

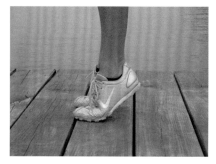

Choice C: Donkey Calf Raise

Stand with your feet shoulder-width apart and bend at your waist. Stabilize yourself by placing your hands on a stool or bench. Lift yourself up on your toes (8 seconds), hold (4 seconds), and slowly return to start (8 seconds). Do five repetitions. To increase the challenge, place a child or a weighted backpack across your hips and your lower back as you lift, hold, and lower.

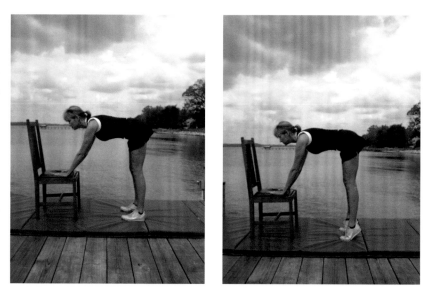

Appendix F

Note: The charts in appendix F can be downloaded from the Web site at www.habitsofhealth.net.

Rate of Perceived Exertion (Borg Scale)

Adapted from Borg, G. V., "Psychological Basis of Perceived Exertion," *Medicine and Science Sports* 14 (1982): 377–81.

EAT Walking Program
Daily Tracking Sheet

| RATE OF PERCEIVED EXERTION ||
Borg Scale	RPE
0	nothing at all
0.5	very, very light
1	very light
2	light
3	moderate
4	somewhat hard
5 – 6	hard
7 – 8	very hard
9	very, very hard
10	maximum exertion

Day	Warm-Up	Time	Cool-Down	Steps	Miles*	Calories
Day 1						
Day 2						
Day 3						
Day 4						
Day 5						
Day 6						
Day 7						
Day 8						
Day 9						
Day 10						
Day 11						
Day 12						
Day 13						
Day 14						

*1 mile = 2,000 steps

EAT Walking Program Weekly Tracking Sheet

Week	Steps per Day		Steps per Week	Miles*	Comments
	Actual	Recommended			
1		1,000/day			
2		1,200/day			
3		1,400/day			
4		1,600/day			
5		1,800/day			
6		2,000/day			
7		2,500/day			
8		3,000/day			
9		3,500/day			
10		4,000/day			
11		4,500/day			
12		5,000/day			
13		5,500/day			
14		6,000/day			

*1 mile = 2,000 steps

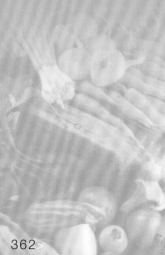

EAT Resistance Program Training Log: Upper Body

Muscle Group	Exercise / Level (level one, level two)	Weight: Body (B) or Pounds (lbs)	Rate of Perceived Exertion (RPE)
Rotation A			
Core			
Chest			
Back			
Shoulders			
Arms			
Rotation B			
Core			
Chest			
Back			
Shoulders			
Arms			

EAT Resistance Program Training Log: Lower Body

Muscle Group	Exercise / Level (level one, level two)	Weight: Body (B) or Pounds (lbs)	Rate of Perceived Exertion (RPE)
Rotation A			
Core			
Thighs			
Gluteals			
Hamstrings			
Calves			
Rotation B			
Core			
Thighs			
Gluteals			
Hamstrings			
Calves			

Note: The charts in appendix G can be downloaded from the Web site at www.habitsofhealth.net.

Appendix G

Sleep Log

The Sleep Log is designed to help you figure out which behaviors are affecting your sleep. To use the log:

• Answer the following questions, from part two of the sleep assessment on page 217, every day for one week.
• Each day, enter your answers in the log on page 367, using the symbols in the key.

1. What time did you get into bed last night?

2. What time did you get out of bed in the morning?

3. What hours did you actually sleep?

4. Did you take a nap? For how long?

5. Did you consume alcohol? How much, and at what time?

6. Did you exercise? How long, and at what time?

7. Did you drink coffee or other caffeinated beverages? How much, and at what time?

8. What hours did you watch television?

9. Did you take any medications? At what time?

To help you get started, take a look at the sample sleep log on the next page.

Sample Sleep Log

TIME	SUN–MON	MON–TUES	TUES–WED	WED–THURS	THURS–FRI	FRI–SAT	SAT–SUN
6:00 PM				E			
7:00 PM	TV					A	
8:00 PM		TV	C		A	A	
9:00 PM		TV	TV				
10:00 PM	F	○	TV	TV	A	A, F	
11:00 PM			○	TV	A	A, F	
MIDNIGHT	○			○			○
1:00 AM	●	●	●		○ ●	○	
2:00 AM				●	●	●	
3:00 AM							●
4:00AM					⊕		
5:00 AM						⊕	
6:00 AM	●				●		
7:00 AM	☀	● ☀	● ☀	● ☀	☀	●	
8:00 AM		C	C				●
9:00 AM	C			C	C	☀	
10:00 AM							☀
11:00 AM	C					C	
NOON						C	C
1:00 PM							
2:00 PM		N					
3:00 PM						E	TV
4:00 PM							TV
5:00 PM		N	E				TV
6:00 PM							

KEY

In Bed = ○	Nap = N⌇⌇N 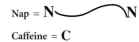	Television = TV	
Asleep = ●—●	Caffeine = C	Alcohol = A	
Awake during the night = ⊕	Exercise = E	Medication = M	
Arise in the morning = ☀	Food after 10:00 p.m. = F		

Sleep Log

TIME	SUN–MON	MON–TUES	TUES–WED	WED–THURS	THURS–FRI	FRI–SAT	SAT–SUN
6:00 PM							
7:00 PM							
8:00 PM							
9:00 PM							
10:00 PM							
11:00 PM							
MIDNIGHT							
1:00 AM							
2:00 AM							
3:00 AM							
4:00 AM							
5:00 AM							
6:00 AM							
7:00 AM							
8:00 AM							
9:00 AM							
10:00 AM							
11:00 AM							
NOON							
1:00 PM							
2:00 PM							
3:00 PM							
4:00 PM							
5:00 PM							
6:00 PM							

	MONDAY	TUESDAY	WEDNESDAY	THURSDAY	FRIDAY	SATURDAY	SUNDAY
How did you feel when you woke up? *							
How did you feel during the day?*							
Were you more alert in the morning or evening?							

*Tired--------------OK----------Refreshed
1   2   3   4   5   6   7   8   9   10

Appendix H

Caffeine in Commonly Consumed Products

COFFEE	CAFFEINE (MILLIGRAMS)
Caribou Cappuccino, 12 oz.	160–200
Decaffeinated, instant, 8 oz.	2
Decaffeinated, brewed, 8 oz.	2
Espresso, 1 fluid oz.	64
Instant, 8 oz.	62
Plain, brewed, 8 oz.	95
Starbucks Caffe Latte, 16 oz.	150

TEA	CAFFEINE (MILLIGRAMS)
Black tea, brewed, 8 oz.	47
Decaffeinated black tea, 8 oz.	2
Green tea, brewed, 8 oz.	30–50
Lipton Brisk Iced Tea, lemon flavored, 12 oz.	10
Nestea, sweetened or unsweetened, 12 oz.	17
Snapple Iced Tea, 16 oz.	18
Sobe Green Tea, 8 oz.	14
Starbucks Tazo Chai Tea Latte, 12 oz.	75

SOFT DRINKS, 12 OZ.	CAFFEINE (MILLIGRAMS)
7Up	0
A&W Creme Soda	29
Barq's Root Beer	23
Cherry Coca-Cola, Diet Cherry Coca-Cola	35
Coca-Cola Classic	35
Code Red Mountain Dew	54
Diet Barq's Root Beer	0
Diet Coke	47
Dr. Pepper, Diet Dr. Pepper	41
Diet Pepsi	35
Diet Wild Cherry Pepsi	38
Fanta	0
Mello Yello	53
Mountain Dew, Diet Mountain Dew	54
Pepsi	38
Sprite, Sprite Zero	0
Sunkist Orange Soda	41
Tab	47
Wild Cherry Pepsi	38

FOODS	CAFFEINE (MILLIGRAMS)
Excedrin, Extra Strength, 2 tablets	130
Foosh Energy Mints, 1 mint	100
Haagen-Dazs Coffee Ice Cream, ½ cup	30
Hershey's Chocolate Bar, 1.55 oz	9
Hershey's Special Dark Chocolate Bar, 1.45 oz	18
Jolt Caffeinated Gum, 1 stick	33
NoDoz Maximum Strength, 1 tablet	200

Resources

www.habitsofhealth.net
An in-depth resource on the Habits of Health, including support, tips, activities, exercises, links, and additional information on creating health. Information on enhanced support, training, and coaching through the bionetwork for those who currently do not have a personal health coach, as well as information on becoming a coach yourself. In addition you can visit the Web site to order the workbook *Living a Longer, Healthier Life: The Companion Guide to Dr. A's Habits of Health* and the DVD *Dr. A's Habits of Health Video Series.*

www.drwayneandersen.com
Find out more about Dr. Andersen and his work to foster optimal health.

www.tsfl.com
Learn how to become part of the Take Shape for Life bionetwork, a powerful support team made up of health-conscious, coach-supported people dedicated to optimizing their health through the Habits of Health. The site also provides information on ordering Medifast's medically formulated portion-controlled meal replacements (PCMRs), antioxidants, and eicosanoids (fish oil); information about becoming a coach; free personal health coaching; and free access to the supportive online community Support in Motion.

www.medifast.com
An online source for ordering Medifast's medically formulated portion-controlled meal replacements (PCMRs) and dietary supplements, antioxidants, and eicosanoids (fish oil) for those who do not wish to take part in free personal health coaching. The site also provides free access to the supportive online community My Medifast.

ALZHEIMER'S ASSOCIATION
www.alz.org
Valuable information on ways to protect your brain.

AMERICAN COLLEGE OF SPORTS MEDICINE
www.acsm.org
Information on movement and musculoskeletal health.

AMERICA ON THE MOVE
www.americaonthemove.org
Nonprofit initiative dedicated to helping people avoid weight gain by increasing their level of activity.

THE AMERICAN INSTITUTE OF STRESS
www.stress.org/americas
Information and problem-solving on stress-related health issues.

CANADIAN FITNESS EDUCATION SERVICES
www.canadianfitness.net
Educational courses on exercise.

CANADIAN COUNCIL OF FOOD AND NUTRITION
www.nin.ca
Information and advocacy on food and nutrition issues.

THE COOPER INSTITUTE
www.cooperinstitute.org
Promotes healthy eating and other healthy habits.

JOHNS HOPKINS HEALTH SITE
www.hopkinsmedicine.org
An excellent resource for information on all aspects of health.

MAYO CLINIC
www.mayoclinic.com
Information to help you live a healthier life.

NATIONAL HEART, LUNG, AND BLOOD INSTITUTE
www.nhlbi.nih.gov
Information on lowering risk for disease.

THE OBESITY SOCIETY
www.obesity.org
A source of information for weight-challenged individuals.

NATIONAL SLEEP FOUNDATION
www.sleepfoundation.org
Education on the importance of sleep and sleep issues.

WORLD HEALTH ORGANIZATION
www.who.int
Information on prevention and treatment of disease at the global level.

www.mypyramid.gov
Information to help you understand the food pyramid.

www.nutrition.gov
U.S.-based nutrition resource.

Index

*A lowercase **b** following a page number indicates a text box; **s** indicates a sidebar.*

Leider, Richard, 265, 268, 273
Levine, James A., 181, 182s, 188s
libido, 253
life expectancy, 9, 280, 290, 291
lighting, affect of, on appetite, 69
lipid profile, 46, 318
liver function, 6, 7b, 58
longevity, 282b, 286–288, 292, 296
low-density lipoprotein (LDL), 46, 47, 63, 248, 250, 253, 258, 318
low-glycemic diet, 63, 65, 70, 75b, 77, 81, 99, 128, 134–136, 150, 152, 162–164, 166, 234
  color-coded system, 93
L-tyrosine, 176
lutein, 247, 262
lycopenes, 247, 262

macronutrients, 132, 152
magnesium, 251, 262, 317
manganese, 252
margarine vs. butter, 111, 112s
massage, therapeutic, 240
meal and fueling frequency, 62–63, 66, 84, 90–92, 119, 132, 150, 176
meal planning
  Phase I, 78, 83–84, 118–119, 161
  transitional phase, 158–169
meats
  alternatives to, 80
  fat content, 79–80, 102–103
  processed, 67, 101–102
  wild, 79–80, 102
medicine, third era of, 276–277
Medifast, xx, 74, 76, 77, 158
meditation, 313–315
melatonin, 214, 215s, 216, 218
menus, sample
  Phase I, 122–128
  transition week 4, 160
metabolic equivalents, 181
metabolic syndrome, xvii–xviii, 12, 58
Michner, James A., 274
micronutrients, 132s
Mifflin-St. Jeor calculation, 155
migraines, 252
mindless eating, 141
minerals, 250–252
molybdenum, 253
motivation, problem-oriented vs. outcome-oriented, 19–23, 152
multivitamins, 247, 261
musculoskeletal system, 195–196, 315
music
  ergogenic benefits, 174, 191, 205
  stress-reducing benefits, 238

napping, 219
National Institute of Health, 319
National Weight Control Registry, xvi, 29b, 149
nature, enjoying, 240, 273
NEAT System, 185–194
Nelson, Mark, 22b
nerve growth factor (NGF), 312
neuropeptides, 311
neurotransmitters, 214, 311
niacin. See vitamins: B complex
Nicklaus, Jack, 32–33
noise pollution, 238
non-exercise activity thermogenesis (NEAT), 175, 180–182
non-sickness, defined, 12, 13s
non-steroidal anti-inflammatory drugs (NSAIDs), 252
Norman, Greg, 32–33
nutrient-deficient food, 244–245
nutritional intervention, 94
nuts. See seeds and nuts

obesity
  childhood, 100
  and sleep, 212–213, 215
  in the United States, 7, 15, 225–226
oils
  cooking and salad, 39s, 68, 112–113, 234–235, 257, 316
  hydrogenated, 68
omega fats, 101b, 112–113, 235, 246, 261, 316
optimal health
  defined, 12s, 23
  steps to achieving, xix–xxiii
oral health, 295
organic food, 96
osteoporosis, 104, 197, 251
oxidative stress, 232, 281
oxygen free radicals, 102, 111, 132, 232, 248, 254, 281, 283b, 308

pancreatic health, 12, 38, 133
pantothenic acid. See vitamins: B complex
para-aminobezoic acid (PABA), 249
Parkinson's disease, 252
Pauling, Linus, 245
PCMRs. See portion-controlled meal replacements (PCMRs)
pedometers, 183b
perchlorethylene, 237b
personal trainers, 206
pharmaceutical companies, marketing of, 14s
phosphatidylserine, 255, 317

Acknowledgments

This book could not have been possible without the help of so many individuals.

First, I thank all the people who have taken this journey themselves and served as my teachers. Your stories, your experiences, your ideas have blazed the path to optimal health. These stories, woven throughout this book, are validation that reaching and maintaining optimal health is possible in our obesigenic world. To those of you who are leading the way by becoming health coaches and *health* care professionals, now too numerous to mention by name, you've shown enormous courage in stepping out to fuel this bionetwork and provide safe harbor for others who desire to create health in their lives. I am eternally grateful.

Three individuals were instrumental in moving this book from idea to reality. First, Vaughn Feather, who believed and insisted that this book needed to be written. Second, my dear friend Dan Bell, who provided guidance, encouragement, and support, and has been an endless source of information and advice. And finally, my close friend Robert Fritz, who has been my mentor and taught me the craft of creating, and who encouraged me to write this book myself, in my own voice.

A number of incredibly brilliant health professionals have joined the health movement and contributed to the genesis of this book. Thanks to my medical colleagues: Lawrence Cheskin, MD, FACP; Lisa M. Davis, PhD, PA-C, CNS, LDN; Joe Pecararo, MD, FACP; Mark Nelson, MD, FACP; Mark Oldendorf, MD, FACP; Robert Hambly, MD; Ariel D. Soffer, MD, FACC; Yousef Elyaman, MD; John S. Urse, DO, FAOAO; Carla Myers, DO; Ken Gatto, DO; Scott Corliss, DO; Lori Lynn Andersen, RN, MSHS; Joni Rampolla, RD, LDN; Greg Freitag, MS, CSCS; Kim Ruby, BS, CN; Christina Winsey-Rudd, DC; Roger Russo, DC; J. C. Dornick, DC; Dan Van Zandt, DC; and Bob Cochran, MPE. Thanks, too, to three unique physicians who helped mold me as a young physician: Dr. Tom Moody, Dr. Tom Hetzel, and Dr. Joe Civetta.

A special thanks to Brad MacDonald, chairman of the board of Medifast Inc. and co-founder of Take Shape for Life (TSFL), for believing in this big idea of getting people healthy and for providing the infrastructure to fuel the growth of this new health movement. I also thank Mike McDevitt, Meg McDonald, Rick Logsdail, Jaime Elwood, Brendan Connors, and Herman and Porsche Dunst for their support of the infrastructure that has allowed this idea to take flight, and the TSFL staff, who have work so hard to help us build our coaching organization. That starts with the tireless efforts of an amazing young woman, Allison Bell, and her staff, Erin Bents, Kristin Fuhrer, Austin Sandkuhler, Takki Williams, and Allan Cannington. Thanks too to Rod Heckman for his business acumen, as well as to Sarah Graves and Emily Trainor. The spirit of optimal health and fellowship is alive and well in TSFL as a result of the addition of Janet Cronstedt to our team. She and her support staff, Brian Walker, Roland Dobbins, Swan Gilyard, Francine Varona, Nasifa Bishop, and Denise Lazo, have gone way beyond the call of duty. I must personally single out the individual who's been instrumental in carrying the banner of optimal health to the private, corporate, and governmental arena for us, my dear friend General Leo Williams III.

Special thanks go to my personal trainer, J. D. Adamson, for helping me on my own journey to optimal health and to chef Joe Blanchard, CEC, CCA, for creating the wonderful recipes for this text. I would also like to thank my friend Kevin McCarthy for his contribution to helping us get America healthy through a simple yet powerful system of self-discovery that helps people organize their lives around what matters most.

Thanks as well to the special group of people who have helped craft this book into its final state. Charlie Dorris, for your insights and your ability to see the big picture. Dede Cummings, for designing and implementing my vision into a wonderfully crafted finished product with the exact look and feel I'd hoped for. You're amazing! Thanks too to Carolyn Kasper, for helping Dede make all this work; to our proofreader, Jon Potter; our indexer, Thomas Kozachek; to Linda Shaffer, for the cover photography; and Aleta Coursen, for the graphics; and to Ellen Keelan, my editor, who immersed herself in this project with an intensity, fervor, and professionalism that a writer can only dream of, who toiled long and hard to sculpt a finished product that would help me bring my message home. Thanks too to the always gracious Mary Bell for volunteering her time to review the manuscript. And once again, I thank Robert Fritz for his ability to use structural dynamics as a weapon of mass effectiveness to guide the creation of this book and lead the whole creative movement! Thank you, Rosalind, for sharing him with me!

Last but far from least, I thank my family, who has sacrificed the most throughout this adventure. First, my wife, Lori, who has contributed professionally from her vast nursing and coaching experience helping people reach optimal health, with a special caring and touch that can only come from the heart. But that is only the beginning of my gratitude, for without her support, encouragement, partnership, sage advice, and willingness to abandon every comfort, I would never have begun this journey. To my two precious daughters, Savannah and Erica, who even at their young age have the wisdom to understand how important it was that this book be written! And of course to my Mom, whom I love so much, and to my other two moms, Marilyn and Sharon, whom I love as my own.

Dr. Wayne Scott Andersen
October 2008